Pediatric Otolaryngology for Primary Care

2ND EDITION

Scott R. Schoem, MD, MBA, FAAP
David H. Darrow, MD, DDS, FAAP
Editors

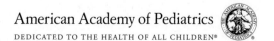

American Academy of Pediatrics
DEDICATED TO THE HEALTH OF ALL CHILDREN®

American Academy of Pediatrics Publishing Staff

Mary Lou White, *Chief Product and Services Officer/SVP, Membership, Marketing, and Publishing*

Mark Grimes, *Vice President, Publishing*

Carrie Peters, *Editor, Professional/Clinical Publishing*

Theresa Wiener, *Production Manager, Clinical and Professional Publications*

Linda Smessaert, MSIMC, *Senior Marketing Manager, Professional Resources*

Mary Louise Carr, MBA, *Marketing Manager, Clinical Publications*

Published by the American Academy of Pediatrics

345 Park Blvd

Itasca, IL 60143

Telephone: 630/626-6000

Facsimile: 847/434-8000

www.aap.org

The American Academy of Pediatrics is an organization of 67,000 primary care pediatricians, pediatric medical subspecialists, and pediatric surgical specialists dedicated to the health, safety, and well-being of infants, children, adolescents, and young adults.

The recommendations in this publication do not indicate an exclusive course of treatment or serve as a standard of medical care. Variations, taking into account individual circumstances, may be appropriate.

Statements and opinions expressed are those of the authors and not necessarily those of the American Academy of Pediatrics.

Any websites, brand names, products, or manufacturers are mentioned for informational and identification purposes only and do not imply an endorsement by the American Academy of Pediatrics (AAP). The AAP is not responsible for the content of external resources. Information was current at the time of publication.

The publishers have made every effort to trace the copyright holders for borrowed materials. If they have inadvertently overlooked any, they will be pleased to make the necessary arrangements at the first opportunity.

This publication has been developed by the American Academy of Pediatrics. The contributors are expert authorities in the field of pediatrics. No commercial involvement of any kind has been solicited or accepted in development of the content of this publication. Disclosures: Dr Bly (Chapter 13) disclosed a consulting relationship with Spiway, LLC, and cofounder relationships with Edus Health, Inc, and EigenHealth, Inc. Dr Papsin (Chapter 2) disclosed a speakers bureau relationship with Cochlear Americas Corporation.

Every effort has been made to ensure that the drug selection and dosage set forth in this text are in accordance with the current recommendations and practice at the time of publication. It is the responsibility of the health care professional to check the package insert of each drug for any change in indications and dosage and for added warnings and precautions.

Every effort is made to keep *Pediatric Otolaryngology for Primary Care* consistent with the most recent advice and information available from the American Academy of Pediatrics.

Special discounts are available for bulk purchases of this publication. Email Special Sales at aapsales@aap.org for more information.

Printed in the United States of America

9-435/0420   1 2 3 4 5 6 7 8 9 10

MA0965

ISBN: 978-1-61002-400-6

eBook: 978-1-61002-401-3

Cover and publication design by Peg Mulcahy

Library of Congress Control Number: 2019944503

Contributors

Joan C. Arvedson, PhD, CCC-SLP, BCS-S
Speech-Language Pathologist
Children's Hospital of Wisconsin–Milwaukee
Clinical Professor
Department of Pediatrics
Medical College of Wisconsin
Milwaukee, WI

Cristina M. Baldassari, MD, FACS, FAAP
Assistant Professor
Department of Otolaryngology
Eastern Virginia Medical School
Department of Sleep Medicine
Children's Hospital of The King's Daughters
Norfolk, VA

Randall A. Bly, MD
Assistant Professor
Department of Otolaryngology–Head and Neck Surgery
University of Washington School of Medicine
Seattle, WA

Charles M. Bower, MD, FAAP
Professor, Otolaryngology–Head and Neck Surgery
University of Arkansas for Medical Sciences
Arkansas Children's Hospital
Little Rock, AR

Lisa Ann Brock, RN, BSN, CBS, IBCLC-RLC
Pediatric RN Lactation Consultant
Cleveland, WI

Christen Caloway, MD
Assistant Professor
Department of Otolaryngology–Head and Neck Surgery
Rutgers New Jersey Medical School
Newark, NJ

Simon Carr, MD, FRCS (ORL-HNS)
Clinical Fellow
The Hospital for Sick Children (SickKids)
Toronto, Ontario, Canada

David H. Chi, MD
Division Chief, Department of Pediatric Otolaryngology
UPMC Children's Hospital of Pittsburgh
Pittsburgh, PA

Sukgi S. Choi, MD, MBA
Department of Otolaryngology and Communication Enhancement
Harvard Medical School
Boston, MA

David H. Darrow, MD, DDS, FAAP
Professor of Otolaryngology and Pediatrics
Director, Center for Hemangiomas and Vascular Birthmarks
Eastern Virginia Medical School
Norfolk, VA

Conor M. Devine, MD
Assistant Professor of Clinical Otorhinolaryngology
Perelman School of Medicine at the University of Pennsylvania
Philadelphia, PA

Alexandra G. Espinel, MD, FAAP
Assistant Professor of Otolaryngology and Pediatrics
Children's National Health System
Washington, DC

Christopher R. Grindle, MD, FAAP
Assistant Professor of Pediatric Otolaryngology
Connecticut Children's Medical Center
University of Connecticut School of Medicine
Hartford, CT

Christopher Hartnick, MD, FAAP
Professor, Department of Otolaryngology
Harvard Medical School
Massachusetts Eye and Ear
Boston, MA

Dorsey Ann Heithaus, MA
Pediatric Audiologist
Cincinnati Children's Hospital Medical Center
Cincinnati, OH

Amy Hughes, MD
Assistant Professor of Otolaryngology
Division of Otolaryngology
Connecticut Children's Medical Center
Hartford, CT

Ian N. Jacobs, MD, FAAP
Associate Professor of Otolaryngology
Perelman School of Medicine at the University of Pennsylvania
Director, Center for Pediatric Airway Disorders
Children's Hospital of Philadelphia
Philadelphia, PA

Adam B. Johnson, MD, PhD
Assistant Professor of Pediatric Otolaryngology
Director of Velopharyngeal Dysfunction
University of Arkansas for Medical Sciences
Arkansas Children's Hospital
Little Rock, AR

David L. Mandell, MD, FAAP
Affiliate Associate Professor
Charles E. Schmidt College of Medicine
Florida Atlantic University
Boca Raton, FL
Clinical Associate Professor, Division of Otolaryngology
Nova Southeastern University Dr. Kiran C. Patel College of
    Osteopathic Medicine
Fort Lauderdale, FL
Voluntary Associate Professor, Department of Otolaryngology

Miller School of Medicine
University of Miami
Miami, FL
Center for Pediatric Otolaryngology–Head and Neck Surgery
Boynton Beach, FL

Stephen Maturo, MD
Pediatric Otolaryngologist
ENT Residency Director, Walter Reed National Military Medical Center
Uniformed Services University of the Health Sciences
Bethesda, MD

Kara D. Meister, MD
Clinical Assistant Professor of Otolaryngology–Head and Neck
Surgery, Pediatrics
Lucile Packard Children's Hospital
Stanford University
Palo Alto, CA

Anna K. Meyer, MD, FACS, FAAP
Associate Professor, Otolaryngology–Head and Neck Surgery
Division of Pediatric Otolaryngology
University of California, San Francisco
San Francisco, CA

Stephanie Moody Antonio, MD, FACS
Associate Professor of Otolaryngology–Head and Neck Surgery
Eastern Virginia Medical School
Norfolk, VA

Nicole Murray, MD, FAAP
Director, Connecticut Children's Medical Center for Airway, Voice, and
    Swallowing Disorders
Assistant Director, Pediatric Otolaryngology
Connecticut Children's Medical Center/UConn Health Otolaryngology
Hartford, CT

T.J. O-Lee, MD
Director, Pediatric Otolaryngology
Loma Linda University School of Medicine
Loma Linda, CA

Blake Papsin, MD, MSc, FRCSC, FACS, FAAP
Otolaryngologist-in-Chief, The Hospital for Sick Children (SickKids)
Professor of Otolaryngology–Head and Neck Surgery
Faculty of Medicine
University of Toronto
Toronto, Ontario, Canada

Sanjay R. Parikh, MD, FACS
Professor of Otolaryngology–Head and Neck Surgery
University of Washington
Medical Director, Bellevue Clinic and Surgery Center
Seattle Children's Hospital
Seattle, WA

Maria T. Peña, MD, FAAP
Division of Otolaryngology
Children's National Hospital
Professor of Otolaryngology and Pediatrics
The George Washington University Medical Center
Washington, DC

Eileen Raynor, MD, FACS, FAAP
Associate Professor of Pediatric Otolaryngology
Department of Head and Neck Surgery and Communication Sciences
Duke University School of Medicine
Durham, NC

Corrie E. Roehm, MD, FACS, FAAP
Director, The Hearing Center at Dell Children's
Clinical Associate Professor
Dell Medical School
University of Texas at Austin
Austin, TX

Kristina W. Rosbe, MD, FACS, FAAP
Professor of Otolaryngology and Pediatrics
Chief, Division of Pediatric Otolaryngology
Benioff Children's Hospital
University of California, San Francisco
San Francisco, CA

Tara L. Rosenberg, MD
Surgical Director, Vascular Anomalies Center
Assistant Professor of Otolaryngology/Head and Neck Surgery
Division of Pediatric Otolaryngology
Texas Children's Hospital
Baylor College of Medicine
Houston, TX

Scott R. Schoem, MD, MBA, FAAP
Professor, University of Connecticut Department of Allied Health
    Sciences
Director, Pediatric Otolaryngology
Connecticut Children's Medical Center
Hartford, CT

Anthony Sheyn, MD
Assistant Professor of Otolaryngology–Head and Neck Surgery
Director of Resident Research
University of Tennessee Health Science Center
    Department of Otolaryngology
Le Bonheur Children's Hospital
Chief of Otolaryngology–Head and Neck Surgery
St. Jude Children's Research Hospital
Memphis, TN

Sally R. Shott, MD, FAAP
Professor
Department of Pediatric Otolaryngology–Head and Neck Surgery
Cincinnati Children's Hospital Medical Center
University of Cincinnati
Cincinnati, OH

Elizabeth A. Shuman, MD
Resident Physician
Department of Otolaryngology–Head and Neck Surgery
University of California, San Francisco
San Francisco, CA

Steven Sobol, MD, MSc, FAAP
Associate Professor of Otorhinolaryngology–Head and Neck Surgery
Perelman School of Medicine at the University of Pennsylvania
Philadelphia, PA

Tulio A. Valdez, MD, MSc
Associate Professor of Otolaryngology–Head and Neck Surgery
Division of Pediatric Otolaryngology
Stanford University
Palo Alto, CA

Mark S. Volk, MD, DMD
Associate in Otolaryngology
Department of Otolaryngology and Communication Enhancement
Boston Children's Hospital
Assistant Professor, Department of Otolaryngology
Harvard Medical School
Boston, MA

Daniel L. Wohl, MD, FACS, FAAP
Adjunct Associate Professor, Pediatric Otolaryngology
Department of Surgery
University of Florida College of Medicine–Jacksonville
Jacksonville, FL

Karen B. Zur, MD
Director, Pediatric Voice Program
Associate Director, Center for Pediatric Airway Disorders
Children's Hospital of Philadelphia
Perelman School of Medicine at the University of Pennsylvania
Philadelphia, PA

*To our first and most important teachers, Scott's parents,
Florence and Melvin Schoem, and David's parents, Vivienne
and Stanley Darrow, who taught us to live every day fully,
laugh often, listen to others, and love sincerely.*
Scott R. Schoem, MD, MBA, FAAP
David H. Darrow, MD, DDS, FAAP

"Every home is a university and the parents are the teachers."
Mahatma Gandhi (The Wit and Wisdom of Gandhi)

Contents

Foreword

As a primary care pediatrician and child advocate, I remember working through the Virginia state legislature and Department of Health to ensure that children with cleft lip and palate were automatically eligible for early intervention services. The physicians by my side in this effort were my pediatric otolaryngology colleagues; they understood how this spectrum of disability would affect the developmental trajectory of the children with cleft lip and palate. Pediatric physicians, both medical and surgical, formed a team that could effectively advocate for children.

Pediatricians encounter otolaryngology concerns with their patients on a daily basis. From common diagnoses such as recurrent otitis media to rare congenital anomalies, pediatricians look to their pediatric otolaryngology specialists as a trusted source of quality patient care, surgical expertise, evidence-based practice, and the best outcomes for children.

This book serves as a valuable reference for any pediatrician in practice. The authors are dedicated pediatric surgical specialists whose experience in the field of otolaryngology provides a broad overview and a practical approach to children with many diagnoses. Guidelines for evaluation, referral, and management blend the best of pediatric otolaryngology specialists with the pediatric medical home.

Our pediatric otolaryngologists still stand side by side with our primary care pediatricians to promote the best care for children.

Colleen A. Kraft, MD, MBA, FAAP
2018 President, American Academy of Pediatrics

Preface

Readers of this second edition of our textbook may note the change in title from *Pediatric Otolaryngology* to *Pediatric Otolaryngology for Primary Care.* This change reflects the emphasis we have placed in the current edition on providing primary care clinicians with practical information and suggestions for intervention and referral. In this edition, we believe we have created a comprehensive reference that still allows clinicians to rapidly locate material relevant to the needs of their patients. The reader will find fewer citations within the text and selected readings following each chapter.

The current edition has been further updated to incorporate new knowledge gained from basic science and clinical investigations over the past decade. We have also added 3 new chapters, one addressing care of the child with a tracheotomy, another addressing the assessment and management of feeding issues and ankyloglossia in children, and a third on complications of eustachian tube dysfunction (ie, retractions, perforations, and cholesteatoma). Where possible, we have also included recent clinical practice guidelines that have helped to establish best practices for primary providers of pediatric care.

The success of a work such as this is dependent on the excellence of its authors, and we are greatly indebted to our contributors for their expertise and effort. Special thanks are due to Carrie Peters, our editor at the American Academy of Pediatrics, who has kept us on task and seen the manuscript through to fruition. We also wish to thank our families for their patience and understanding in allowing us the time to complete this textbook. But perhaps our deepest appreciation is for the many pediatric primary care clinicians who have trusted us with their patients and who have served as partners and mentors in their care.

Scott R. Schoem, MD, MBA, FAAP
David H. Darrow, MD, DDS, FAAP

Ear and Temporal Bone

CHAPTER 1

Neonatal Hearing Screening, Hearing Loss, and Treatment for Hearing Loss

Anna K. Meyer, MD

Introduction

Hearing impairment in infants and children is a common and serious disability that can have far-reaching implications for cognitive, psychosocial, and academic development. Hearing in the earliest years is essential to the development of speech and language, and even mild impairment can impede this process. Unfortunately, primary care residencies and medical schools provide little education about the diagnosis of hearing loss, counseling of families, and interventions that are available. The most important aspect of pediatric hearing loss is early identification and intervention. Universal newborn hearing screening (UNHS) programs have markedly improved the ability of health care professionals to diagnose congenital hearing loss at a younger age. However, children who have late-onset or progressive loss are still at risk for delays in diagnosis. Recognizing children who have problems with speech acquisition and hearing impairment is essential to ensure early referral to audiologists and otolaryngologists.

Once a hearing loss is identified, the next key step is identifying the best intervention strategy for each child and family. Interventions can range from sign language to cochlear implantation. Many of the interventions depend on the type and cause of hearing loss. Primary care clinicians (PCCs) should have an understanding of the common causes of hearing loss and the equipment and resources that will assist a hearing-impaired child in developing the best possible auditory perception and speech, as well as maximizing social and academic performance.

> **Pearl:** Early identification of and intervention for childhood hearing loss are essential for the best outcomes in speech and language, as well as cognitive, social, and academic functioning.

Epidemiology

The estimated incidence of permanent childhood hearing loss identified in the newborn period is 1 to 3 per 1,000 screened neonates. The prevalence of hearing loss in older children and adolescents is as high as 3.1%. Hearing loss is slightly more common among boys, with a ratio of 1.2 to 1. Ethnic and socioeconomic variation exists, with a higher prevalence of hearing loss among Hispanic Americans, blacks, and children living in lower-income households.

A tremendous shift in the common etiologies of pediatric hearing impairment has occurred since the advent of antibiotics and immunizations. While the early 20th century was dominated by hearing loss caused by childhood infection, the last 50 years have seen a relative increase in the proportion of hearing loss due to inherited causes. In developed countries, it is estimated that 20% of all pediatric hearing loss and 50% of congenital loss is genetic. An ever-growing number of gene mutations have been linked to hearing loss; approximately 80% of hereditary hearing loss is autosomal recessive and 15% is autosomal dominant. Many syndromes are associated with hearing loss, the most common of which is Down syndrome.

Approximately 25% to 50% of hearing loss is acquired. Causes of acquired congenital pediatric hearing loss include maternal infections or toxins taken during pregnancy, maternal diabetes, and birth-related problems. Recently, congenital cytomegalovirus (CMV) has been estimated as the etiology in more than 20% of patients with hearing loss identified at birth. Acquired causes of childhood hearing loss include ear infections, ototoxic medications, meningitis, viral illnesses, trauma, and noise exposure.

The etiology cannot be identified in all cases; 25% to 50% of children will never have a cause identified.

> **Pearl:** Hearing impairment is more common than all other diseases screened for in the newborn period combined.

■ Presenting Symptoms

One of the greatest challenges in infants is recognizing symptoms of hearing loss. Nearly two-thirds of children identified as having hearing loss are initially suspected by their parents of having impaired hearing. While audiologic evaluation should be initiated whenever a parent or caregiver has concerns about hearing or speech development, a lack of parental concern is not a reliable indicator of intact hearing in an infant or a child. For example, children with moderate hearing loss may respond when their parent yells or may startle at a loud noise, and parents may interpret this as normal hearing, although careful questioning will reveal that the children struggle with quieter speech and sounds. On average, the time between suspicion and diagnosis of hearing loss is 9 months. **Table 1-1** lists expected hearing, speech, and language milestones for young children. Those who do not meet these milestones should be evaluated for hearing loss.

Preschoolers and older children are somewhat easier to assess for symptoms of hearing loss, but subtle indicators can still be overlooked. Often, impaired hearing can be interpreted as ignoring or not listening. Children should be observed for the following symptoms of possible hearing loss:

- Turning up the volume of the radio or television
- Responding inappropriately to questions
- Having difficulty understanding what people are saying
- Not replying when called
- Problems with articulation or difficulty for others to understand the child's speech
- Speech/language delays
- Decline in previous language skills
- Ear pain/aches or head noise complaints
- School performance problems
- Behavioral problems

In addition, PCCs should be aware of high-risk indicators of hearing loss in children (**Box 1-1**) and should ensure that these children have been appropriately evaluated.

A family history of hearing loss affecting first- and second-degree relatives should be elicited as well as a determination of common origin from ethnically isolated locations or consanguinity.

> **Pearl:** All children who have a speech delay should undergo evaluation for hearing loss.

▪ Physical Examination

A complete physical examination should be performed in all children with hearing loss because nearly every organ system can have abnormalities associated with hearing loss. The head and face should be evaluated for any features that could be consistent with a

Table 1-1. Normal Hearing, Speech, and Language Development

	Birth to 3 mo	4 to 6 mo	7 to 12 mo	12 to 24 mo
Expressive language	◆ Smiles or coos[a] ◆ Cries differently for different needs[a]	◆ Makes vowel babbling sounds[a] ◆ May begin consonant sounds p, b, m ◆ Laughs ◆ Vocalizes excitement or displeasure ◆ Entertains oneself with gurgling sounds	◆ Babbles many consonants and vowels ◆ Says "mama" or "dada" or other words by first birthday ◆ Repeats some sounds made by others ◆ Uses voice to get attention	◆ Uses more words each month ◆ Names common objects ◆ Puts 2 words together
Receptive language	◆ Startles or awakens to loud noises ◆ May turn head in direction of sound ◆ Changes sucking behavior in response to sound ◆ May seem to recognize parent's voice	◆ Turns toward familiar sounds ◆ Responds to tone of voice ◆ Smiles when spoken to[a] ◆ Notices sound-making toys[a] ◆ Pays attention to music	◆ Responds to name ◆ Listens when spoken to ◆ Turns and looks in direction of sounds ◆ Understands simple requests	◆ Points to familiar objects when named ◆ Listens to stories, songs, and rhymes ◆ Follows simple commands ◆ Points to body parts when asked ◆ Points to pictures in book when named

[a] Hearing-impaired children can be very responsive to facial expressions and visual stimuli and will also make sounds, which can fool parents and health care providers into believing that hearing is intact.

Box 1-1. Acquired Causes of Pediatric Hearing Loss		
Prenatal	**Perinatal**	**Postnatal**

♦ Congenital infection
  — Cytomegalovirus
  — Rubella
  — Toxoplasmosis
  — Herpes
  — Syphilis
  — Varicella
♦ Teratogens
  — Alcohol
  — Cocaine
  — Methyl mercury
  — Thalidomide
♦ Ototoxic medications
  — Aminoglycosides
  — Loop diuretics
  — Quinine,
    chloroquine
♦ Gestational diabetes
  or diabetes mellitus
	♦ Prematurity
	♦ Low birth weight
	♦ Birth hypoxia/low
	  Apgar score
	♦ Hyperbilirubinemia
	♦ Sepsis
	♦ NICU admission
	♦ Ototoxic medications
		♦ Infection
		  — Mumps
		  — Measles
		  — Varicella
		  — Lyme disease
		  — Meningitis
		♦ Recurrent acute
		  otitis media or
		  persistent OME
		♦ Head trauma
		♦ Noise exposure
		♦ Ototoxic medications
		♦ Neurodegenerative
		  disorders

Abbreviations: NICU, neonatal intensive care unit; OME, otitis media with effusion.

craniofacial syndrome associated with hearing loss (**Table 1-2**). For example, the hair should be examined for a white forelock, which suggests Waardenburg syndrome. The external ear should be thoroughly inspected for abnormalities, including low-set ears, abnormal shape, preauricular pits and tags, and branchial cleft anomalies. The ear canal should be evaluated for infection, stenosis, or atresia and the presence of obstructing foreign bodies or cerumen. The tympanic membrane should be visualized in its entirety to examine for perforations, areas of retraction, tympanosclerosis (scar of the tympanic membrane), and squamous debris that could be consistent with cholesteatoma. This is especially important because many PCCs rely on the "light reflex," which is an unreliable indicator of disease of the tympanic membrane and middle ear. Reliance on the light reflex may mislead PCCs to examine only the anterior-inferior portion of the eardrum. Pneumatic otoscopy should always be performed to assess for the presence of middle-ear effusion, as well as the integrity of the tympanic membrane. The eyes should be evaluated for the presence of colobomas of the lids, iris, or retina and for heterochromia of the irises. The maxilla and mandible should be assessed for hypoplastic

Table 1-2. Common Syndromes Associated With Hearing Loss

Name	Inheritance	Gene	Phenotype
Down	Sporadic	Trisomy 21	SNHL, CHL, or MHL; classic facies, intellectual disability, congenital heart disease; intestinal, thyroid, and skeletal problems
Stickler	Autosomal dominant and autosomal recessive	COL2A, COL9A1, COL11A, COL11A2	Congenital high-frequency SNHL, Pierre Robin syndrome (micrognathia and cleft palate), myopia
Treacher Collins	Autosomal dominant	TCOF1	CHL, microtia, external auditory canal atresia, ossicular malformation, cleft palate, micrognathia, hypoplastic zygomas, cleft palate, coloboma
Crouzon	Autosomal dominant	FGFR2	CHL or MHL, ear malformations, craniosynostosis
Waardenburg	Autosomal dominant	EDN3, EDNRB MITF, PAX3, SNAI2, SOX10	Dystopia canthorum, congenital SNHL, heterochromia irises, white forelock
Branchio-oto-renal	Autosomal dominant	EYA1	SNHL, MHL, or CHL; external ear abnormalities, preauricular pits, branchial cleft anomalies, renal abnormalities
Pendred	Autosomal recessive	SLC26A4	SNHL stable or progressive, enlarged vestibular aqueduct with or without cochlear aplasia, goiter
Usher	Autosomal recessive	CDH23, CLRN, GPR98, MYO7A, PCDH15, USH1, USH1G, USH2A	Type 1: congenital or progressive SNHL, progressive vision loss, with or without vestibular dysfunction
Alport	X-linked: 80% Autosomal recessive: 15% Autosomal dominant: 5%	COL4A, COL4A4, COL4A5	Progressive SNHL, progressive renal failure, anterior lenticonus and perimacular flecks

Abbreviations: CHL, conductive hearing loss; MHL, mixed hearing loss; SNHL, sensorineural hearing loss.

or dysmorphic growth. The nose should be evaluated for bilateral nasal patency, and if obstruction is suspected, endoscopic evaluation for choanal atresia should be performed. The neck should be examined for any pits that could be consistent with branchial cleft anomalies. A complete cranial nerve examination also should be performed. In children who are old enough to cooperate, vestibular testing may be performed because hearing loss and balance problems may be associated.

> **Pearl:** The light reflex is not a reliable indicator of middle-ear or tympanic membrane disease.

■ Diagnosis

UNIVERSAL NEWBORN HEARING SCREENING

In 1993, an expert panel at the National Institutes of Health recommended that all infants be screened for hearing loss. A great improvement in the early detection of and intervention in congenital hearing loss subsequently occurred with the advent of the UNHS program, and currently 95% of newborns are screened in the United States. In addition, agencies such as the National Center for Hearing Assessment and Management and state-based early hearing detection and intervention (EHDI) programs have markedly improved identification of and education about pediatric hearing loss. Before the advent of UNHS, the average age at identification of congenital hearing loss was 2.5 to 3 years; that has now dropped to 14 months. The goal of UNHS is not only to have all neonates screened for hearing loss before discharge or by 1 month of age but also to ensure that appropriate follow-up is achieved. Newborns who fail hearing screening should undergo a follow-up evaluation by 3 months of age, and those with identified hearing loss should receive appropriate hearing rehabilitation and services by 6 months of age. Despite the great success that has occurred with initial newborn hearing screening, half of those who fail screening tests do not undergo follow-up testing. Children who are identified with hearing loss and receive intervention by 6 months of age usually have normal language development by age 5 years; children who experience delays in identification and intervention have difficulty catching up to their hearing peers.

Universal newborn hearing screening cannot identify all children with hearing loss because many with mild hearing loss will be missed, and a proportion of children who pass UNHS will go on to develop hearing loss later in life. Those children often are not identified until the preschool or school years. Because of the risk of delayed diagnosis in these children, in 2007 the Joint Committee on Infant Hearing (JCIH) updated its guidelines to improve identification of newborns at risk for late-onset hearing impairment (**Box 1-2**).

The PCC plays an essential role in the ongoing screening for hearing loss. After UNHS, the next formalized hearing evaluation may not occur until the beginning of school. Guidelines from the American Academy of Audiology recommend screening in preschool,

---

Box 1-2. 2007 Joint Committee on Infant Hearing Risk Indicators Associated With Permanent Congenital, Delayed Onset, or Progressive Hearing Loss

- Caregiver concern about hearing, speech, language, or developmental delay
- Family history of permanent childhood hearing loss
- Neonatal intensive care of more than 5 days or any of the following regardless of length of stay: extracorporeal membrane oxygenation, assisted ventilation, exposure to ototoxic medications (gentamicin, tobramycin) or loop diuretics (furosemide/Lasix), and hyperbilirubinemia that requires exchange transfusion
- In utero infections, such as cytomegalovirus, herpes, rubella, syphilis, and toxoplasmosis
- Craniofacial anomalies, including those that involve the pinna, ear canal, ear tags, ear pits, and temporal bone anomalies
- Physical findings, such as white forelock, that are associated with a syndrome known to include a sensorineural or permanent conductive hearing loss
- Syndromes associated with hearing loss or progressive or late-onset hearing loss, such as neurofibromatosis, osteopetrosis, and Usher syndrome; other frequently identified syndromes include Waardenburg, Alport, Pendred, and Jervell and Lange-Nielsen
- Neurodegenerative disorders, such as Hunter syndrome, or sensory motor neuropathies, such as Friedreich ataxia and Charcot-Marie-Tooth syndrome
- Culture-positive postnatal infections associated with sensorineural hearing loss, including confirmed bacterial and viral (especially herpesviruses and varicella) meningitis
- Head trauma, especially basal skull/temporal bone fracture that requires hospitalization
- Chemotherapy

Derived from American Academy of Pediatrics Joint Committee on Infant Hearing. Year 2007 position statement: principles and guidelines for early hearing detection and intervention programs. *Pediatrics*. 2007;120(4):898–921.

---

kindergarten, and grades 1, 3, 5, and either 7 or 9, whereas the JCIH recommends hearing screening for newborns as well as during routine well-child visits at ages 4, 5, 6, 8, and 10. Primary care clinicians should be vigilant in screening for signs of developing hearing loss. They should provide parents with information about hearing, speech, and language milestones; identify and treat middle-ear disease; and provide ongoing developmental surveillance. They should also be aware of and assess neonates for any of the risk factors for late-onset hearing loss.

Hospitals and clinics use 2 types of newborn hearing screening. Many use otoacoustic emissions (OAEs) testing. This test measures the function of the external auditory canal, tympanic membrane, middle ear, and outer hair cells of the cochlea but does not assess the inner hair cells of the cochlea or the cochlear nerve. Other hospitals use automated auditory brain stem response (ABR) testing, which assesses the entire hearing pathway, with a sensitivity down to 30 decibels (dB) (normal hearing is considered ≤20 dB). Screening OAEs and automated ABR provide only a pass or fail report and do not require the interpretation of an audiologist. False-positive results can occur because of amniotic fluid in the middle ear. Neither test determines the degree of hearing loss and both can miss mild hearing loss (<30 dB). One type of hearing loss, auditory neuropathy/dyssynchrony spectrum disorder (ANSD), may not be detected by UNHS programs using OAEs. It is actually a range of disorders in which sound enters the inner ear normally, but the transmission of sound from the cochlea to the brain is abnormal. Children who are admitted to the neonatal intensive care unit (NICU) are at higher risk for ANSD and thus should always be screened with automated ABR and not OAEs alone. In addition, children who are readmitted during the newborn period for conditions associated with hearing loss, such as hyperbilirubinemia requiring exchange transfusion or sepsis, should undergo repeated hearing screening by automated ABR.

> **Pearl:** All newborns should be screened for hearing loss by discharge or 1 month of age; those who fail the hearing screening should undergo follow-up evaluation by 3 months of age; and those with identified hearing loss should receive appropriate hearing rehabilitation and services by 6 months of age.

AUDIOLOGIC EVALUATION

Neonates who fail UNHS should undergo a timely formal audiologic evaluation, including an otoscopic inspection, child and family history, assessment of middle-ear function, and OAE and diagnostic ABR testing. Every child with identified permanent hearing loss should be referred to the state EHDI program and requires evaluation by an otolaryngologist.

AUDITORY BRAIN STEM RESPONSE TESTING

The automated ABR used in UNHS gives only a pass or fail reading and does not assess the degree of hearing loss. Diagnostic ABR is used to assess newborn hearing after the neonate has failed UNHS. The ABR is an electrophysiologic measurement of the function of the entire hearing pathway, including the brain stem. It is performed by placing earphones or probes in the ears, which give clicks and tones, and electrodes on the head that measure the waveform response to the sounds emitted. The results can provide frequency range and dB response level information. A quiet room is needed for testing. Auditory brain stem response can be performed in sleeping infants or with sedation. Generally, children younger than 6 months do not require sedation.

OTOACOUSTIC EMISSIONS

Whether the initial hearing screening was OAEs or automated ABR, OAEs will be performed at the audiologic evaluation. Otoacoustic emissions are performed with an ear probe that, like ABR, delivers clicks and tone bursts. The probe also contains a microphone that detects acoustic signals generated by the cochlea in response to sound. The advantages of OAEs are that they can be performed quickly in children of any age who are awake or asleep. Otoacoustic emissions do not quantify the degree of hearing loss and do not assess the function of the auditory nerve or brain stem. In addition, middle-ear or tympanic eardrum pathology will affect the accuracy of this test.

Both ABR and OAEs measure only the integrity of the auditory pathway and are not a direct measure of the ability to hear. Hearing cannot be confirmed until the child is old enough to undergo audiometric testing.

AUDIOMETRY

Audiometry is ideally performed in a sound booth in which extraneous noise is eliminated. Children vary in their ability to cooperate with behavioral audiometric testing, and various tests exist for different ages.

Audiometry measures the hearing in several ways. Bone conduction transmits sound through the skull directly to the cochlea. Air conduction transmits sound through the ear canal to the tympanic membrane, ossicles, and cochlea. These measurements allow the audiologist to determine if hearing loss is *conductive* (caused by pathology in the ear canal, tympanic membrane, middle ear, or ossicles) or *sensorineural* (caused by pathology of the cochlea or eighth nerve). Hearing thresholds greater than 20 dB are considered hearing impairment.

Visual Reinforcement Audiometry

Infants as young as 6 months may be able to provide behavioral hearing responses. For visual reinforcement audiometry, the infant is seated in the caregiver's lap and is trained to turn toward a toy or light when he or she hears a sound. Some children may tolerate wearing earphones, and individual ear hearing data can be obtained. Most young children will not wear earphones and, thus, the hearing is assessed in "the sound field," meaning that only the hearing of both ears together can be measured. This allows for accurate measurement of hearing in only the ear that hears better, so unilateral hearing loss cannot be ruled out.

Play Audiometry

Once children are 2 years of age, they may be tested by training them to respond to auditory stimuli by play activities (eg, dropping a block in a box when a sound is heard). Children of this age can usually wear headphones, and individual ear hearing levels can be measured.

Conventional Audiometry

Children older than 4 years can undergo audiometry testing in the same way that adults do—by wearing headphones and raising their hand when they hear auditory stimuli.

Tympanometry

Tympanometry assesses the mobility of the tympanic membrane by creating positive and negative pressure in the ear canal. Tympanometry results can provide information about the integrity of the tympanic membrane and the condition of the middle ear and ossicles.

> **Pearl:** Testing of hearing is individualized to the age of the child.

◼ Medical Evaluation

OTOLARYNGOLOGY EVALUATION

All children with confirmed hearing loss should be referred to an otolaryngologist as soon as possible. The otolaryngologist will review the history and perform a thorough physical examination, as outlined earlier. In addition, the otolaryngologist will counsel the family about the consequences of hearing loss and pursue diagnostic evaluations to potentially determine the cause. The most suitable type of treatment for the hearing loss will then be determined. Hearing aids cannot be distributed without clearance from an otolaryngologist.

RADIOGRAPHIC EVALUATION

Radiographic imaging is among the highest yielding studies in the investigation of hearing loss etiology. As many as 40% of children with hearing loss have an identifiable etiology on computed tomography (CT) or magnetic resonance imaging (MRI). Computed tomography is most helpful at identifying middle- and inner-ear abnormalities, while MRI is used most often to identify the cochlear nerve and intracranial masses that can lead to hearing loss. Emerging evidence indicates that there may be long-term risks of malignancy from CT scans performed in young children. Therefore, some otolaryngologists favor MRI or are opting to limit these examinations or use a sequential approach to testing in which other high-yield tests (eg, genetic testing) are performed before a CT scan is obtained. Because progressive sensorineural hearing loss (SNHL) is associated with the anatomical abnormality of wide or enlarged vestibular aqueduct (EVA), children with worsening of their baseline hearing loss should undergo CT or MRI to assess for EVA if prior imaging was not performed. Almost certainly, the best approach to testing is to engage in an informed discussion with parents or caregivers to come to a mutually acceptable decision about which tests to perform.

Children who have ear anomalies as well as hearing loss, dysmorphic features, a family history of deafness, or a maternal history of gestational diabetes or diabetes mellitus should undergo a renal ultrasound. The ultrasound may aid in the diagnosis of syndromic hearing loss, such as branchio-oto-renal syndrome, CHARGE (Coloboma, Heart defects, choanal Atresia, Retarded growth, and Genital and Ear anomalies) syndrome, and diabetic embryopathy.

GENETIC TESTING

Although imaging remains the highest-yield modality for investigating the cause of hearing loss, the number of genes associated with hearing loss is rapidly expanding. The most common mutations that cause bilateral SNHL occur in the *GJB2* gene (codes for the connexin 26 gap junction protein). The International Pediatric Otolaryngology Group consensus recommendations on hearing loss in pediatric patients suggest that otolaryngologists should consider using genetic testing as their first evaluation and only proceed with imaging or laboratory testing if the genetic test result is negative. Testing a panel of genes associated with hearing loss has become more affordable and available, including better coverage by insurance.

The interpretation of genetic tests and the understanding of the ramifications of the diagnosis of a syndrome are complex and require the expertise of geneticists and genetic counselors. A genetics team should always be engaged when evaluating for the presence of a syndrome, and it is also highly useful for pretest and posttest counseling about genetic testing results.

OPHTHALMOLOGIC EVALUATION

While hearing loss can be associated with abnormalities in every system of the body, the highest association is with ophthalmologic disorders. Syndromic children are especially likely to have ocular anomalies, and all should undergo evaluation by an ophthalmologist. In addition, nonsyndromic children with hearing loss are at particular risk for decreased learning and function if they also have visual impairment; thus, it is wise to ensure that their vision is fully intact.

> **Pearl:** Many otolaryngologists opt for sequential use of the highest-yield tests to limit radiation and reduce unnecessary evaluations.

CARDIOLOGIC EVALUATION

Electrocardiography is used to assess the presence of prolonged QT, a life-threatening cardiac arrhythmia that can lead to sudden death. Prolonged QT with congenital severe to profound SNHL can be associated with a very rare syndrome called Jervell and Lange-Nielsen syndrome. Electrocardiography is recommended in all children with bilateral profound SNHL, especially those who have a personal history of syncope or a family history of sudden death in childhood.

LABORATORY TESTS

Historically, a large array of laboratory tests were performed to look for rare causes of hearing loss. These include a complete blood cell count, serum chemistry, blood glucose, thyroid function test, TORCH (Toxoplasmosis, Other, Rubella, CMV, Herpes simplex titers), fluorescent treponemal antibody absorption testing for syphilis, autoimmune serologies, and urinalysis. Cost-benefit analyses have suggested that these studies should be selectively ordered based on a thorough history and physical examination findings, and perhaps only after other high-yield tests have been performed. Cytomegalovirus has emerged as a common cause of both congenital and delayed-onset SNHL. Though fewer than half of cases of SNHL caused by CMV are present at birth, it may be beneficial to perform CMV testing (saliva or urine culture) within the first 3 weeks after birth in children who do not pass newborn hearing screening, as diagnostic testing after this critical period is limited because of the high rate of postnatal CMV exposure.

■ Types of Hearing Loss

Several types of hearing loss exist. Conductive hearing loss (CHL) occurs whenever there is a disruption of function of the external ear, external auditory canal, tympanic membrane, middle ear, or ossicles. In children, the most common causes of CHL are otitis media with effusion (OME), foreign body in the external auditory canal, and cerumen impaction. Several syndromes are also associated with CHL, particularly those with external auditory canal atresia such as Treacher Collins syndrome. Disruptions in the function of the cochlea, cranial nerve VII, or brain stem can all cause SNHL. The level and quality of sound heard may be diminished. Mixed hearing loss (MHL) is a combination of CHL and SNHL and often occurs in syndromic children. Hearing loss can also be defined as stable or progressive, congenital or delayed onset, and genetic or nongenetic. As mentioned earlier, ANSD is a special type of hearing loss in which the transmission of sound from the cochlea to the brain is altered. It is heterogenous and can include abnormalities ranging from the transmission of sound from the inner hair cells of the cochlea to the auditory nerve, discoordinated neuron function or hypoplasia of the auditory nerve, or dysfunction of the auditory nuclei in the brain stem. Etiologies include genetic mutations (otoferlin gene), events associated with hypoxemia (prematurity, ventilator dependence), hyperbilirubinemia, and neurologic disorders. In children with this type of hearing loss, hearing may range from normal to profound SNHL on audiometric testing. They typically have more difficulty understanding speech, especially with background noise, than children with similar levels of hearing who do not have ANSD. Children with ANSD may experience fluctuations in hearing, and their hearing may improve, worsen, or stay the same over time. Because of the complexity of this disorder, children with ANSD should be cared for by pediatric audiologists and otolaryngologists who are knowledgeable about this disorder.

Table 1-3 defines the degrees of hearing loss in terms of dB lost. **Figure 1-1** gives a pictorial account of the types of sounds that are missed at different levels of hearing loss.

■ Causes of Hearing Loss

GENETIC

Genetic causes account for at least 50% of congenital SNHL and approximately 20% of all pediatric hearing loss. Genetic causes can be divided into nonsyndromic (80%) and syndromic (20%). More than 300 genes have been associated with pediatric hearing loss. Seventy-five percent to 80% of nonsyndromic hearing loss is autosomal recessive. Therefore, most children with genetic hearing loss are born to parents with normal hearing. The remaining distribution of nonsyndromic hereditary hearing loss is 20% autosomal dominant,

Table 1-3. Levels of Hearing Loss	
Degree of Hearing Loss	**Hearing Loss Range (dB)**
Normal	-10 to 15
Slight	16 to 25
Mild	26 to 40
Moderate	41 to 55
Moderately severe	56 to 70
Severe	71 to 90
Profound	≥91

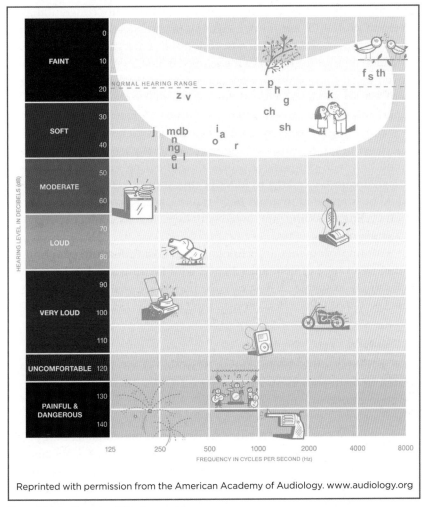

Reprinted with permission from the American Academy of Audiology. www.audiology.org

Figure 1-1. Audiogram of familiar sounds.

2% to 5% X-linked, and 1% mitochondrial. Remarkably, mutations in a single gene, *GJB2,* account for about half of all hereditary SNHL in the United States. *GJB2* encodes the protein connexin 26, which is involved in the gap-junction system of the inner ear. Hearing loss from mutations in the *GJB2* gene is autosomal recessive and can vary from mild to profound and be stable or progressive.

Pendred syndrome is the most common form of syndromic hearing loss. Children with Pendred syndrome have SNHL, EVA with or without cochlear aplasia, and goiter. Most cases are caused by mutation in the *SLC26A4* gene. Hearing loss is usually congenital and severe to profound, but milder loss and progressive loss are possible. Goiter does not present until late childhood. Enlarged vestibular aqueduct syndrome (EVAS), which is SNHL and EVA without goiter, is even more common than Pendred syndrome and may account for 5% to 15% of all SNHL. The etiology is multifactorial, with environmental and genetic causes. Children with EVAS may be born with normal hearing or have congenital hearing loss. They are at risk of experiencing progressive hearing loss, especially from trauma. Thus, all children with progressive or late-onset hearing loss should be evaluated with CT or MRI to identify this abnormality. They also should be counseled to avoid head trauma, wear protective helmets when cycling or skiing, and avoid activities such as contact sports and scuba diving.

With improvements in technology and cost reduction, panel testing of a range of genes associated with hearing loss has become increasingly available. A host of gene panels are available, including GeneDx, OtoSCOPE, OtoGenome, and OtoSeq.

ACQUIRED

Most acquired causes of childhood hearing loss are infectious or related to birth complications (see **Box 1-1**). Vaccinations against common causes of congenital hearing loss have nearly eliminated some infectious etiologies, such as rubella. In developed countries, congenital CMV is currently the most common infectious etiology and is estimated to cause 20% of congenital hearing loss. Congenital CMV is also a major contributor to delayed and progressive hearing loss in childhood, and a quarter of childhood hearing loss is likely due to CMV. However, confirmatory diagnosis requires blood samples obtained in the first 3 weeks after birth and because this rarely occurs, most suspected cases of CMV-related hearing loss cannot be verified or treated. More recently, polymerase chain reaction analysis of archived newborn heel stick blood spots has allowed the detection of congenital CMV, though the yield is poor. Treatment with valganciclovir in this critical period may prevent the development or limit progression of hearing loss. Some are now advocating adding CMV testing to the battery of newborn screening measures to allow for early antiviral treatment. Several states have passed legislation mandating or offering CMV testing.

During the perinatal period, the most common causes of acquired hearing loss are related to other postnatal morbidities. Admission to the NICU, while not a direct risk, is a measure of serious perinatal morbidity and is associated with a 10-fold increase in SNHL. Many of the risk factors, such as low Apgar scores and prematurity, are most likely caused by hypoxemic injury to the inner ear and cochlear nerve. These children are at particular risk for auditory neuropathy/dyssynchrony and require continued surveillance for progressive hearing loss.

Conductive hearing loss because of acute otitis media or OME is the most common cause of hearing loss in infants and young children. Bacterial meningitis, though rare with the advent of vaccination for *Streptococcus pneumoniae* and *Haemophilus influenzae* type b, is the most frequent cause of acquired SNHL in this age group. The most common etiologies of new hearing loss in older school-aged children are likely silent congenital CMV infection and noise trauma, although many older children, especially those with unilateral hearing loss, may have had unrecognized hearing loss since birth or early childhood.

> **Pearl:** Identifying the cause of hearing loss can help families process the diagnosis and make treatment decisions. However, some families will opt to not obtain this information.

▨ Treatment for Sensorineural Hearing Loss

AMPLIFICATION

No medical treatment exists for SNHL. The first step for these children is amplification. All children with bilateral SNHL and many with unilateral SNHL are candidates for amplification. Even those with profound loss on ABR may still experience some benefit and, at the very least, need to undergo a trial with hearing aids before being considered for cochlear implantation. Often, considerable time delay occurs between identification of a hearing loss and fitting of hearing aids. This can be because of cost issues, access to audiologic services, or parental concern about the use of hearing aids. Primary care clinicians should emphasize to parents the vital importance of hearing-impaired children's wearing hearing aids, and that it is essential for excellent speech and language development and good school performance. Social recognition by peers of "differentness" does not usually occur until 5 or 6 years of age; therefore, this may reassure some parents about the appearance of wearing hearing aids. As children get older, they may decide not to wear their aids for various reasons, including lack of perceived benefit and social issues. Primary care clinicians and caregivers should respect the concerns of these children, while at the same time continuing to assess whether they are having difficulties in school or in communicating by not wearing the aids. Some families may request smaller devices, but because the ear canal is constantly growing, children can only wear behind-the-ear (BTE) hearing aids, not the smaller aids available to adults.

Hearing aids are fitted by creating a properly sized mold for the external ear and canal. The hearing aid rests over and behind the ear. The amplification is adjusted to optimize hearing while avoiding pain from sound pressure on the tympanic membrane.

Types of Hearing Amplification

BEHIND THE EAR (BTE)

Most children wear BTE hearing aids. Some who cannot tolerate wearing a device on the ear use a body aid. The advantages of BTE aids are that they are the most durable; as the child grows only the ear mold must be replaced; they are less likely to produce feedback; and they can be coupled to assistive technology. Adolescents whose ears are fully grown may use smaller aids that are partly or completely in the ear canal. However, these aids cost more, cannot be coupled to other devices, and are more easily damaged.

CONTRALATERAL ROUTING OF SIGNAL

Children with severe to profound unilateral hearing loss are unlikely to gain significant benefit from BTE aids. Contralateral routing of signal (CROS) systems have a microphone on the impaired ear that transmits the sound signal to a device worn on the normal-hearing ear. Some children do not tolerate this because they do not wish to wear an aid in the normal-hearing ear. Children with severe to profound hearing loss in one ear and hearing that can be aided in the other ear can use a similar system called the BiCROS (Bilateral microphones with Contralateral Routing Of Signal).

BONE-ANCHORED HEARING AIDS

Several types of hearing loss are not suitable for wearing BTE aids. Children with microtia or external auditory canal atresia with CHL or MHL cannot wear traditional aids. In addition, some children who have chronic ear drainage that cannot be treated by surgery cannot wear aids in the ear. Children with single-sided severe to profound SNHL also will not benefit from BTE aids. For these children, a bone-anchored hearing aid (BAHA) may be used. This involves the surgical implantation of a titanium implant in the temporal bone behind the auricle. Two options exist for sound transmission from an external processor. The classic type involves a titanium strut that is attached to the bone-anchored implant and protrudes through the skin and directly connects to the external sound processor (**Figure 1-2**). A more recent type has a magnet attached to the bone-anchored implant beneath the skin (**Figure 1-3**). The external sound processor has a second magnet that rests on the skin over the internal magnet. For both types, sound is transmitted from the sound processor to the implant and then through the bone directly to the cochlea, bypassing the external and middle ear. The quality of the sound is better with the classic type than with the magnet, but minor irritation or infection at the strut is common, so families can choose the type they prefer. In the United States, children cannot obtain this implant until they are 5 years of age when the skull has grown sufficiently thick to support the implant. Until then, they can wear a headband (soft band) that holds the sound processor firmly against the skull.

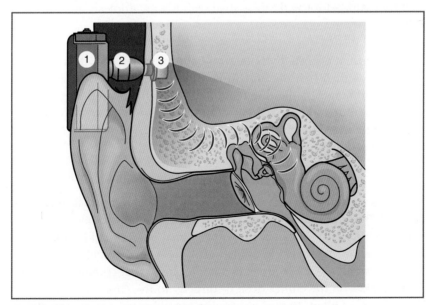

Figure 1-2. Bone-anchored hearing aid via transcutaneous strut: (1) external sound processor; (2) titanium strut; (3) osseointegrated implant.

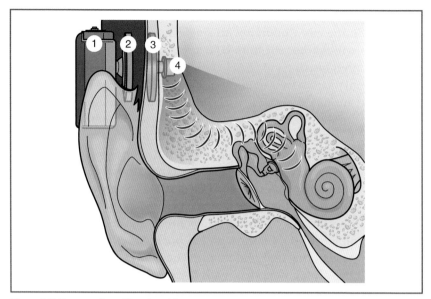

Figure 1-3. Bone-anchored hearing aid via magnet: (1) external sound processor; (2) external magnet; (3) internal magnet; (4) osseointegrated implant.

Some children prefer the soft band to surgery and opt to continue using it instead of undergoing surgery, though most find the hearing quality better with the BAHA.

SPEECH THERAPY

Many children, especially those who have experienced a delay in diagnosis of their hearing impairment, have significant issues with speech and language development. Speech therapy can be helpful for these children. Many schools offer brief sessions 1 or 2 times per week, but children with significant delays may require more intensive therapy outside of school.

SCHOOL ACCOMMODATIONS

Children with hearing impairment should be seated nearest to the teacher. Because many teachers move about the classroom, and background noise can interfere with optimal hearing aid perfor-mance, an FM (frequency modulation) system is often helpful. With an FM system, the teacher wears a microphone that communicates to a speaker on the child's desk or directly to the child's hearing aid or cochlear implant. Closed captioning for films and videos can also be beneficial. Children with hearing impairment should always have an Individualized Education Program to ensure they are receiving the services they require.

> **Pearl:** Early intervention and multidisciplinary collaboration are necessary for the best outcomes for children with hearing impairment.

COCHLEAR IMPLANTS

Cochlear implantation has revolutionized the care of children with severe to profound hearing loss. Numerous studies have shown a clear benefit of implantation over amplification or other modes of communication. It cannot be underestimated that time is of the essence when evaluating infants with congenital SNHL for implantation. Children who do not receive an implant until after their first birthday are at increasing risk for poor speech and language development, whereas children who receive implants at or near 12 months of age have a greater potential to function at the level of their normal-hearing peers. Children who have experienced late-onset hearing loss after the development of language (postlingually deaf) are also excellent candidates. While implants were initially placed in only 1 ear, research supports bilateral implantation in children. Children who are prelingually deaf are assessed for candidacy based on their ABR results as well as failure to develop auditory skills. Older children are evaluated by audiometry as well as by several more specific tests that assess the development of speech and language. All children must undergo a 3-month hearing aid trial to determine if they may benefit from hearing aids and to assess if they and their parents will adhere to wearing an aid device regularly. All children evaluated for cochlear implantation must undergo imaging studies, usually MRI with or without CT, to evaluate the inner ear anatomy and confirm the presence of a cochlear nerve. Children with abnormalities of the inner ear are still candidates for implantation, but modifications in surgical technique and expectations of outcome by parents may be necessary.

Counseling families about expectations for implantation is paramount. While many children have excellent outcomes, it is not possible to predict how someone will perform with an implant. Children with developmental delay, autism spectrum disorder, or other cognitive issues may not perform as well. This does not preclude them from receiving an implant, but it is important for parents to tailor their expectations. In addition, families must understand that the aural rehabilitation following implantation is intensive and requires a long-term commitment. The cochlear implant team should determine that adequate resources will be available to ensure maximal benefit from the implant. Educational programs for the hearing impaired are varied in their emphasis and quality, and children undergoing implantation should participate in programs that promote listening and speaking instead of signed communication, as their ultimate outcome depends considerably on the quality of these programs. Continuing assessment and dialogue should occur among audiologists, otolaryngologists, speech pathologists, the school, and family to ensure maximal benefit from the implant.

Children with SNHL are at an increased risk of developing meningitis; undergoing cochlear implantation increases this risk. The 13-valent pneumococcal conjugate vaccine (PCV13, Prevnar 13) and the 23-valent pneumococcal polysaccharide vaccine (PPSV23, Pneumovax 23) should be administered. Children cannot undergo PPSV23 vaccination until they are 24 months old; thus, children receiving the implant prior to that age must undergo immunization after implantation.

> **Pearl:** Children with congenital hearing loss who are candidates for cochlear implantation ideally should receive an implant by their first birthday.

▓ Treatments for Conductive Hearing Loss

Children with OME that has not resolved after 3 months are candidates for bilateral myringotomies and pressure-equalization tubes. Depending on the degree of hearing loss and presence of speech delay, developmental delay, intellectual disability, or MHL, the length of time that OME with hearing loss should be observed varies. In general, children who have or are at risk for speech or cognitive delay should have tubes placed earlier, while those who do not can be observed longer.

Children who use cotton-tipped swabs to clean their ears are at risk for cerumen impaction, as well as retention of part of the swab in their ear. These should be removed promptly to restore hearing.

External auditory canal atresia, tympanic membrane perforation, and ossicular pathologies can lead to CHL that may benefit from surgery or hearing amplification.

■ Natural History and Prognosis

Immunizations and antibiotics have contributed substantially to decreasing many causes of pediatric hearing loss. Before the advent of vaccines, mumps and rubella were leading causes of pediatric hearing loss. In the developing world, congenital rubella syndrome contributes heavily to the burden of SNHL, especially in countries without vaccination programs. The proportion of hearing loss due to other causes has shifted to genetic mutations and complications in the neonatal period.

Even children with mild hearing loss are at risk for delays in speech and language development. In particular, they may have difficulty acquiring new words and may require visual and auditory input to develop language at the rate of their peers. The more severe the hearing loss, the greater the risk for deficient speech acquisition and poor academic performance. Infants with severe to profound loss will develop no spoken language at all without amplification or cochlear implantation. These children may use sign language, but because 90% of children with hearing loss are born to hearing parents, tremendous effort will be required for parents and the child to learn this new language.

Historically, sign language was an essential form of communication for people with severe to profound hearing loss. Children who were prevented from learning sign language and relied on lipreading and acquiring oral speech were often exhausted by the intensity of the therapy required. Children born into deaf families easily learn sign language in the same way that hearing children learn oral language. However, for a host of factors, deaf children who sign lag their hearing peers and children who have received cochlear implants. The median reading level of deaf adults is fourth grade. In addition, exclusive use of sign language can isolate individuals from the world community and limit vocational opportunities. Children with developmental delay or autism spectrum disorder and those with severe to profound loss who are not candidates for cochlear implantation may never develop spoken language.

For those children, sign language is an essential communication modality.

Unilateral hearing loss offers additional insight into the natural history of pediatric hearing impairment, as these children are less likely to be helped. Thirty-five percent of children with unilateral loss failed at least 1 grade, 50% exhibited some difficulty in educational progress, and 20% were believed by teachers to have a behavioral problem. Functional MRI studies have shown that children with unilateral hearing loss utilize their frontal lobe, in addition to their auditory cortex, when performing auditory tasks, lending evidence to why they may struggle in school.

Children who are identified with hearing loss early and receive appropriate intervention in a timely manner are still at risk for academic and social problems. Ongoing assessment and collaboration among schools, parents, speech therapists, and PCCs are essential to improving developmental and academic achievement.

■ Selected References

American Academy of Pediatrics Joint Committee on Infant Hearing. Year 2007 position statement: principles and guidelines for early hearing detection and intervention programs. *Pediatrics.* 2007;120(4):898–921

American Speech-Language-Hearing Association. How does your child hear and talk? http://asha.org/public/speech/development/chart.htm. Accessed September 5, 2019

Bess FH, Tharpe AM, Gibler AM. Auditory performance of children with unilateral sensorineural hearing loss. *Ear Hear.* 1986;7(1):20–26

Driver S, Jiang D. Paediatric cochlear implantation factors that affect outcomes. *Eur J Paediatr Neurol.* 2017;21(1):104–108

Fowler KB, Boppana SB. Congenital cytomegalovirus (CMV) infection and hearing deficit. *J Clin Virol.* 2006;35(2):226–231

Jerry J, Oghalai JS. Towards an etiologic diagnosis: assessing the patient with hearing loss. *Adv Otorhinolaryngol.* 2011;70:28–36

Katbamna B, Crumpton T, Patel DR. Hearing impairment in children. *Pediatr Clin North Am.* 2008;55(5):1175–1188, ix

Korver AM, Admiraal RJ, Kant SG, et al; on behalf of the DECIBEL-collaborative study group. Causes of permanent childhood hearing impairment. *Laryngoscope.* 2011;121(2):409–416

Mehra S, Eavey RD, Keamy DG Jr. The epidemiology of hearing impairment in the United States: newborns, children, and adolescents. *Otolaryngol Head Neck Surg.* 2009;140(4):461–472

Misono S, Sie KC, Weiss NS, et al. Congenital cytomegalovirus infection in pediatric hearing loss. *Arch Otolaryngol Head Neck Surg.* 2011;137(1):47–53

National Institute on Deafness and Other Communication Disorders. Enlarged vestibular aqueducts and childhood hearing loss. https://www.nidcd.nih.gov/health/enlarged-vestibular-aqueducts-and-childhood-hearing-loss. Updated February 2017. Accessed September 5, 2019

NIH Consensus Development Conference. Early identification of hearing impairment in infants and young children. *Int J Pediatr Otorhinolaryngol.* 1993;27(2):201–202

Shah RK, Lotke M. Hearing impairment clinical presentation. Medscape. http://emedicine.medscape.com/article/994159-clinical. Updated July 14, 2017. Accessed September 5, 2019

Smith RJ, Bale JF Jr, White KR. Sensorineural hearing loss in children. *Lancet.* 2005; 365(9462):879–890

Toriello HV, Reardon W, Gorlin RJ. *Hereditary Hearing Loss and Its Syndromes.* 2nd ed. New York, NY: Oxford University Press; 2004

Traxler CB. The Stanford Achievement Test, 9th Edition: National Norming and Performance Standards for Deaf and Hard-of-Hearing Students. *J Deaf Stud Deaf Educ.* 2000;5(4):337–348

Wang RY, Earl DL, Ruder RO, Graham JM Jr. Syndromic ear anomalies and renal ultrasounds. *Pediatrics.* 2001;108(2):e32

CHAPTER 2

Management and Treatment of Patients With Acute and Chronic Otitis Media

Simon Carr, MD, and Blake Papsin, MD

▓ Introduction

Otitis media (OM) is a broad term given to any inflammatory process within the middle ear. Multiple diagnoses can be included under this general term, but typically they are classified as acute or chronic, based on the period from onset of the disease. A disease that persists for more than 3 months usually is considered chronic. Otitis media can be subclassified as suppurative, nonsuppurative, or recurrent (**Box 2-1**). The main focus of this chapter is the management and treatment of patients with acute OM (AOM) and chronic OM (COM), including chronic suppurative OM (CSOM) and OM with effusion (OME). Current guidelines are reviewed, and advances in epidemiology and pathogenesis are included, as well as the facts necessary to make a definitive diagnosis, provide adequate management, and prevent complications.

Acute OM and COM are probably the most common ear diseases that primary care clinicians (PCCs), as well as pediatric otolaryngologists, encounter in their daily clinical practice. Sometimes, distinguishing each condition can be a challenging process for the PCC or specialist. This can lead to overdiagnosis, inappropriate use of antibiotics, and overtreatment, which, in turn, can have a significant effect on children's health and the direct cost of health care. Therefore, it is important to recognize and classify each condition accordingly and understand the pathophysiology and treatment options available.

Acute OM is defined by the American Academy of Pediatrics (AAP) and American Academy of Family Physicians (AAFM) as an infection of the middle ear with acute onset, along with effusion and signs of middle-ear inflammation, such as otalgia, and distinct erythema of the tympanic membrane (TM). The presence of

---

Box 2-1. Classification of Otitis Media

Acute Otitis Media
- ◆ Suppurative
- ◆ Nonsuppurative
- ◆ Recurrent (≥3 episodes)

Chronic Otitis Media
- ◆ Suppurative
- ◆ Nonsuppurative
- ◆ Otitis media with effusion

middle-ear inflammation can be indicated by any of the following: bulging of the TM, limited or absent mobility of the TM with pneumatic otoscopy, air-fluid level behind the TM, or otorrhea. Acute OM is the most common diagnosis given to a febrile child, and it is commonly overdiagnosed (often because the TM cannot be visualized owing to the presence of cerumen, so the diagnosis becomes speculative). The high incidence and high rate of spontaneous recovery from uncomplicated AOM suggest that it is a natural event and part of the gradual maturation of the child's immune system. On the other hand, an untreated complex AOM can lead to complications such as acute mastoiditis, subperiosteal abscess, and, much more uncommonly, meningitis, brain abscess, or thrombophlebitis of the sigmoid sinus, among others.

Chronic suppurative OM is defined as a TM perforation with chronic ear drainage. Signs of middle-ear inflammation are usually present. If not treated successfully with medical or surgical intervention, CSOM can lead to complications similar to those of AOM. In reality, the presence of a low-pressure exit pathway for the infection through the ear canal results in a decreased incidence of complications occurring centrally (ie, the brain and meninges), although structures of the middle ear remain at risk for complications (ie, the facial nerve and ossicles).

Otitis media with effusion is more common than AOM and is defined as middle-ear effusion (MEE) without signs or symptoms of an acute infection. Otitis media with effusion can occur spontaneously because of eustachian tube (ET) dysfunction or may be the result of, or sequela to, AOM. Even though both disorders require MEE for diagnosis, the main difference is the absence of acute signs and symptoms of middle-ear inflammation in OME. Otitis media with effusion differs from CSOM because there is no TM perforation. Otitis media with effusion commonly resolves spontaneously within 3 months (if there is no reinfection), but if persistent and untreated, conductive hearing loss (CHL) can occur, which may affect behavior and delay communicative development.

> **Pearl:** *Acute otitis media* refers to an acute infection or inflammation in the middle ear with local or systemic signs and symptoms and the presence of an effusion in the middle ear.

▮ Epidemiology of Otitis Media

Despite advances in public health and medical care, OM is still prevalent globally and the incidence in North America has actually increased over the past 2 decades. The overall use of antibiotics has also remained high during this interval. In 2006, 9 million children aged 0 to 17 years were reported to have had an ear infection; of those, 8 million visited a PCC or obtained a prescription drug for treatment.

Otitis media occurs in all age groups but is considerably more common in children between the ages of 6 months and 3 years. This is presumably because of immunologic and anatomical factors. Children with significant predisposing factors (eg, cleft palate, Down syndrome) acquire infections more frequently. Generally, by age 3 years, nearly all children have experienced an episode of OM. Males are more susceptible to OM (no specific causative factors identified), and there is a very high incidence of middle-ear infections in Native Americans. Overall, mortality is rare and it is uncommon in countries where treatment of complications is available. However, morbidity is high and may be significant for infants who develop complications and in those in whom persistent effusion results in communicative deficits (perceptive and productive).

Otitis media is most commonly associated with exposure to large numbers of other children (often with upper respiratory infections [URIs]) via child care or crowded households, decreased breastfeeding, and exposure to secondhand smoke. Seasonal increase in the incidence of OM also has been reported, most commonly in winter, fall, and spring. An increased incidence of AOM and COM has been found in children who live in low socioeconomic conditions, who have poor medical care, or both (these factors are often nested). However, these factors are not well established; they may represent an increased exposure to other children with URIs. Farjo et al, among others, have shown a well-established relationship between attending child care and an increased incidence of OM in children younger than 3 years. Casselbrant et al reported a strong genetic predisposition to OM, with a higher incidence in children who have older siblings or parents with a significant history of OM.

Pearl: Acute otitis media is the second most frequent diagnosis made by primary care clinicians and is the most common indication for antibiotic use in children in North America.

▦ Pathogenesis of Otitis Media

The pathogenesis of OM is multifactorial. Immunologic and environmental factors have an important role, and any imbalance between them can predispose the host to OM. Age, genetic predisposition, and atopy are host factors that can impair immune response, whereas older siblings, child care, and season of the year are environmental factors related to microbial load (**Figure 2-1**). For the inflammatory process to develop in the middle ear, the pathogens must adhere to the nasopharyngeal epithelium, enter the middle-ear cavity through the ET, and be able to overcome the defensive mechanisms of the middle ear.

The ET provides clearance of secretions and pressure regulation to the middle ear. It is also the port of entry for middle-ear pathogens from the nasopharynx. Abnormal function of the ET is the cornerstone of the pathogenesis of OM. Dysfunction of the ET can be caused by a URI, with decreased mucus clearance and increased obstruction, which predisposes the child to bacterial growth and subsequent middle-ear inflammation. Infants and children are predisposed to MEE and OM secondary to a more horizontal and functionally less mature ET.

Other conditions associated with ET dysfunction and MEE are presented in **Box 2-2**. Children with craniofacial anomalies affecting ET function, such as cleft palate or craniofacial disorders, have a statistically higher incidence of OM at all ages, especially during the first 2 years after birth. These patients need to be followed up until adolescence because the incidence of acquired cholesteatoma in children, especially teenagers, with cleft lip and

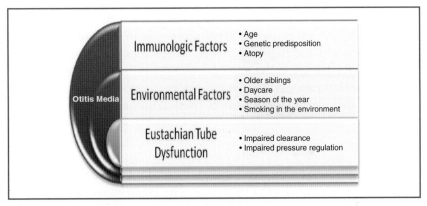

Figure 2-1. Factors involved in otitis media pathogenesis.

Box 2-2. Risk Factors Associated With Middle-Ear Effusion

Craniofacial Disorders
♦ Cleft palate
♦ Midface deformity
♦ Down syndrome
♦ Apert syndrome
Immunodeficiencies
♦ Hypogammaglobulinemia
♦ IgA deficiency
♦ DiGeorge syndrome
♦ HIV
♦ Drug-induced immunodeficiency
Allergy
Nasal Obstruction
♦ Sinusitis
♦ Adenoid hypertrophy
♦ Nasopharyngeal tumor
♦ Ciliary dysfunction

palate is approximately 200 times the baseline rate. Children with congenital or acquired immunodeficiency are at a higher risk secondary to decreased middle-ear clearance; such conditions include hypogammaglobulinemia, IgA deficiency, DiGeorge syndrome, mucopolysaccharidoses, HIV, and drug-induced immunodeficiency (eg, chemotherapy, steroids).

Allergy, nasal obstruction (eg, sinusitis, adenoid hypertrophy, nasal or rare pediatric nasopharyngeal tumors), ciliary dysfunction, prolonged nasal intubation or nasogastric tube placement, and possibly gastroesophageal reflux are other conditions associated with an increased incidence of MEE. Gastroesophageal reflux is common in children and, therefore, has been implicated in the pathophysiology of OM. In 20% of cases, pepsin has been found in the middle ear of patients with OM and is considered an independent risk factor for OM. A role for allergy in the etiology of OM has long been postulated. However, no data support the use of antihistamine-decongestant combinations in treating OME. Also, there is an increased incidence in patients exposed to secondhand smoke and in those who use a pacifier.

Children attending child care centers are predisposed to antibacterial-resistant organisms in their nasopharynx, leading to AOM that may be refractory to antibacterial treatment. The environment at child care centers facilitates the development and spread of resistant organisms because of the large number of children, frequent close person-to-person contact, and wide use of antibiotics. Crowded living conditions, poor sanitation, and inadequate medical care have all been associated with OM.

Increasing evidence shows that biofilm formation may play a role in the inflammatory changes observed in the middle ear of patients with OME. There is also accumulating evidence that gastric acid may act as a cofactor in the inflammatory process by facilitating biofilm formation. In fact, the common factor of inflammation suggests that diverse types of insult can influence different stages of the immune cascade that results in persistent MEE.

> **Pearl:** The pathogenesis of acute otitis media is multifactorial. Immunologic and environmental factors play an important role, and any imbalance between them can predispose the host to otitis media.

■ Acute Otitis Media

Acute OM is the second most frequent diagnosis made by PCCs and is the most common indication for antibiotic use in children in North America. In general, most children have at least 1 episode of AOM by age 1 year, with a peak incidence between ages 6 and 11 months. Approximately 10% to 20% of children have recurrent episodes of AOM by 1 year of age, and 80% have had at least 1 episode by 3 years of age. As many as 45% of children experience persistent effusion 1 month after an episode of AOM, but this number decreases to 10% after 3 months.

MICROBIOLOGY OF AOM

The pathogens most frequently associated with AOM are *Streptococcus pneumoniae* (30%–50%), *Haemophilus influenzae* (20%–30%), *Moraxella catarrhalis* (10%–20%), and group A streptococci (1%–5%) (**Table 2-1**). Block et al found that children aged 7 to 24 months with recurrent episodes of AOM who were vaccinated with heptavalent pneumococcal vaccine had 2-fold more gram-negative bacteria than *S pneumoniae*. Anaerobic bacteria play a minor role in the pathogenesis of AOM.

Table 2-1. Microbiology of Acute Otitis Media	
Population	**Most Common Pathogens**
Neonates	Streptococcus pneumoniae Haemophilus influenzae Staphylococcus aureus Escherichia coli Group B Streptococcus
Infants	S pneumoniae H influenzae S aureus E coli Group B Streptococcus
Children	S pneumoniae H influenzae Moraxella catarrhalis
Immunocompromised	Mycobacterium tuberculosis Mycoplasma pneumonia Chlamydia trachomatis

The exact percentage of bacterial resistance for any particular organism varies with the geographic area and the population studied. The incidence of penicillin-resistant pneumococcus in the United States ranges from 10% to 40% and is more than 80% in Korea and the Middle East. Beta-lactamase is produced by 20% to 50% of *H influenzae* and nearly all *M catarrhalis*. Possible clinical factors in the development of bacterial resistance to antibiotics include multiple and prolonged courses and incomplete or inappropriate administration.

Viruses have been suspected increasingly of causing AOM, possibly by acting alone or as bacterial co-pathogens. Viral AOM is most frequently caused by respiratory syncytial virus or rhinovirus, but influenza virus, adenovirus, enterovirus, and parainfluenza viruses have also been isolated from middle-ear fluid. Viral infection can substantially worsen clinical and bacteriologic outcomes of AOM.

Pearl: The pathogens most frequently associated with acute otitis media are *Streptococcus pneumoniae*, *Haemophilus influenzae*, and *Moraxella catarrhalis*.

▨ Assessment and Diagnosis of AOM

PRESENTING SYMPTOMS

Clinical history alone is poorly predictive of the presence of AOM, especially in younger children. Children with AOM usually have a rapid onset of signs and symptoms such as otalgia or pulling of the ear in an infant, irritability, otorrhea, or fever. These findings, except for otorrhea, are nonspecific and frequently manifest during an uncomplicated viral URI. However, these symptoms in combination with the presence of MEE and inflammation in the physical examination increase the likelihood of an AOM diagnosis.

Less common signs and symptoms in children are hearing loss, dizziness, and tinnitus. Fever is present in up to two-thirds of children with AOM, but fever (temperature above 40°C) is uncommon and may represent bacteremia or other complications. A protruding ear with swelling behind the ear may represent mastoiditis with a developing subperiosteal abscess.

The diagnosis of AOM, particularly in infants and young children, is often made with a degree of doubt, most frequently because of the inability to confirm the presence of MEE. Common factors that increase uncertainty include the inability to clear the external auditory canal of cerumen, a narrow ear canal, or inability to maintain an adequate seal for successful pneumatic otoscopy or tympanometry. Despite all efforts made by the PCC to differentiate AOM from OME or a normal ear, uncertainty is almost always unavoidable.

A definitive diagnosis of AOM meets all 3 of these criteria: rapid onset, presence of MEE, and signs and symptoms of middle-ear inflammation. The PCC should maximize diagnostic strategies, particularly to establish the presence of MEE, and should consider the certainty of diagnosis in determining management.

> **Pearl:** A definitive diagnosis of acute otitis media meets all 3 of these criteria: rapid onset, presence of middle-ear effusion, and signs and symptoms of middle-ear inflammation.

PHYSICAL EXAMINATION

A complete head and neck examination is essential for diagnosis. To establish a definitive diagnosis of AOM, it is important to identify MEE and inflammatory changes of the TM. Therefore, the physical examination of a child with AOM should include otoscopy and pneumatic otoscopy. For an adequate visualization of the TM, the ear canal should be cleared of any cerumen obscuring the TM, and the otoscope lighting must be adequate. Depleted batteries and dim lights will make the PCC's job even more difficult and will sometimes alter perceptions of the image. For an accurate pneumatic otoscopy, a speculum of proper shape and diameter must be selected to obtain a good seal in the external auditory canal. At the same time, if necessary, it is important to appropriately restrain the child to permit an adequate examination.

A normal eardrum, such as the one shown in **Figure 2-2**, will provide the opportunity to identify landmarks such as the annulus, pars flaccida, pars tensa, malleus handle and lateral process, umbo, light reflex, and long process of the incus. The eardrum is quite translucent and does not really appear to be any color except perhaps gray. Also, it is important to distinguish normal variants from pathology. A crying child can have increased TM vascularity, which can be easily

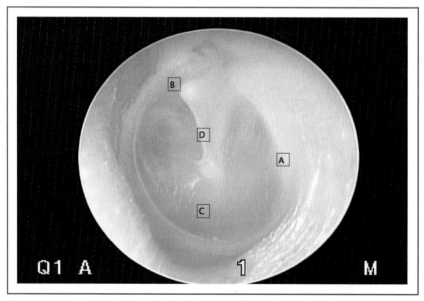

Figure 2-2. Normal left eardrum. A, Annulus. B, Pars flaccida. C, Pars tensa. D, Malleus.

misidentified because of an erythematous and bulging TM and lead to an incorrect diagnosis and treatment. As the child quiets down, the TM erythema becomes less intense and fades away, while the TM erythema in a patient with AOM persists.

The findings on otoscopy indicating the presence of MEE and inflammation associated with AOM include erythema, opacification, and fullness or bulging of the TM, along with loss of TM landmarks, such as the malleus handle, the light reflex, and pars flaccida (**Figure 2-3**). Bulging of the TM is often evident, and it has the highest predictive value for the presence of MEE. Reduced or absent mobility of the TM during the pneumatic otoscopy is additional evidence of fluid in the middle ear.

> **Pearl:** The findings on otoscopy associated with acute otitis media include erythema, opacification, and fullness or bulging of the tympanic membrane, along with loss of tympanic membrane landmarks.

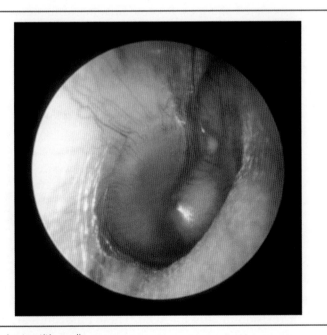

Figure 2-3. Acute otitis media.

DIAGNOSTIC TESTS

Hearing Evaluation

Pure tone audiometry or visual reinforcement audiometry can be used to diagnose the CHL associated with AOM in young children. Tympanometry is a simple, objective, and quantitative method of assessing TM mobility and middle-ear function, with similar sensitivity but lower specificity than that of pneumatic otoscopy. One must keep in mind that impedance tympanometry does not provide a diagnosis but merely confirms what the PCC suspects based on the physical examination findings. Tympanometry should never be used without confirmatory otoscopy. Tympanometry results can be classified with quantitative measures or by pattern curves (A, B, C1, C2) (**Figure 2-4**). The presence of type B or C2 curves has 94% sensitivity for MEE but only 62% specificity. Acoustic reflectometry can also be used to diagnose MEE, but studies are heterogeneous, and performance is poorer than that of pneumatic otoscopy or tympanometry.

OTHER DIAGNOSTIC PROCEDURES

Other diagnostic procedures, such as lateral neck radiography, immunologic evaluation, and fiber-optic nasopharyngeal examination, are useful in identifying predisposing factors, such as adenoid hypertrophy and associated allergies. Routine imaging of the temporal bone is not warranted unless patients have developed complications. Computed tomography (CT) with intravenous (IV) contrast is the imaging modality of choice in screening for complications of AOM. Magnetic resonance imaging with gadolinium is useful when intracranial involvement is suspected.

> **Pearl:** Tympanometry is useful to identify presence of middle-ear effusion when diagnosis is unclear. Further imaging studies are not necessary unless the patient has developed a complication.

▦ Treatment Options for AOM

Evidence-based clinical practice guidelines were published in 2013 with a minor revision in 2014 for AOM. These guidelines are mostly recommendations and options supported by published evidence on

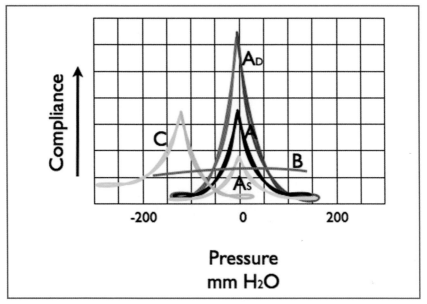

Figure 2-4. Tympanogram classification. A, Normal. As, Stiffened tympano-ossicular system. Ad, Disarticulation. B, Middle-ear effusion, tympanic membrane perforation, or impacted cerumen. C, Negative middle-ear pressure.

the management of this condition. Current recommendations are available to pediatricians, family physicians, otolaryngologists, physician assistants, nurse practitioners, and emergency department physicians (referred to as *clinicians*) who treat these conditions on a routine basis.

■ 2014 Guidelines for AOM

KEY ACTION STATEMENT 1

A (Grade B Evidence) (Recommendation)—Clinicians should diagnose AOM in children who present with moderate to severe bulging of the TM or new onset of otorrhea not caused by acute otitis externa.

B (Grade C Evidence) (Recommendation)—Clinicians should diagnose AOM in children who present with mild bulging of the TM and recent (less than 48 hours) onset of ear pain (holding, tugging, rubbing of the ear in a nonverbal child) or intense erythema of the TM.

C (Grade B Evidence) (Recommendation)—Clinicians should not diagnose AOM in children who do not have MEE (based on pneumatic otoscopy and/or tympanometry).

KEY ACTION STATEMENT 2

A (Grade B Evidence) (Strong Recommendation)—The management of AOM should include an assessment of pain. If pain is present, the clinician should recommend treatment to reduce pain.

KEY ACTION STATEMENT 3

A (Grade B Evidence) (Strong Recommendation)—Severe AOM: The clinician should prescribe antibiotic therapy for AOM (bilateral or unilateral) in children 6 months and older with severe signs or symptoms (ie, moderate or severe otalgia for at least 48 hours or temperature 39°C [102.2°F] or higher).

B (Grade B Evidence) (Recommendation)—Nonsevere bilateral AOM in young children: The clinician should prescribe antibiotic therapy for bilateral AOM in children 6 months through 23 months of age without severe signs or symptoms (ie, mild otalgia for less than 48 hours and temperature lower than 39°C [102.2°F]).

C (Grade B Evidence) (Recommendation)—Nonsevere unilateral AOM in young children: The clinician should either prescribe antibiotic therapy or offer observation with close follow-up based on joint decision-making with the parent(s)/caregiver for unilateral AOM in children 6 to 23 months of age without severe signs or symptoms (ie, mild otalgia for less than 48 hours and a temperature lower than 39°C [102.2°F]). When observation is used, a mechanism must be in place to ensure follow-up and begin antibiotic therapy if the child's condition worsens or fails to improve within 48 to 72 hours of onset of symptoms.

D (Grade B Evidence) (Recommendation)—Nonsevere AOM in older children: The clinician should either prescribe antibiotic therapy or offer observation with close follow-up based on joint decision-making with the parent(s)/caregiver for AOM (bilateral or unilateral) in children 24 months or older without severe signs or symptoms (ie, mild otalgia for less than 48 hours and a temperature lower than 39°C [102.2°F]). When observation is used, a mechanism must be in place to ensure follow-up and begin antibiotic therapy if the child's condition worsens or fails to improve within 48 to 72 hours of onset of symptoms.

KEY ACTION STATEMENT 4

A (Grade B Evidence) (Recommendation)—Clinicians should prescribe amoxicillin for AOM when a decision to treat with antibiotics has been made and the child has not received amoxicillin in the past

30 days or the child does not have concurrent purulent conjunctivitis or the child is not allergic to penicillin.

B (Grade C Evidence) (Recommendation)—Clinicians should prescribe an antibiotic with additional β-lactamase coverage for AOM when a decision to treat with antibiotics has been made, and the child has received amoxicillin in the past 30 days or has concurrent purulent conjunctivitis or has a history of recurrent AOM unresponsive to amoxicillin.

C (Grade B Evidence) (Recommendation)—Clinicians should reassess the patient if the caregiver reports that the child's symptoms have worsened or failed to respond to the initial antibiotic treatment within 48 to 72 hours and determine whether a change in therapy is needed.

KEY ACTION STATEMENT 5

A (Grade B Evidence) (Recommendation)—Clinicians should not prescribe prophylactic antibiotics to reduce the frequency of recurrent AOM.

B (Grade B Evidence) (Option)—Clinicians may offer tympanostomy tubes for recurrent AOM (3 episodes in 6 months or 4 episodes in 1 year with 1 episode in the preceding 6 months).

KEY ACTION STATEMENT 6

A (Grade B Evidence) (Recommendation)—Clinicians should recommend pneumococcal conjugate vaccine to all children according to the schedule of the Advisory Committee on Immunization Practices of the Centers for Disease Control and Prevention, American Academy of Pediatrics (AAP), and American Academy of Family Physicians (AAFP).

B (Grade B Evidence) (Recommendation)—Clinicians should recommend annual influenza vaccine to all children according to the schedule of the Advisory Committee on Immunization Practices, AAP, and AAFP.

C (Grade B Evidence) (Recommendation)—Clinicians should encourage exclusive breastfeeding for at least 6 months.

D (Grade C Evidence) (Recommendation)—Clinicians should encourage avoidance of tobacco smoke exposure.

Medical management of AOM includes observation versus immediate antibiotic treatment. The approach for watchful waiting in selected cases is based on the evidence that most children recover uneventfully from AOM without the use of antibiotics. The decision to observe or treat with antibiotics is based on the child's age, the diagnosis of certainty, and the severity of the disease. In cases in which the child may not be able to return for care, observation is not recommended. A definitive diagnosis of AOM meets all 3 of the following criteria: rapid onset, signs of MEE, and signs and symptoms of middle-ear inflammation. An AOM episode is considered severe if the child presents with moderate to severe otalgia or a temperature at or above 39°C orally (39.5°C rectally). A child with a nonsevere AOM episode presents with mild otalgia and a temperature below 39°C orally (39.5°C rectally) or no fever.

A more aggressive approach is recommended for younger children as well as children with underlying medical conditions (eg, Down syndrome, cochlear implant, craniofacial abnormalities). Children younger than 6 months with an AOM episode should be treated with antibiotics regardless of whether the diagnosis of AOM is certain or uncertain (**Table 2-2**). Children between the ages of 6 months and 2 years can be observed if they have an uncertain diagnosis with a nonsevere illness; otherwise, they should be treated with antibiotics. Children 2 years and older usually can be observed unless they have a certain diagnosis with severe illness. If observation is considered, the clinician should always explain to parents or caregivers the degree of diagnostic certainty and take into account their preference. Observation should only be considered when there is ready access to adequate follow-up care. Also, if observation results

Table 2-2. Criteria for Initial Antibacterial-Agent Treatment or Observation in Children With Acute Otitis Media

Age	Certain Diagnosis	Uncertain Diagnosis
<6 mo	Antibacterial therapy	Antibacterial therapy
6 mo to 2 y	Antibacterial therapy	Antibacterial therapy if severe illness; observation option[a] if nonsevere illness
≥2 y	Antibacterial therapy if severe illness; observation option[a] if nonsevere illness	Observation option[a]

[a] Observation is an appropriate option only when follow-up can be ensured and antibacterial agents started if symptoms persist or worsen. Nonsevere illness is mild otalgia and fever <39°C in the past 24 hours. Severe illness is moderate to severe otalgia or fever ≥39°C. A certain diagnosis of AOM meets all 3 criteria: rapid onset, signs of middle-ear effusion, and signs and symptoms of middle-ear inflammation.

From Rosenfeld RM. Observation option toolkit for acute otitis media. *Int J Pediatr Otorhinolaryngol.* 2001;58(1):1–8, with permission from Elsevier.

in clinical failure after 48 to 72 hours, antibacterial therapy should be considered as the next step.

Pain management (grade B evidence level: strong recommendation) is an important issue to address in the medical management of AOM, because pain is present in most cases and can be persistent in children younger than 2 years even after 3 to 7 days despite antibiotic treatment. Analgesics provide pain relief within 24 hours and should be used whether or not antibiotics are prescribed, and they should be continued as long as needed. Acetaminophen or ibuprofen should form the mainstay of analgesia in AOM. A study published in 2008 assessed the efficacy of local anesthetic eardrops. The 2014 guidelines concluded that local anesthetic eardrops (lidocaine, benzocaine, procaine) offered additional, but brief, benefit over acetaminophen in children older than 5 years.

A Cochrane review assessed the effectiveness of topical analgesia in AOM and included studies that compared anesthetic drops with placebo and with naturopathic drops. The authors concluded that there is limited evidence that eardrops are effective at 30 minutes, and that it is unclear if the findings were the result of or the natural course of AOM. The 2014 guidelines state that naturopathic drops are comparable to amethocaine/phenazone drops in children older than 6 years.

Ototopical antibiotics are of no value in cases in which the TM is intact. Suppurative OM (ie, OM of the external canal or drainage through a TM perforation or tympanotomy tube can be treated with ototopical agents, such as ofloxacin and ciprofloxacin, with or without steroids. Although often prescribed, there is no proven benefit from oral decongestants and antihistamines in the management of AOM. These agents may relieve accompanying nasal symptoms only.

Amoxicillin remains the drug of choice in the treatment of uncomplicated AOM (**Box 2-3**). This drug remains efficient against *S pneumoniae*, has a favorable pharmacodynamic profile, is safe and low cost, and has an acceptable taste and a narrow microbiological spectrum. High doses of amoxicillin (80–90 mg/kg/d) can be used effectively in the case scenario in which resistant *S pneumoniae* strains or highly resistant *S pneumoniae* strains are the main pathogens.

High-dose amoxicillin-clavulanate (90 mg/kg/d amoxicillin component) is recommended as second-line empirical therapy in nonresponding patients treated initially with amoxicillin or other antibacterial agents, or in patients for whom additional coverage for

Box 2-3. Choice of Antibiotic in the Management of Acute Otitis Media

First-line Therapy

1. Amoxicillin (80–90 mg/kg/d for 7–10 d)
   Empirical treatment of AOM in children who received antibiotics during previous months; in otitis-prone children; in child care attendants
   Empirical treatment of AOM in areas with high prevalence of pneumococcal penicillin resistance
2. Amoxicillin-clavulanate (90 mg/kg/d amoxicillin component, with 6.4 mg/kg/d clavulanate for 7–10 d)
   Empirical treatment of AOM in neonates
   Empirical treatment of AOM in immunocompromised patients
   Empirical treatment of AOM in areas with high prevalence of β-lactamase-producing organisms
   Empirical treatment of AOM in patients who received antibiotics for AOM during preceding month

Second-line Therapy[a]

1. Amoxicillin/clavulanate (90 mg/kg/d amoxicillin component, with 6.4 mg/kg/d clavulanate for 7–10 d)
2. Intramuscular ceftriaxone (50 mg/kg/d for 3 d)

Abbreviation: AOM, acute otitis media.

[a] Therapeutic failure is considered if no improvement occurs after 72 hours of starting first-line therapy.

Adapted from American Academy of Pediatrics Subcommittee on Management of Acute Otitis Media. Diagnosis and management of acute otitis media. *Pediatrics*. 2004;113(5):1451-1465; and Segal N, Leibovitz E, Dagan R, Leiberman A. Acute otitis media—diagnosis and treatment in the era of antibiotic resistant organisms: updated clinical practice guidelines. *Int J Pediatr Otorhinolaryngol*. 2005;69(10): 1311-1319.

β-lactamase–producing *H influenzae* and *M catarrhalis* is desired (see **Box 2-3**). Child care attendance and previous antibiotic treatment are risk factors for the presence of bacterial species likely to be resistant to amoxicillin. In cases of non–IgE-mediated penicillin allergy, cefuroxime (50 mg/kg/d) in 2 divided doses may be used.

In situations in which the patient cannot tolerate the oral route, a single intramuscular dose of parenteral ceftriaxone (50 mg/kg) has been shown to be effective for the initial treatment of AOM (see **Box 2-3**). In selected cases, macrolides (azithromycin 10 mg/kg/d on day 1 followed by 5 mg/kg/d for 4 days as a single daily dose) or clarithromycin (15 mg/kg/d in 2 divided doses) can be an option. However, resistance to macrolide antibiotics from the 2 main common pathogens involved in AOM—*S pneumoniae* and *H influenzae*—is common.

The optimal duration of antibiotic treatment of AOM remains uncertain. The usual course of treatment remains 7 to 10 days in most cases. Despite the uncertainty of the antibiotic duration, the time course of clinical response should be 48 to 72 hours. Parents should expect improvement of symptoms within this period; if not, reassessment is necessary. Failure to improve clinically to a second-line treatment will result in the need to consider a different antibiotic, such as parenteral ceftriaxone (50 mg/kg/d once daily for 3 days) (see **Box 2-3**). If no improvement occurs despite outpatient treatment, admission to a hospital and surgical intervention with myringotomy for cultures and antibacterial-agent sensitivity studies of the fluid are warranted to guide effective treatment and decrease the risk of complications. In practice, this is rarely required.

Surgical intervention in a patient with an uncomplicated AOM episode refractory to treatment consists of tympanocentesis and myringotomy with possible placement of a tympanostomy tube. Multiple randomized studies comparing antibiotics with a combination of antibiotics and myringotomy failed to show any benefit from surgical intervention over medical therapy with regard to symptom resolution. Indications for myringotomy include severe otalgia or high fever, impending complications, AOM in newborns, AOM in patients with immunodeficiency, or unsatisfactory response to antibiotic treatment. Tympanocentesis provides adequate drainage as well as fluid for microbiological analysis. However, it is unlikely that acute tympanocentesis will result in a lasting clearance of the middle ear, and in most cases it should be accompanied by tympanostomy tube insertion.

Tympanostomy tube insertion has been advocated in children with recurrent episodes of AOM. In 2003, Rosenfeld and Bluestone reported that children with recurrent AOM who received tympanostomy tubes had 67% fewer episodes than controls. Otorrhea is common after tympanostomy tube insertion and may require treatment with ototopical antibiotic drops. Adenoidectomy also may be considered in patients who have recurrent AOM because it reduces the incidence by 0 to 3 episodes per child-year. This procedure also reduces the need for future tympanostomy tube insertion for children 2 years or older who have recurrent AOM. In practice, adding adenoidectomy to the treatment of AOM usually occurs at surgery for repeated tympanostomy tube insertion and in the presence of nasal symptoms.

> **Pearl:** Most children recover well from acute otitis media, even without antibacterial therapy. In most patients, the choice of treatment is empirical and should be based on the available local epidemiologic information regarding the most common pathogens and their susceptibility patterns.

▨ Natural History and Complications of AOM

The natural history of most children who experience AOM is clinical resolution within 4 to 7 days of diagnosis. Once the patient has shown clinical improvement, follow-up is based on the usual clinical course of AOM. No therapy is needed for persistent middle-ear fluid after resolution of acute symptoms. Middle-ear effusion is a common sequela of AOM, and approximately 60% to 70% of children will have fluid 2 weeks after resolution of symptoms; after 3 months, only 10% have fluid. The presence of MEE is not an indication for ototopical or systemic antibiotics because neither will hasten the resolution of the effusion.

Complications of AOM are rare, and the diagnosis depends on a high index of suspicion because antibiotic therapy can mask signs and symptoms. If complications are left untreated, they may rapidly progress with life-threatening consequences. Complications can be classified as intratemporal or extratemporal, which can be further subdivided into intracranial and extracranial. Intratemporal complications are more common and include acute TM perforation, mastoiditis, subperiosteal abscess, facial nerve paralysis, and labyrinthitis. Extratemporal intracranial complications consist of meningitis, extradural/subdural/intracerebral abscesses, sigmoid sinus thrombosis, and otic hydrocephalus. Extratemporal extracranial complications occur when abscess formation spreads beyond the mastoid to the sternocleidomastoid (Bezold), submandibular space (Citelli), and root of zygoma (Luc).

Increased pressure within the middle-ear space can lead to TM rupture during an AOM episode. Most of these TM perforations heal spontaneously within 1 to 2 weeks. Patients who develop mastoiditis have a protruding ear associated with erythema, tenderness, and swelling of the mastoid bone. Fluctuance in this area can suggest coalescent mastoiditis, which involves demineralization of the bone by osteoclastic activity, and the diagnosis can be confirmed with a CT scan of the temporal bone with contrast. Medical treatment with IV antibiotics is preferable in the presence of mastoiditis. In the absence of coalescent mastoiditis, 75% to 90% of cases can be treated with IV antibiotics along with myringotomy or tympanostomy tube insertion. However, a cortical mastoidectomy and tympanostomy tube placement are advocated in patients in whom a coalescence develops or an intracranial complication has occurred or is imminent.

Subperiosteal abscess is the most common extracranial complication of AOM. Patients present with a purulent collection lateral to the mastoid cortex. Intravenous antibiotics, tympanostomy tube placement, and incision and drainage of the collection are the treatments of choice, either alone or more commonly in combination. Cortical mastoidectomy is rarely required and, again, is only indicated in cases in which the mastoid has coalesced (as evidenced by erosion of the mastoid air cell system on CT) or intracranial complications have occurred or are likely. Acute OM is the most common cause of facial nerve paralysis in children; however, this is an uncommon complication of AOM, with an incidence of 0.005%. Treatment consists of IV antibiotics and early myringotomy with placement of a tympanostomy tube. Complete recovery from facial nerve paralysis occurs in more than 95% of cases. The authors have found that with acute facial nerve paralysis caused by AOM, early tympanostomy tube placement leads to faster return of function than late tube placement. Protection of the eye during the paralysis is key to successful overall management.

When, very rarely, patients with AOM present with acute sensorineural hearing loss and vertigo, labyrinthitis is suspected. This occurs when the infection progresses from the middle ear and mastoid to the inner ear. Labyrinthitis can also be a sequela of meningitis, the most common intracranial complication of AOM. Meningitis presents with lethargy, altered mental status, and fever. A lumbar puncture is necessary for diagnosis and to guide treatment. Other intracranial complications of AOM include sigmoid sinus thrombosis, otitic hydrocephalus, and brain abscess (such as epidural, subdural, and intracranial abscesses). This complication can occur more commonly in children with cochlear anomalies. Interestingly, before universal infant hearing screening was instituted, a cochlear anomaly was commonly first identified in children with labyrinthitis or meningitis complicating an episode of AOM.

> **Pearl:** The natural course of acute otitis media is spontaneous resolution. However, the primary care clinician or specialist must be aware of the potential complications of acute otitis media and bear in mind that if left untreated, it may rapidly progress, with potentially life-threatening consequences.

▓ Prevention of AOM

Several environmental control measures based on nonrandomized controlled trials have been taken to prevent the onset of AOM episodes. Prolonging breastfeeding, limiting pacifier use, and eliminating exposure to tobacco smoke and child care have been postulated as reducing the incidence of AOM. The benefits of antibiotic prophylaxis in the prevention of recurrent AOM by decreasing the number of episodes per month must be balanced against the risk of drug-induced side effects and the disadvantage of promoting antibiotic resistance. This practice has fallen out of favor. Reduction of upper airway infections by changing child care attendance patterns, limiting crowded environments, avoiding full-time child care attendance, or postponing child care until age 6 months is often recommended. Intranasal fluticasone administered during viral URIs has no effect and might even increase the incidence of AOM.

Influenza vaccines given to children older than 2 years have demonstrated more than 30% efficacy in the prevention of AOM during the influenza season, but no efficacy has been found in younger children. The introduction of the 7-valent pneumococcal conjugate vaccine (PCV7) had a major role in decreasing the number of episodes of *S pneumoniae* AOM secondary to the serotypes included in the vaccine. It also had a major role in reducing the nasopharyngeal carriage of vaccine-type *S pneumoniae,* particularly antibacterial-resistant organisms, preventing its spread to contacts in the community. Although the vaccine decreased AOM episodes caused by *S pneumoniae* serotypes by 56% to 67%, it was associated with a shift in serotype distribution from PCV7 types to non-PCV7 types, as well as in bacterial pathogens such as *H influenzae* and *Moraxella*. Future studies will determine if PCV13 has a greater protective role than PCV7 administration.

In 2010, the United States Food and Drug Administration approved the 13-valent vaccine PCV13, which included 6 additional serotypes than PCV7. As a result of the PCV7/PCV13 program in the United States, there was a reported decrease in hospital admissions for AOM and complications of AOM between 2000 and 2012. The observed reduction was from 3.965 to 2.618 per 100,000 persons, which equated to a relative risk reduction of 34%. The most pronounced decrease was observed in those aged 1 year or younger, with a decrease from 22.647 to 8.715 per 100,000 persons. In addition, a significant decrease in AOM-related health care utilization occurred during this period. Tawfik et al observed a reduction in AOM-related office visit rates in children younger than 2 years from 1.42 per child-year in 2008 to 0.82 per child-year in 2011. A significant decrease occurred in 2010, which they attributed to the advent of PCV13.

These results also were observed in Israel and Europe. However, in a large series from the United Kingdom, Thorrington et al observed a reduction in otitis media, but could not confirm a beneficial effect of the PCV7/PCV13 program.

Talathi et al compared PCV7 with PCV13 with respect to the incidence of AOM in the United States and demonstrated that although there had been a reduction in AOM, there was no significant difference between the 2 vaccines.

Le Saux reported that although there may be increased effectiveness of PCV13 in preventing AOM, this has not been conclusively demonstrated. However, its primary benefit is to prevent invasive, life-threatening infections in children.

> **Pearl:** Recurrent episodes of otitis media can be prevented by applying environmental control measures such as decreased exposure to child care centers and secondhand smoke and by using prophylactic antibiotics. Vaccines are known to be effective in preventing acute otitis media.

■ Chronic Otitis Media

SUPPURATIVE

Chronic Suppurative Otitis Media

Chronic suppurative OM is defined as a perforated TM with persistent drainage from the middle ear lasting more than 12 weeks. Chronic suppurative OM most commonly follows an episode of acute infection but can also occur after trauma or iatrogenic injury (tympanostomy tubes). During an acute infection, a TM perforation can develop secondary to irritation, subsequent inflammation of the middle-ear mucosa, and the resulting increased pressure behind an intact drum. Chronic suppurative OM is also associated with granulation tissue, which can develop into polyps within the middle-ear space. The cycle of inflammation, ulceration, infection, and granulation tissue formation may continue, destroying surrounding bony margins and ultimately leading to complications, such as a chronic draining ear or cholesteatoma.

> **Pearl:** Chronic suppurative otitis media is defined as a perforated tympanic membrane with persistent drainage from the middle ear; it develops most commonly after an episode of acute otitis media but also can occur after trauma or placement of tympanostomy tubes.

MICROBIOLOGY OF CSOM

Understanding the unique microbiology of CSOM allows creation of a treatment plan with the greatest efficacy and least morbidity. *Pseudomonas aeruginosa, Staphylococcus aureus, Proteus* species, *Klebsiella pneumoniae,* and diphtheroids are the predominant bacteria cultured from chronically draining ears. Anaerobes and fungi can also be found within the MEE.

Pseudomonas aeruginosa is the most commonly recovered organism from the chronically draining ear (48%–98%). *Pseudomonas aeruginosa* can be found in areas of necrotic or diseased epithelium of the middle ear and can produce proteases, lipopolysaccharide, and other enzymes that inhibit normal immunologic defense mechanisms. Pseudomonal infections commonly resist macrolides, extended-spectrum penicillin, and first- and second-generation cephalosporins. They have been associated with biofilm formation and therefore can complicate treatment plans, especially in children.

Staphylococcus aureus is the second most common organism isolated from chronically draining ears (15%–30%). The remainder of infections are caused by a large variety of gram-negative organisms. *Klebsiella* (10%–21%) and *Proteus* (10%–15%) species are slightly more common than other gram-negative organisms. Approximately 5% to 10% of infections are polymicrobial in etiology, often demonstrating a combination of gram-negative organisms and *S aureus.* Anaerobes *(Bacteroides, Peptostreptococcus,* and *Peptococcus)* and fungi *(Aspergillus, Candida)* complete the spectrum of colonizing organisms in CSOM.

> **Pearl:** *Pseudomonas aeruginosa, Staphylococcus aureus, Proteus* species, *Klebsiella pneumoniae,* and diphtheroids are the most common bacteria cultured from chronically draining ears.

■ Assessment and Diagnosis of CSOM

PRESENTING SYMPTOMS

Patients with CSOM present with otic drainage lasting longer than 3 months and a premorbid history of recurrent AOM with perforation, traumatic perforation, or placement of ventilation tubes. Additionally, they commonly present with hearing loss in the affected ear and occasionally can report fever, vertigo, and pain. A history of persistent CSOM after appropriate medical treatment or unilateral CSOM should alert the PCC or specialist to the possibility of an underlying cholesteatoma.

PHYSICAL EXAMINATION

Patients with CSOM generally have a TM perforation associated with otorrhea that can range from clear or serous to purulent or foul smelling. Physical examination findings can also reveal signs of external auditory canal and middle-ear inflammation. Granulation tissue can be found in the ear canal or middle-ear space. The middle-ear mucosa that can be visualized through the TM perforation is commonly polypoid, pale, or edematous. It will easily bleed if touched.

An acutely perforated TM is often erythematous and thickened, with otorrhea discharging through the perforation. Other findings of the TM can include tympanosclerosis, retraction pockets, or areas of atelectasis (collapse of the TM). Tympanosclerosis appears as white and thickened areas of the TM (**Figure 2-5**) but uncommonly affects hearing independently. Retraction pockets can be located anywhere in the TM and may represent areas of atelectasis or result from persistent negative middle-ear pressure. Retraction pockets in the superior quadrant, especially if filled with debris, can be associated with a pars flaccida cholesteatoma.

DIAGNOSTIC TESTS

Hearing Evaluation

An audiogram with impedance should be obtained in patients with CSOM to evaluate for any associated hearing loss and corroborate the presence of a perforation. Most patients present with CHL secondary to middle-ear inflammation (eg, fluid, polyps, adhesions) or ossicular chain erosion. Although rare, some patients present with mixed hearing loss, indicating more extensive damage to the inner ear.

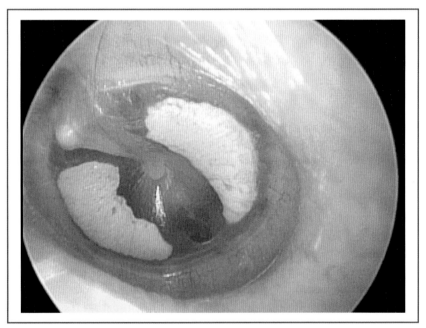

Figure 2-5. Tympanosclerosis appears as white and thickened areas of the tympanic membrane.

OTHER DIAGNOSTIC PROCEDURES

The otorrhea in CSOM can be treated successfully in most cases with ototopical antibiotic drops. The most common cause of treatment failure when using ototopical antibiotic drops is improper administration. The drops will only affect material with which they are in contact, so gentle retraction of the pinna posteriorly and light tragal pressure ensure admixture of the drops with the infected otorrhea and significantly increase their effectiveness. However, in the unusual case in which medical therapy fails with properly administered antibiotic drops, then a culture of ear drainage should be obtained for sensitivity. The test results can lead to modification of systemic therapy and guide treatment successfully.

A CT scan of the temporal bone also can be considered when CSOM is unresponsive to treatment, is quickly and repeatedly recurrent, or is unilateral. The results can provide information about any occult cholesteatoma, foreign body, intratemporal and intracranial complications, or other diseases to be considered, such as Langerhans cell histiocytosis or a rare neoplasia. A fine-cut CT scan can provide more details about the temporal bone anatomy and reveal any complications of the disease, such as ossicular erosion, bone erosion, petrous apex involvement, coalescent mastoiditis, and subperiosteal abscess. Magnetic resonance imaging can be performed when intracranial complications are suspected.

> **Pearl:** Chronic suppurative otitis media can present with a serous or purulent ear drainage, signs of middle-ear inflammation, and granulation tissue. An audiogram can reveal hearing loss secondary to drainage occluding the ear canal or resulting from ossicular erosion.

■ Treatment Options for CSOM

Treatment of CSOM is aimed at controlling otorrhea, restoring the integrity of the TM, and improving any associated hearing loss. Control of the ear discharge can be temporary, so patients may opt to undergo surgical intervention to treat the structural changes involved and for better long-term results. However, if proper control of otorrhea is achieved, early closure of the TM is not always necessary and can be postponed.

Topical antibiotic therapy, regular and aggressive aural toilet, and control of granulation tissue are frequently the first options for treating CSOM. Unfortunately, there are no available guidelines for the management of CSOM. However, 2 studies offer a guide to evidence-based treatment of otorrhea in children with CSOM. Smith et al demonstrated that topical and systemic antibiotic treatment after aural toilet resulted in better resolution of otorrhea than aural toilet alone. Macfadyen et al reported that topical antiseptics, such as boric acid and alcohol, were less effective at drying discharging ears than topical quinolones. Based on their conclusions, the following are some guidelines for the medical treatment of CSOM in children:

1. It seems probable that topical treatment with antibiotics after aural toilet is more effective than systemic treatment with antibiotics. The importance of adequately cleaning the ear prior to properly instilling drops cannot be overemphasized.

2. It is not clear whether topical quinolones are more effective than other topical antibiotics for the control of CSOM. However, topical quinolones do not carry the potential for ototoxicity associated with aminoglycosides. When possible, topical antibiotic preparations free of potential ototoxicity should be used rather than ototopical preparations that have the potential for otologic injury if the middle ear and mastoid are open.

3. The use of aminoglycoside ear drops should be for short periods, never more than 2 weeks at a time, and only in the presence of active CSOM, where the risk of ototoxicity from pus in the middle-ear cleft probably outweighs that from aminoglycoside drops. The child's parents should be counseled about the risks of using aminoglycosides when the middle ear is exposed.

4. Microbiological guidance should be required, especially if the patient fails to respond after an initial course of treatment.

Aminoglycosides and fluoroquinolones are the most commonly used antibiotic drops. These antibiotics have an appropriate spectrum of activity against the most common organisms involved in CSOM, *Pseudomonas* and *S aureus*. Gentamicin- and tobramycin-containing ophthalmic drops have been widely used off label for the treatment of otologic infections. All aminoglycosides have significant potential ototoxicity, causing vestibular dysfunction or hearing loss. Studies designed to detect hearing loss from use of ototopical aminoglycosides have found that the incidence is very low and dose related, and hearing loss occurs following prolonged courses of treatment. However, because an alternative treatment with equal efficacy exists, the use of aminoglycoside topical antibiotic drops has almost disappeared. Though rare, complications such as vestibular loss or sensorineural hearing loss after aminoglycoside use are indefensible, and almost all otolaryngologists have stopped using them except in unusual circumstances. However, in some countries, such as the United Kingdom, because of the lack of a quinolone-steroid combination drop, gentamicin with hydrocortisone is commonly used for a short course. **Table 2-3** provides more information about topical antibiotics used for CSOM.

The anti-inflammatory effect of steroids is an important advantage when a significant amount of granulation tissue is present on physical examination. Granulation tissue can exacerbate otorrhea and prevent topical antibiotic agents from adequately penetrating the middle ear.

Table 2-3. Antimicrobials Used for Chronic Suppurative Otitis Media			
Antibiotic	**Dosing**	**Contraindications**	**Precautions**
Ciprofloxacin otic suspension	5–10 drops instilled in affected ear twice a day	Hypersensitivity	Headache and pruritus
Tobramycin	5–10 drops instilled in affected ear twice a day	Hypersensitivity	Monitor for auditory or vestibular toxicity
Ciprofloxacin	10–20 mg/kg orally every 12 h	Hypersensitivity	Increased risk of tendinitis and tendon rupture in all ages
Piperacillin	200–300 mg/kg/d IV divided every 4–6 h; not to exceed 24 g/d	Hypersensitivity	Caution in patients with renal impairment and history of seizures
Ceftazidime	1–2 g IV every 8–12 h	Hypersensitivity	Adjust dosage in severe renal insufficiency

Abbreviation: IV, intravenous.

Topical steroids are effective in treating granulation tissue and hastening resolution. A fixed-ratio combination of ciprofloxacin and dexamethasone has been especially popular in North America. When topical steroids are ineffective, silver nitrate can be used along with cautery or an excision technique performed under the microscope.

Aural toilet is an essential part of the medical treatment of CSOM. Ear drainage must be removed from the ear canal to permit better penetration of topical antibiotics. Traditionally, this is performed using the microscope and microinstruments available at an otolaryngologist's office. Aural irrigation with a solution of 50% peroxide and 50% sterile water is an alternative procedure that is generally painless and effective. It should be performed prior to instilling ototopical antibiotics.

Treatment failures are almost always secondary to incomplete penetration of the topical antimicrobials to the middle ear (often because of inadequate instructions given by the prescribing PCC) and almost never because of an antimicrobial resistance to the organisms causing CSOM. In true cases of failure, an underlying cholesteatoma, a foreign body, and other diseases in the differential diagnosis must be ruled out. If the patient has failed to respond to topical antimicrobial therapy, cultures for sensitivities should be performed and a CT scan of the temporal bone should be considered. A trial of systemic antibiotics that exceed the minimal inhibitory concentration of most relevant organisms can be used for 3 to 4 weeks. Most patients experience cessation of otorrhea soon after proper administration of systemic antibiotics. Currently, the most effective and commonly used oral antibiotics in patients with CSOM are fluoroquinolones. These drugs are not approved for use in children because of potential joint injury demonstrated in juvenile experimental animals. However, this side effect has not been reported in the large database available from children with cystic fibrosis treated with high doses of systemic quinolones. Most parents will agree to the off-label use of oral fluoroquinolones if they understand the relative risks and potential benefits of this class of drugs.

Surgical intervention should be considered in the rare instance in which CSOM does not respond to medical therapy. A tympanomastoidectomy can eliminate the infection and stop otorrhea in approximately 80% of cases. Surgical intervention with tympanoplasty is the treatment of choice to close the TM perforation. Controversy exists regarding the best time to perform tympanoplasty in children. Meta-analyses seem to suggest that successful closure of TM perforation is more likely in older children. Vrabec et al reported an improvement in closure rate with advancing age when comparing children grouped by age, as did Tan et al; however, Hardman et al stated that there was no relationship between age and closure rate. Of interest, when the authors looked at index ages of 9, 13, and 15 years, they found a statistically significant relationship between those younger than the index age and those older. They concluded that the presence of a healthy contralateral ear was a more reliable predictor of a successful outcome than age alone, but the outcome can be influenced by age, as young children are more likely to have middle-ear effusions. Children at about age 10 years often prefer the option of surgery to continued water precautions. Therefore, tympanoplasty may reasonably be delayed until then, unless the child has troublesome otorrhea or hearing loss.

> **Pearl:** The initial treatment of chronic suppurative otitis media should include topical antimicrobials, aural toilet, and topical steroids for any associated granulation tissue. Topical antimicrobial treatment failures should be evaluated with culture sensitivities, and patients should be treated with a trial of systemic therapy. Surgical intervention with tympanoplasty or tympanomastoidectomy can be considered in medical therapy failures.

▓ Natural History and Complications of CSOM

If not treated successfully, CSOM can cause CHL from ossicular erosion, and occasionally can result in social stigma secondary to the foul-smelling fluid draining from the affected ear. Other sequelae include acquired cholesteatoma and tympanosclerosis. Complications of CSOM are similar to AOM complications discussed earlier. Chronic suppurative OM without prompt appropriate treatment can progress into a variety of mild to life-threatening complications that can be separated into 2 subgroups: intratemporal and intracranial. Intratemporal complications include petrositis, facial paralysis, and labyrinthitis. Intracranial complications include lateral sinus thrombophlebitis, meningitis, and intracranial abscess.

Prevention of CSOM

In patients with a known TM perforation, CSOM can be prevented by practicing dry ear precautions when washing and swimming, with diligent use of earplugs. Tympanoplasty, a surgical intervention that recreates the TM by sealing the perforation with a graft, is another option to prevent any further drainage and improve hearing, with good long-term results. It is important to refer a patient with CSOM who has symptoms of aural fullness, otalgia, fever, or headaches to an otolaryngologist for further evaluation and management.

Nonsuppurative Otitis Media

OTITIS MEDIA WITH EFFUSION

The lack of acute symptoms with OME makes prevalence difficult to estimate. However, the point prevalence of MEE on a screening test is approximately 20%. Approximately 50% of children will experience OME in the first year after birth, increasing to 60% by age 2 years. About 90% of children develop OME at some time before they reach school age. The incidence seems to peak during the second year after birth, is most prevalent during the winter months, and is associated with URIs. Most OME episodes resolve spontaneously within 3 months; however, 30% to 40% of children have persistent episodes. The recurrence rate within 24 months is 50%.

> **Pearl:** Otitis media with effusion is defined as middle-ear effusion without signs or symptoms of an acute infection. It can be secondary to eustachian tube dysfunction or a sequela to acute otitis media.

MICROBIOLOGY OF OME

In the past, chronic MEE was often thought to be sterile. However, several studies have isolated *S pneumoniae, H influenzae, M catarrhalis,* and group A streptococci in 30% to 50% of children with chronic MEE. Although bacterial isolation from middle-ear fluid is not proof of an active bacterial infectious process, Post et al reported that bacteria may be present in a higher percentage of OME specimens than was previously thought. In chronic OME, anaerobic organisms such as

Peptostreptococcus species, *Prevotella* species, and *Propionibacterium acnes* have been isolated. In a recent study, *Helicobacter pylori* was found in middle ear, tonsillar, and adenoid tissues in patients with OME, indicating a possible role in the pathogenesis of the infection.

> **Pearl:** Otitis media with effusion appears to peak during the second year after birth, is most prevalent during the winter months, and is associated with upper respiratory infections.

■ Assessment and Diagnosis of OME

PRESENTING SYMPTOMS

The presence of fluid in the middle ear without acute signs of MEE inflammation is characteristic of OME. Because patients do not present with acute-onset signs, such as fever, otalgia, or irritability, the diagnosis of OME is usually made by screening or as an incidental finding on routine physical examination. However, some children manifest noninfectious discomfort (commonly, tugging or itching of the ears), hearing loss, clumsiness, or sleep disruption, but most children are referred from school when they fail screening hearing programs. Physical examination along with a formal audiogram can confirm the presence of MEE and mild hearing impairment.

> **Pearl:** Because of the lack of acute symptoms, diagnosis of otitis media with effusion is usually made by screening or as an incidental finding on routine physical examination.

PHYSICAL EXAMINATION

To establish a definitive diagnosis of OME, it is important to identify MEE without inflammatory changes of the TM. Therefore, physical examination should include otoscopy and pneumatic otoscopy if possible. Adequate visualization of the TM should be achieved.

Air-fluid levels or bubbles without signs of middle-ear inflammation are the usual physical examination findings in OME. Air-fluid levels will indicate intermittent aeration of the middle ear through the ET (**Figure 2-6**). Pneumatic otoscopy has a sensitivity of 94% and specificity of 88% for diagnosis of MEE when compared with myringotomy, which is the gold standard. In difficult cases, determination of the presence of MEE can be supplemented by tympanometry or impedance (acoustic reflex measurements).

> **Pearl:** The usual findings on physical examination in otitis media with effusion include air-fluid levels or bubbles without signs of middle-ear inflammation.

DIAGNOSTIC TESTS

Hearing Evaluation

Pure tone audiometry or visual reinforcement audiometry can be used to diagnose the CHL associated with OME in young children. Tympanometry can assess TM mobility and middle-ear function, and the results can be classified with quantitative measures or by pattern curves, as mentioned earlier.

OTHER DIAGNOSTIC PROCEDURES

Other diagnostic procedures, such as lateral neck radiography, immunologic evaluation, and fiber-optic nasopharyngeal examination, may be useful in identifying predisposing factors, such as adenoid hypertrophy and associated allergies, but are not routinely performed. Routine imaging of the temporal bone is not warranted for OME.

▪ Treatment Options for OME

Evidence-based clinical practice guidelines were originally published in 2004 for OME. These guidelines are mostly recommendations and options supported by published evidence on the management of this condition. Current recommendations are from 2016 and are available to pediatricians, family physicians, otolaryngologists, physician assistants, nurse practitioners, and emergency department physicians

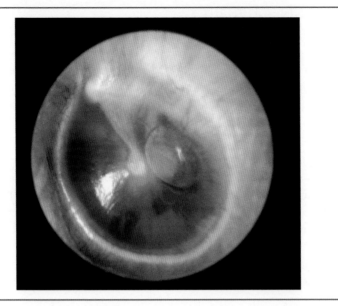

Figure 2-6. Air-fluid levels or bubbles without signs of middle-ear inflammation are usually found in otitis media with effusion. Note the bubble on the right side of the tympanic membrane.

(referred to as *clinicians*) who treat OME on a routine basis. These guidelines offer evidence-based recommendations to make the appropriate diagnosis and provide options available for management.

▓ 2016 Guidelines for OME

KEY ACTION STATEMENT 1

A (Grade A Evidence) (Strong Recommendation)—Pneumatic otoscopy: clinicians should document the presence of middle-ear effusion with pneumatic otoscopy when diagnosing OME in a child.

B (Grade A Evidence) (Strong Recommendation)—Pneumatic otoscopy: clinicians should perform pneumatic otoscopy to assess for OME in a child with otalgia, hearing loss, or both.

KEY ACTION STATEMENT 2

(Grade B Evidence) (Strong Recommendation)—Tympanometry: Clinicians should perform tympanometry in children with suspected OME for whom the diagnosis is uncertain after performing (or attempting to perform) pneumatic otoscopy.

KEY ACTION STATEMENT 3

(Grade C Evidence) (Recommendation)—Failed newborn hearing screen: Clinicians should document in the medical record having counseled parents of infants with OME who fail a newborn hearing screen regarding the importance of follow-up to ensure that hearing is normal when OME resolves and to exclude an underlying sensorineural hearing loss.

KEY ACTION STATEMENT 4

A (Grade C Evidence) (Recommendation)—Identifying at-risk children: clinicians should determine if a child with OME is at increased risk for speech, language, or learning problems from MEE because of baseline sensory, physical, cognitive, or behavioral factors.

B (Grade D Evidence) (Recommendation)—Evaluating at-risk children: clinicians should evaluate children at risk for OME at the time of diagnosis of an at-risk condition and at 12 to 18 months of age (if diagnosed as being at risk prior to this time).

KEY ACTION STATEMENT 5

(Grade A Evidence) (Recommendation)—Screening healthy children: clinicians should not routinely screen children for OME who are not at risk and do not have symptoms that may be attributable to OME, such as hearing difficulties, balance (vestibular) problems, or ear discomfort.

KEY ACTION STATEMENT 6

(Grade C Evidence) (Recommendation)—Patient education: clinicians should educate families of children with OME regarding the natural history of OME, need for follow-up, and possible sequelae.

KEY ACTION STATEMENT 7

(Grade A Evidence) (Strong Recommendation)—Watchful waiting: clinicians should manage the child with OME who is not at risk with watchful waiting for 3 months from the date of effusion onset (if known) or 3 months from the date of diagnosis (if onset is unknown).

KEY ACTION STATEMENT 8

A (Grade A Evidence) (Strong Recommendation Against)—Steroids: clinicians should recommend against using intranasal steroids or systemic steroids for treating OME.

B (Grade A Evidence) (Strong Recommendation Against)—Antibiotics: clinicians should recommend against using systemic antibiotics for treating OME.

C (Grade A Evidence) (Strong Recommendation Against)—Antihistamines or decongestants: Primary care clinicians should recommend against using antihistamines, decongestants, or both for treating OME.

KEY ACTION STATEMENT 9

(Grade C Evidence) (Recommendation)—Hearing test: clinicians should obtain an age-appropriate hearing test if OME persists for more than 3 months or for OME of any duration in an at-risk child.

KEY ACTION STATEMENT 10

(Grade C Evidence) (Recommendation)—Speech and language: clinicians should counsel families of children with bilateral OME and documented hearing loss about the potential impact on speech and language development.

KEY ACTION STATEMENT 11

(Grade C Evidence) (Recommendation)—Surveillance of chronic OME: clinicians should re-evaluate at 3- and 6-month intervals children with chronic OME until the effusion is no longer present, significant hearing loss is identified, or structural abnormalities of the eardrum or middle ear are suspected.

KEY ACTION STATEMENT 12

A (Grade B Evidence) (Recommendation)—Surgery for children younger than 4 years: clinicians should recommend tympanostomy tubes when surgery is performed for OME in a child younger than 4 years; adenoidectomy should not be performed unless a distinct indication (eg, nasal obstruction, chronic adenoiditis) exists other than OME.

B (Grade B Evidence) (Recommendation)—Surgery for children 4 years of age or older: clinicians should recommend tympanostomy tubes, adenoidectomy, or both when surgery is performed for OME in a child 4 years or older.

KEY ACTION STATEMENT 13

(Grade C Evidence) (Recommendation)—Outcome assessment: When managing a child with OME, clinicians should document in the medical record resolution of OME, improved hearing, or improved quality of life.

The initial management of patients with OME is to provide reassurance to parents of the self-limiting nature of OME and the likelihood that surgical treatment will not be required. The child needs monitoring over a 3- to 6-month period to determine if the effusion is persistent and if surgical intervention is needed.

Medical treatment of OME does not provide lasting resolution of symptoms. Multiple studies have reviewed and compared antibiotics versus a combination of antibiotics and oral corticosteroids, but none has found a lasting benefit from these treatments. The role of intranasal corticosteroids has been evaluated and they are not clinically effective. A Cochrane review reported that there was no evidence to support the use of autoinflation, but that because of the low cost and absence of any adverse effects, it is a reasonable treatment to consider while awaiting the natural resolution of OME. There is no recommendation addressing complementary and alternative medicine, as well as allergy management, in the treatment of OME.

A child with OME becomes a surgical candidate when the effusion lasts longer than 3 months with persistent hearing loss; if the effusion is recurrent or persistent in children at risk for speech, language, or learning problems regardless of hearing status; and if there is evidence of structural damage to the TM or middle ear. Ultimately, the decision for surgery must be made on a case-by-case basis with consensus among the PCC, otolaryngologist, and parent or caregiver.

Tympanostomy tube placement is the preferred initial surgery in patients with OME. It results in a 62% relative decrease in effusion prevalence and an absolute decrease in effusion days per child. Myringotomy alone is ineffective for chronic OME. A standard ventilation tube will normally extrude between 6 and 9 months after insertion. Unfortunately, approximately 20% to 50% of children who have received tympanostomy tubes experience OME relapse after tube extrusion. These patients might benefit from adenoidectomy at the time of repeated placement of tympanostomy tubes, especially if symptoms of nasal obstruction are present. Adenoidectomy results in a 50% reduction in the need for future surgeries in children 4 years of age or older. The benefit of adenoidectomy is apparent at age

2 years, greatest at age 3 years, and independent of adenoid size. There is a clear preponderance of benefit over harm when considering the effect of surgery for OME. Surgical and anesthesia costs are offset by reduced OME after tube placement and a reduced need for reoperation after adenoidectomy.

The decision to use short-, medium-, or long-term tympanostomy tubes is usually dictated by the number of previous tube insertions. If a child is expected to require several sets of tubes owing to persistent OME or if the short-term tubes extrude early, then insertion of a long-term tube, with the benefit of avoiding several further general anesthetics, may be more appropriate. Parents must be told that the rate of complication increases with long-term tubes (rate of retained tube, perforation). A Reuter-Bobbin tube is used when there is a shallow middle-ear space (eg, with a severely retracted TM).

Surgical intervention comes with potential risks, including anesthesia, adenoidectomy (bleeding, infection, and velopharyngeal insufficiency), and sequelae of tympanostomy tubes. Anesthesia risks include laryngospasm, bronchospasm, and mortality, which has been reported to be about 1 in 50,000.

Tube insertion can result in a discharging ear in up to 30% of children. It usually responds to antibiotic eardrops; however, if the discharge proves to be refractory to this therapy, tube removal may be required. However, the OME may recur once the tube has been removed, at which point hearing aids could be considered for hearing rehabilitation.

Following extrusion of the tympanostomy tube, the TM usually heals. However, there may be resultant weakness at the site of tube insertion, which may lead to the formation of a retraction pocket. This should be closely monitored to ensure that the pocket does not accumulate keratin, potentially leading to cholesteatoma.

In approximately 2% of children, the TM does not heal after tube extrusion, causing a persistent TM perforation. This risk is greater if several sets of tubes have been placed or if long-term tubes are used; the risk is as high as 15% if the tubes are in place for longer than 3 years. A perforation can enable ventilation of the middle ear, which can be advantageous in certain circumstances, providing that appropriate water precautionary measures are used. However, if there is persistent discharge leading to CSOM, a tympanoplasty should be considered to repair the TM; this procedure usually is performed at 8 years of age or older.

An uncommon complication of tube insertion is the formation of implantation cholesteatoma in which squamous epithelium is pushed into the middle ear by insertion of the tube.

Adenoidectomy has a 0.2% to 0.5% incidence of hemorrhage and a 2% incidence of velopharyngeal insufficiency. Among the surgical treatments for OME, there is a predominance of benefit over harm; however, the potential risks should be explained in detail to parents and caregivers after the decision to intervene surgically is made.

> **Pearl:** Medical treatments have not been proven to be effective in the management of otitis media with effusion. When watchful waiting has failed, insertion of ventilation tubes in children with bilateral hearing impairment associated with otitis media with effusion is effective in restoring hearing thresholds. Adenoidectomy, when performed in conjunction with repeated placement of tympanostomy tubes, reduces the incidence of recurrent otitis media with effusion.

■ Natural History and Complications of OME

As stated earlier, OME will usually resolve spontaneously without the need for any intervention. Children with persistent OME are at risk of developing hearing loss and early language acquisition impairment. Conductive hearing loss may adversely affect binaural processing, sound localization, and speech perception in noise. Primary care clinicians or specialists should ask parents about specific concerns regarding their child's language development. There is evidence that untreated OME may produce lasting effects on behavior and development, particularly attention and hyperactivity. Otitis media with effusion also has a variable but real effect on balance in children, especially when the OME is predominantly unilateral. This added effect often occurs during the period of growth and significant maturation in the balance system, further taxing compensatory mechanisms and increasing the cognitive load.

Damage to the TM and middle ear is common in patients with persistent OME. There is no evidence that treating OME surgically reduces the risk of cholesteatoma formation or permanent damage to the TM.

> **Pearl:** Otitis media with effusion resolves spontaneously in most cases; however, persistent effusion can cause hearing loss and early language acquisition impairment.

Prevention of OME

Behavioral modifications that may help decrease the frequency of OME include breastfeeding whenever possible, limiting pacifier use, avoiding feeding in a supine position, as well as eliminating exposure to tobacco smoke and child care attendance.

Selected References

American Academy of Family Physicians; American Academy of Otolaryngology-Head and Neck Surgery; American Academy of Pediatrics Subcommittee on Otitis Media With Effusion. Otitis media with effusion. *Pediatrics.* 2004;113(5):1412–1429

Belshe RB, Gruber WC. Prevention of otitis media in children with live attenuated influenza vaccine given intranasally. *Pediatr Infect Dis J.* 2000;19(5 Suppl):S66–S71

Ben-Shimol S, Givon-Lavi N, Leibovitz E, Raiz S, Greenberg D, Dagan R. Near-elimination of otitis media caused by 13-valent pneumococcal conjugate vaccine (PCV) serotypes in southern Israel shortly after sequential introduction of 7-valent/13-valent PCV. *Clin Infect Dis.* 2014;59(12):1724–1732

Block SL, Hedrick J, Harrison CJ, et al. Community-wide vaccination with the heptavalent pneumococcal conjugate significantly alters the microbiology of acute otitis media. *Pediatr Infect Dis J.* 2004;23(9):829–833

Bolt P, Barnett P, Babl FE, Sharwood LN. Topical lignocaine for pain relief in acute otitis media: results of a double-blind placebo-controlled randomised trial. *Arch Dis Child.* 2008;93(1):40–44

Casselbrant ML, Mandel EM, Fall PA, et al. The heritability of otitis media: a twin and triplet study. *JAMA.* 1999;282(22):2125–2130

Cohen R, Levy C, Bingen E, Koskas M, Nave I, Varon E. Impact of 13-valent pneumococcal conjugate vaccine on pneumococcal nasopharyngeal carriage in children with acute otitis media. *Pediatr Infect Dis J.* 2012;31(3):297–301

Farjo RS, Foxman B, Patel MJ, et al. Diversity and sharing of *Haemophilus influenzae* strains colonizing healthy children attending day-care centers. *Pediatr Infect Dis J.* 2004;23(1):41–46

Flynn CA, Griffin GH, Schultz JK. Decongestants and antihistamines for acute otitis media in children. *Cochrane Database Syst Rev.* 2004;(3):CD001727

Foxlee R, Johansson A, Wejfalk J, Dawkins J, Dooley L, Del Mar C. Topical analgesia for acute otitis media. *Cochrane Database Syst Rev.* 2006;(3):CD005657

Friedmann I. The pathology of otitis media. *J Clin Pathol.* 1956;9(3):229–236

Gates GA, Klein JO, Lim DJ, et al. Recent advances in otitis media. 1. Definitions, terminology, and classification of otitis media. *Ann Otol Rhinol Laryngol Suppl.* 2002;188:8–18

Graham JM, Scadding GK, Bull PD, eds. *Pediatric ENT.* Heidelberg, Germany: Springer-Verlag Berlin Heidelburg; 2007

Greenberg D, Hoffman S, Leibovitz E, Dagan R. Acute otitis media in children: association with day care centers—antibacterial resistance, treatment, and prevention. *Paediatr Drugs.* 2008;10(2):75–83

Hardman J, Muzaffar J, Nankivell P, Coulson C. Tympanoplasty for chronic tympanic membrane perforation in children: systematic review and meta-analysis. *Otol Neurotol.* 2015;36(5):796–804

Harris L, Cushing SL, Hubbard B, Fisher D, Papsin BC, James AL. Impact of cleft palate type on the incidence of acquired cholesteatoma. *Int J Pediatr Otorhinolaryngol.* 2013;77(5):695–698

Kaplan SL, Center KJ, Barson WJ, et al. Multicenter surveillance of *Streptococcus pneumoniae* isolates from middle ear and mastoid cultures in the 13-valent pneumococcal conjugate vaccine era. *Clin Infect Dis.* 2015;60(9):1339–1345

Kay DJ, Nelson M, Rosenfeld RM. Meta-analysis of tympanostomy tube sequelae. *Otolaryngol Head Neck Surg.* 2001;124(4):374–380

Laursen BB, Danstrup CS, Hoffmann S, Nørskov-Lauritsen N, Christensen ALB, Ovesen T. The effect of pneumococcal conjugate vaccines on incidence and microbiology associated with complicated acute otitis media. *Int J Pediatr Otorhinolaryngol.* 2017;101:249–253

Leibovitz E, Piglansky L, Raiz S, Press J, Leiberman A, Dagan R. Bacteriologic and clinical efficacy of one day vs. three day intramuscular ceftriaxone for treatment of nonresponsive acute otitis media in children. *Pediatr Infect Dis J.* 2000;19(11):1040–1045

Lentsch EJ, Goudy S, Ganzel TM, Goldman JL, Nissen AJ. Rate of persistent perforation after elective tympanostomy tube removal in pediatric patients. *Int J Pediatr Otorhinolaryngol.* 2000;54(2-3):143–148

Le Saux N. Pneumococcal conjugate vaccines for preventing otitis media. *Paediatr Child Health.* 2016;21(2):89–90

Lieberthal AS, Carroll AE, Chonmaitree T, et al. The diagnosis and management of acute otitis media [published correction appears in *Pediatrics* 2014;133(2):346]. *Pediatrics.* 2013;131(3):e964–e999

Macfadyen C, Gamble C, Garner P, et al. Topical quinolone vs. antiseptic for treating chronic suppurative otitis media: a randomized controlled trial. *Trop Med Int Health.* 2005;10(2):190–197

Marom T, Tan A, Wilkinson GS, Pierson KS, Freeman JL, Chonmaitree T. Trends in otitis media-related health care use in the United States, 2001-2011. *JAMA Pediatr.* 2014;168(1):68–75

Ochi JW, Wheelbarger L, Dautenhahn LW. Chronic otitis media in ancient American Indians. *Pediatrics.* 2018;141(4):e20172308

O'Reilly RC, He Z, Bloedon E, et al. The role of extraesophageal reflux in otitis media in infants and children. *Laryngoscope.* 2008;118(Suppl 116):1–9

Park SY, Moore MR, Bruden DL, et al. Impact of conjugate vaccine on transmission of antimicrobial-resistant *Streptococcus pneumoniae* among Alaskan children. *Pediatr Infect Dis J.* 2008;27(4):335–340

Perera R, Glasziou PP, Heneghan CJ, McLellan J, Williamson I. Autoinflation for hearing loss associated with otitis media with effusion. *Cochrane Database Syst Rev.* 2013;(5): CD006285

Post JC, Hiller NL, Nistico L, Stoodley P, Ehrlich GD. The role of biofilms in otolaryngologic infections: update 2007. *Curr Opin Otolaryngol Head Neck Surg.* 2007;15(5): 347–351

Roberts JE, Rosenfeld RM, Zeisel SA. Otitis media and speech and language: a meta-analysis of prospective studies. *Pediatrics.* 2004;113(3 Pt 1):e238–e248

Roland PS, Stewart MG, Hannley M, et al. Consensus panel on role of potentially ototoxic antibiotics for topical middle ear use: introduction, methodology, and recommendations. *Otolaryngol Head Neck Surg.* 2004;130(3 Suppl):S51–S56

Rosenfeld RM. Diagnostic certainty for acute otitis media. *Int J Pediatr Otorhinolaryngol.* 2002;64(2):89–95

Rosenfeld RM, Bluestone CD. Clinical efficacy of surgical therapy. In: Rosenfeld RM, Bluestone CD, eds. *Evidence-Based Otitis Media.* 2nd ed. Hamilton, Ontario: BC Decker; 2003:227–240

Rosenfeld RM, Kay D. Natural history of untreated otitis media. *Laryngoscope.* 2003; 113(10):1645–1657

Rosenfeld RM, Shin JJ, Schwartz SR, et al. Clinical practice guideline: otitis media with effusion (update). *Otolaryngol Head Neck Surg.* 2016;154(1 Suppl):S1–S41

Segal N, Leibovitz E, Dagan R, Leiberman A. Acute otitis media-diagnosis and treatment in the era of antibiotic resistant organisms: updated clinical practice guidelines. *Int J Pediatr Otorhinolaryngol.* 2005;69(10):1311–1319

Smith AW, Hatcher J, Mackenzie IJ, et al. Randomised controlled trial of treatment of chronic suppurative otitis media in Kenyan schoolchildren. *Lancet.* 1996;348(9035): 1128–1133

Talathi S, Gupta N, Sethuram S, Khanna S, Sitnitskaya Y. Otitis media in fully vaccinated preschool children in the pneumococcal conjugate vaccine era. *Glob Pediatr Health.* 2017;4:2333794X1774966

Tamir SO, Roth Y, Dalal I, Goldfarb A, Grotto I, Marom T. Changing trends of acute otitis media bacteriology in central Israel in the pneumococcal conjugate vaccines era. *Pediatr Infect Dis J.* 2015;34(2):195–199

Tan HE, Santa Maria PL, Eikelboom RH, Anandacoomaraswamy KS, Atlas MD. Type I tympanoplasty meta-analysis: a single variable analysis. *Otol Neurotol.* 2016;37(7): 838–846

Tawfik KO, Ishman SL, Altaye M, Meinzen-Derr J, Choo DI. Pediatric acute otitis media in the era of pneumococcal vaccination. *Otolaryngol Head Neck Surg.* 2017;156(5): 938–945

Teele DW, Klein JO, Rosner B. Epidemiology of otitis media during the first seven years of life in children in greater Boston: a prospective, cohort study. *J Infect Dis.* 1989;160(1):83–94

Thorrington D, Andrews N, Stowe J, Miller E, van Hoek AJ. Elucidating the impact of the pneumococcal conjugate vaccine programme on pneumonia, sepsis and otitis media hospital admissions in England using a composite control. *BMC Med.* 2018;16(1):13

Vrabec JT, Deskin RW, Grady JJ. Meta-analysis of pediatric tympanoplasty. *Arch Otolaryngol Head Neck Surg.* 1999;125(5):530–534

Williams RL, Chalmers TC, Stange KC, Chalmers FT, Bowlin SJ. Use of antibiotics in preventing recurrent acute otitis media and in treating otitis media with effusion: a meta-analytic attempt to resolve the brouhaha. *JAMA.* 1993;270(11):1344–1351

Zielhuis GA, Heuvelmans-Heinen EW, Rach GH, van den Broek P. Environmental risk factors for otitis media with effusion in preschool children. *Scand J Prim Health Care.* 1989;7(1):33–38

Facial Paralysis

David H. Chi, MD

▓ Introduction

Facial paralysis is a significant condition because of its cosmetic and functional effects. The physical inability to move one side of the face is difficult to disguise. Moreover, facial motion is essential for ocular protection. Secondary corneal injury from drying may occur because of the inability to close the eye. Speech and emotional expression may also be affected. The challenge for primary care clinicians is to determine the extent of the injury, identify the cause of the disorder, and decide whether medical or surgical intervention is required.

▓ Anatomy

Basic knowledge of the anatomy and function of the facial nerve is essential in understanding facial paralysis (**Figure 3-1**). The nerve carries fibers that perform many functions. The main function is from

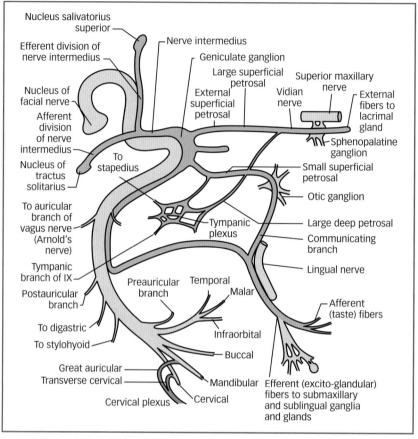

Figure 3-1. Branches of the facial nerve and its connections.

the special visceral efferent fibers that supply motor innervation to the facial musculature as well as to the stapedius, posterior belly of the digastric, and stylohyoid muscles. Special visceral afferent fibers provide the sensation of taste to the anterior two-thirds of the tongue and hard palate. General visceral efferent fibers provide parasympathetic innervation to the lacrimal, submandibular, and sublingual glands. General somatic afferent fibers provide cutaneous sensory innervation to the skin of the concha and a small area behind the ear.

History

A thorough history is essential in evaluating children with facial paralysis. Important information includes the duration and onset of paralysis (sudden vs gradual). Other factors include the severity of the paralysis. The term *paresis* means a partial weakness rather than a complete paralysis. Paresis is usually associated with a good prognosis for recovery as long as the underlying cause is addressed. The primary care clinician (PCC) also should inquire about associated symptoms. Severe otalgia and recent development of vesicular ear lesions suggest herpes zoster oticus. Ipsilateral facial numbness, altered taste, and decreased tearing occur frequently with Bell palsy. Hearing loss and vertigo may indicate tumors of the internal auditory canal or brain stem.

Recurrent episodes of facial palsy may be present with a tumor but also can occur with Bell palsy. Approximately 7% of patients with Bell palsy may have recurrent facial paralysis. Other aspects of the patient's history include recent head trauma, otologic surgeries, and autoimmune disorders.

> **Pearl:** Paresis, or partial weakness instead of full paralysis, is associated with a good prognosis and full recovery can be expected.

Physical Examination

A complete head and neck examination with emphasis on the ear is essential. The external ear should be assessed for vesicular lesions. The external ear canal and tympanic membrane may demonstrate evidence of otitis, cholesteatoma, or tumor. Children with a history of trauma may exhibit hemotympanum (blood behind an intact eardrum), eardrum perforation, or otorrhea. Clear fluid may be indicative of cerebrospinal fluid. Battle sign (mastoid ecchymosis) or raccoon eyes may occur with a skull base fracture. A cheek or neck mass suggests a tumor, especially if the onset of facial paresis has been gradual and segmental paresis is present.

A thorough neurologic examination should be performed. All branches of the facial nerve should be assessed and the 2 sides compared. The patient should be asked to maximally raise the eyebrows, close the eyes tightly, wrinkle the nose, pucker, and smile widely (**Figure 3-2**). A challenge in the physical examination of newborns and very young children is that cooperation is limited, so the PCC may need to observe spontaneous facial motion, such as while the infant is crying or playing. In addition, the young child has good

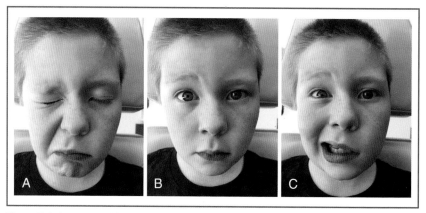

Figure 3-2. An 11-year-old boy with left complete facial paralysis. A, Incomplete closure of the left eye with maximal eye closure. B, No forehead movement with eyebrow elevation. C, No left cheek movement with maximal smile.

facial muscular tone, which may cause the PCC to underestimate the degree of paresis. Multiple cranial neuropathies suggest extensive trauma, infection, extensive neoplasm, or systemic neurologic disease. The House-Brackmann classification is the most commonly used and accepted scale to determine the severity of facial paresis (**Table 3-1**).

An important early distinction is to identify the facial nerve deficit as a *central* or *peripheral* lesion. Central problems usually can be determined by means of a thorough neurologic examination, as most brain lesions are not isolated to the facial nerve. Because the upper face is innervated bilaterally from facial nerve tracts from the brain cortex, a cortical lesion results in facial paralysis of the lower face only.

> **Pearl:** A thorough history and physical examination are required in all patients to determine the prognosis.

▦ Pathophysiology

Understanding the degree of injury is important in predicting facial nerve recovery. The Sunderland classification scheme is based on the histologic changes and physiologic implications (**Table 3-2**).

Table 3-1. Facial Nerve Grading System		
Grade	Description	Characteristics
I	Normal	Normal facial function in all areas

II	Mild dysfunction	Gross: slight weakness noticeable on close inspection; may have very slight synkinesis
		At rest: normal symmetry and tone
		Motion
		    Forehead: moderate-to-good function
		    Eye: complete closure with minimum effort
		    Mouth: slight asymmetry

III	Moderate dysfunction	Gross: obvious but not disfiguring difference between 2 sides; noticeable but not severe synkinesis, contracture, and/or hemifacial spasm
		At rest: normal symmetry and tone
		Motion
		    Forehead: slight-to-moderate movement
		    Eye: complete closure with effort
		    Mouth: slightly weak with maximum effort

IV	Moderately severe dysfunction	Gross: obvious weakness and/or disfiguring asymmetry
		At rest: normal symmetry and tone
		Motion
		    Forehead: none
		    Eye: incomplete closure
		    Mouth: asymmetry with maximum effort

V	Severe dysfunction	Gross: only barely perceptible motion
		At rest: asymmetry
		Motion
		    Forehead: none
		    Eye: incomplete closure
		    Mouth: slight movement

VI	Total paralysis	No movement

From House JW, Brackmann DE. Facial nerve grading system. *Otolaryngol Head Neck Surg.* 1985;93(2):146–147. Reprinted by permission of SAGE Publications.

First-degree injury, or neurapraxia, occurs with increased intraneural pressure such as a compression injury. Continuity of the axon is preserved, and the injury prevents conduction of an action potential. No Wallerian degeneration occurs. With relief of compression, complete recovery is expected.

Injury	Histologic Findings	Physiologic Injury	Potential for Recovery
First degree	Neurapraxia	Increased intraneural pressure	Complete recovery
Second degree	Axonotmesis	Increased intraneural pressure and nerve ischemia	Good-to-complete recovery
Third degree	Neurotmesis	Loss of endoneural tubes	Incomplete recovery, synkinesis
Fourth degree	Partial transection	Disruption of endoneural tubes and perineurium	Poor recovery, synkinesis
Fifth degree	Complete transection	Disruption of entire nerve	None

Table 3-2. Sunderland Classification of Peripheral Nerve Injuries

Derived from Sunderland S. A classification of peripheral nerve injuries producing loss of function. *Brain.* 1951;74(4):491–516.

Second-degree injury, or axonotmesis, occurs when trauma leads to obstruction of vascular flow and subsequent ischemia and breakdown of axons. If trauma is relieved, recovery requires axons to regenerate, which may take weeks to months. The endoneural tubes are intact and no crossover to other axons is expected. Usually, the typical pathological processes that occur with Bell palsy or herpes zoster oticus are limited to first- or second-order injuries, and satisfactory recovery occurs in affected individuals.

With third-degree injury, or neurotmesis, pressure is of enough severity or duration that endoneural sheaths are disrupted. Spontaneous recovery often is incomplete, and synkinesis is expected, as regenerating axons may cross. Synkinesis results from miswiring of nerves after trauma. For example, during voluntary smiling, contraction of the eye muscle may occur with simultaneous involuntary squinting.

Fourth- or fifth-degree injury occurs when partial or complete transection takes place, most often from external trauma. Fourth-degree injury occurs with partial disruption of the nerve. In addition to disruption of the endoneurium, perineural disruption occurs. The only structure holding the nerve together is the epineurium. Recovery potential is poor. Fifth-degree injury occurs when the nerve is completely disrupted. No spontaneous recovery will occur.

DIAGNOSTIC TESTING

Because of the proximity of the seventh and eighth cranial nerves in the posterior fossa, pure tone and speech audiometry is recommended in all cases of facial paralysis. Radiographic imaging assists in delineating the site of the lesion along the facial nerve. Computed tomography (CT) is optimal for assessing temporal bone trauma, cholesteatoma, and otitis media. Magnetic resonance imaging helps in the assessment of suspected tumors or infections.

When other, less common causes of facial paralysis are suspected, laboratory studies should be considered to evaluate for Lyme disease, diabetes, and autoimmune disorders.

Electrophysiologic tests are useful in establishing the prognosis of facial nerve recovery. Tests are complementary and indicated when complete paralysis is present. They do not have a role in clinically evident partial paresis because recovery is expected. Electromyography (EMG) records spontaneous, evoked, and voluntary electrical responses of motor end plates. In the acute setting, presence of voluntary active motor units indicates an intact nerve with incomplete injury. In a denervated muscle, spontaneous involuntary contractions appear as fibrillation potentials. However, they do not develop until 14 to 21 days after facial nerve injury, thus limiting the role of EMG until this period during which voluntary active potentials are absent. With recovery or regeneration, return of neural activity may be predicted by polyphasic potentials, which may be present even though clinically evident facial motion is absent.

Other clinically relevant tests to assess the prognosis for return of function are the nerve excitability test (NET), maximal stimulation test (MST), and electroneuronography (ENoG). These 3 tests can be performed 3 days after the onset of paralysis once Wallerian degeneration has occurred. Even a completely transected nerve will conduct distally stimulated impulses for 48 to 72 hours. Thus, these tests have limited applicability during the first 3 days. The NET is used to measure the current threshold for a barely perceivable facial motor response. The paralyzed side is compared with the unaffected side. Differences of greater than 3.5 mA are considered significant and indicative of nerve fiber degeneration and potentially incomplete recovery. In MST, facial muscle contraction is elicited with the highest electrical current that the patient can tolerate. The response is expressed as the difference between the result for the normal side and that for the paralyzed side and is graded as minimal, moderate, severe, or no response.

Electroneuronography, or evoked EMG, is the recording of compound action potentials from the facial musculature in response to transcutaneous electrical stimulation of the facial nerve at the level of the stylomastoid foramen. Responses from the 2 sides are compared. The percentage response on the affected side compared with that on the unaffected side is proportional to the degree of degeneration. Surgical decompression is recommended in patients who have more than 90% degeneration because of the high likelihood that recovery will be incomplete with medical management alone. The advantage of ENoG over NET or MST is that the response is quantitated and less dependent on the subjective observations of the tester in visualizing responses.

▮ Differential Diagnoses

The presentation and etiology of facial paralysis are variable (**Box 3-1**). Clinical management of paralysis is determined on the basis of etiology and predicted clinical recovery. Regardless of the cause, an important aspect of facial paralysis is eye care because the most common and significant complication is corneal desiccation. Educating parents about the importance of eye moisturization is essential. Treatment measures include ophthalmic lubricants, eyelid taping at night, and use of moisture chambers. Long-term surgical options are gold weights, canthoplasties, and eyelid springs.

> **Pearl:** Corneal desiccation is the most common and significant complication of facial paralysis, regardless of etiology. Eye care is essential in prevention.

BELL PALSY

Bell palsy is the most common etiology and defined as spontaneous facial paralysis without other disease or injury that may account for the paralysis. However, the PCC must be careful not to quickly

Box 3-1. Differential Diagnoses of Facial Paralysis

Infectious

Bell palsy
Acute/chronic otitis media or
mastoiditis
Herpes zoster oticus
Lyme disease
AIDS

Trauma

Birth trauma
Temporal bone fractures
Penetrating trauma
Surgical injury

Congenital

Möbius syndrome
CULLP
Oculoauriculovertebral syndrome

Tumors

Cholesteatoma
Facial neuroma
Schwannoma
Parotid tumors
Malignancy: carcinoma, sarcoma

Autoimmune

Guillain-Barré syndrome
Sarcoidosis

Idiopathic

Melkersson-Rosenthal syndrome

Abbreviation: CULLP, congenital unilateral lower lip palsy.

diagnose Bell palsy, because it is a diagnosis of exclusion once other possible etiologies have been considered and ruled out.

This condition affects patients of all ages, with peak incidence between the ages of 20 and 40 years. The annual incidence is between 30 and 45 per 100,000. A family history of Bell palsy exists in 8% of patients.

The typical presentation is sudden onset or a gradually progressive facial nerve paralysis over a 24- to 48-hour period. Approximately 20% of individuals report ipsilateral ear pain or numbness preceding paralysis. Approximately 30% of patients have paresis only, all of whom are expected to fully recover. The remaining 70% of patients develop complete paralysis. In 1 of the largest series, including patients who did not receive specific therapy, 85% began to recover within 3 weeks of onset. The remaining 15% exhibited partial recovery within 3 to 6 months. Approximately 71% achieved normal facial function, 13% had minor sequelae, and 16% had diminished function.

Although the cause of Bell palsy is considered unknown, edema of the facial nerve is thought to be the underlying factor. This swelling leads to progressive neural ischemia and further edema. Some evidence exists that an underlying factor is viral in origin, as 30% to 50% of patients report a viral prodrome. In addition, samples of endoneural fluid have shown evidence of herpes simplex virus in patients who underwent decompression surgery for Bell palsy.

Medical management of Bell palsy includes the use of corticosteroids to reduce inflammation on the facial nerve. A meta-analysis based primarily on studies in adults has demonstrated the benefit of steroid therapy. Recent Cochrane reviews also support the use of steroids to increase the likelihood of complete recovery. Acyclovir also may be beneficial if treatment is initiated within 3 days of onset.

A recent randomized, double-blind, placebo-controlled study supported the use of prednisolone compared with a placebo and with acyclovir. Surgical management for Bell palsy is indicated in individuals who have complete paralysis and in whom ENoG testing shows greater than 90% degeneration. Decompression involves a middle fossa approach to decompressing the labyrinthine segment. Evidence to support decompression is based on patients who presented within 14 days of onset. Among those who underwent surgical decompression, 91% achieved a House-Brackmann grade I or II; by comparison, only 41% who opted for medical treatment achieved grade I or II. The authors reported no difference in results if decompression was performed after 14 days.

> **Pearl:** Bell palsy is the most common cause of facial paralysis, but other etiologies must be ruled out prior to making this diagnosis.

OTITIS MEDIA

Facial palsy can occur secondary to acute otitis media and mastoiditis. Palsy is secondary to inflammation and neural edema along the course of the nerve. The incidence of palsy with acute otitis media is approximately 1 in 20,000 cases.

Treatment involves myringotomy with or without a tympanostomy tube, culture of middle ear fluid, and antibiotics. The prognosis is excellent, and recovery of facial function is rapid by resolving the underlying inflammation.

Facial paralysis with chronic otitis media and cholesteatoma has a more guarded outcome and requires more extensive surgery than myringotomy alone. Temporal bone CT is recommended to evaluate the extent of involvement and assess for other intratemporal complications. Surgery consists of tympanomastoidectomy to remove granulation or cholesteatoma that may be contributing to inflammation or erosion of the facial nerve. Prognosis is good as long as the onset of paralysis is rapid, and diagnosis and treatment are prompt.

HERPES ZOSTER OTICUS (RAMSAY HUNT SYNDROME)

The incidence of herpes zoster oticus (Ramsay Hunt syndrome) is approximately 5 cases per 100,000 annually. The condition is secondary to a latent varicella zoster infection involving the seventh nerve ganglia. Reactivation of the infection results in facial paralysis, severe otalgia, and vesicular lesions in the skin of the external auditory canal and concha. Some patients also experience sensorineural hearing loss and vertigo.

The prognosis for patients with Ramsay Hunt syndrome is worse than that for those with Bell palsy. Patients are more likely to have complete clinical paralysis, complete electrical denervation, and incomplete recovery with synkinesis. Treatment consists of antiviral drugs (acyclovir or valacyclovir) and steroid therapy.

LYME DISEASE

This multisystem inflammatory illness is caused by the tick-borne spirochete *Borrelia burgdorferi*. The infection is categorized as early localized, early disseminated, or late. Erythema migrans, the early localized presentation, is a painless, reddish lesion with concentric circles that have a white center zone. Early disseminated disease occurs when the spirochete spreads hematogenously. Neurologic symptoms include cranial neuropathy such as facial paralysis. Late Lyme disease manifests as polyarthralgia, arthritis, or polyneuritis.

The diagnosis is made based on the enzyme-linked immunosorbent assay and Western blot techniques. Careful interpretation is necessary as a negative result can occur with disease when IgM has not had a chance to develop. Positive test results also may reflect prior exposure but be unrelated to the patient's current complaints. Treatment consists of appropriate antibiotic therapy. The prognosis for patients with facial palsy is excellent, with permanent dysfunction in 11% of children.

MELKERSSON-ROSENTHAL SYNDROME

Facial paralysis is recurrent and associated with recurrent facial edema and fissured tongue. This condition typically begins during the second decade after birth. Facial swelling may vary in degree from ipsilateral isolated lip swelling to bilateral complete edema. Biopsy of the lip reveals noncaseating epithelioid cell granuloma with surrounding histiocytes, plasma cells, and lymphocytes. The etiology of Melkersson-Rosenthal syndrome is unknown.

KAWASAKI DISEASE

This multisystem condition may involve mucous membranes, skin, coronary arteries, and lymph nodes. Facial paralysis is 1 of the neurologic sequelae. The median age at onset of disease is 13 months. Prognosis of the palsy is good, with typical resolution in less than 3 months.

TRAUMA

The facial nerve is vulnerable to various mechanisms of trauma, including blunt trauma resulting from temporal bone fractures. The most common mechanisms of pediatric fractures are motor vehicle crashes and falls.

The initial physical examination is important in establishing a prognosis, although it may be limited if the child has other injuries and critical care issues prevent evaluation of function. If paresis alone is present, the prognosis is excellent without any surgical intervention. In addition, delayed-onset facial paralysis is associated with good recovery of function.

If the patient has complete paralysis on initial examination, high-resolution temporal bone CT (**Figure 3-3**) along with electrophysiologic testing are essential to determine the prognosis and potential need for surgical intervention.

Classically, temporal bone fractures are classified as longitudinal or transverse relative to the axis of the petrous bone. Longitudinal fractures have been associated with facial nerve injury in 20% of cases, while transverse fractures have been associated with such injuries in 50% of cases. Newer classification schemes have been proposed to help predict the likelihood of facial nerve and inner ear injury with temporal bone fractures. One such scheme—otic capsule sparing vs otic capsule violating—may be more predictive of facial nerve injury.

Penetrating trauma with complete facial paralysis should be repaired as soon as the child is in medically stable condition and other potential vascular injuries have been evaluated. This injury typically necessitates end-to-end anastomosis or cable grafting. Repair

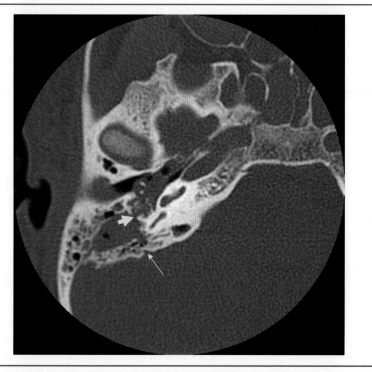

Figure 3-3. Temporal bone computed tomographic scan of fracture through the facial nerve resulting in transection of the nerve. Long arrow depicts the fracture through the nerve. Short arrow depicts the fracture line.

within 3 days of injury also allows for distal stimulation of the nerve, which assists in nerve identification because the anatomy is often distorted from penetrating trauma. If facial nerve injury is medial to the lateral canthus, it should be observed, as multiple cross-innervations from other nerve fibers are present.

Trauma also may occur iatrogenically during ear or parotid gland surgery. The frequency of facial nerve injury during otologic surgery has been reported to range from 0.6% to 3.6%. The most common site of injury is near the second genu at the tympanic segment. Knowledge of the surgical anatomy and identification of the facial nerve in the operative field are the best ways to avoid injury. When facial nerve injury is suspected during surgery, the surgeon should explore and electrically stimulate the injury site to verify nerve integrity. In addition, decompression proximal and distal to the injury should be performed. If more than 50% of the circumference of the nerve has been disrupted, the nerve should be repaired. Facial nerve monitoring is useful in surgical localization of the nerve, but it does not ensure injury prevention. The trend toward routine monitoring is increasing for ear surgery, such as tympanomastoidectomy or cochlear implantation. Regarding parotidectomy, a recent meta-analysis demonstrated that immediate postoperative facial weakness was reduced with facial nerve monitoring. However, monitoring did not influence the final outcome of permanent facial paralysis.

If facial paralysis is noted after surgery, the ear packing should be removed and facial function reassessed after a short period of observation. Incomplete and delayed paralysis indicates that facial nerve integrity has been maintained, and the prognosis is good. Treatment with systemic steroids should be started. If complete facial paralysis is evident immediately after surgery, the prognosis is worse and surgical exploration is warranted.

Repair of facial nerve trauma depends on the extent of the injury. When less than 50% of the diameter of the nerve is involved, the nerve should be decompressed proximal and distal to the site. In patients with more extensive injury, the nerve may be anastomosed without tension. When the injury involves a section of nerve and the nerves cannot be anastomosed without tension, nerve grafting is used. Donor nerves include the greater auricular, sural, or median antebrachial cutaneous nerves.

> **Pearl:** The most common site of facial nerve injury during surgery is near the second genu of the tympanic segment.

TUMORS

Neoplastic lesions may present as facial paralysis. Factors that suggest a mass lesion and warrant further radiographic imaging are slowly progressive facial paralysis, unilateral middle ear effusion, multiple cranial neuropathies, recurrent paralysis, parotid tumor, cutaneous malignancy, or ipsilateral hearing loss.

Tumors causing facial paralysis in children are rare. They may be benign or malignant, but the most common cause is facial schwannoma. The tumor may occur anywhere along the course of the facial nerve. Malignant tumors that may cause facial paralysis include leukemia, rhabdomyosarcoma, and neuroblastoma.

NEONATAL FACIAL PARALYSIS

The incidence of neonatal facial paralysis ranges from 0.05% to 0.23%. A key issue is identifying the paralysis as congenital or traumatic. Traumatic palsy occurs secondary to intrauterine positioning or injury during delivery.

The history and physical examination usually are sufficient to differentiate between traumatic and congenital palsy. Trauma is usually associated with a prolonged or difficult delivery, with potential forceps use. The physical examination may also demonstrate hemotympanum or facial or periauricular ecchymoses. No cases of nerve transection from birth trauma have been reported. Congenital facial paralysis is often associated with other facial anomalies such as maxillary defects or auricular anomalies. In addition, other cranial nerve deficits or dysmorphic features of the chest, limbs, and cardiovascular or genitourinary systems may be presenting findings. Möbius syndrome is a rare condition associated with unilateral or bilateral palsy, often sparing the lower half of the face. Also, abducens palsy often is present. The cause of this syndrome is unknown, with potential explanations including agenesis of facial musculature or the facial nucleus. Hemifacial microsomia or oculoauriculovertebral syndrome is estimated to occur in 1 in 5,600 live births and has a variable presentation of ocular, auricular, mandibular, and facial nerve anomalies. Facial weakness occurs in approximately 20% to 25% of these children. Congenital unilateral lower lip palsy is apparent on physical examination as the infant is unable to depress the lower lip with crying. The incidence is 1 in 120 to 160 newborns. The condition may be associated with ear anomalies and congenital cardiac defects in 10% of children.

Although the history and physical examination may help differentiate between traumatic and congenital causes, in ambiguous cases, CT of the temporal bone is warranted. Electrophysiologic studies also may help to clarify etiologies. The results of electroneuronography testing are abnormal at birth in those with congenital paralysis.

The prognosis for recovery from neonatal traumatic facial paralysis is excellent, with greater than 90% of patients experiencing spontaneous return of function. Because of this anticipated outcome with traumatic paralysis, surgery is reserved for those in whom there is evidence of electrophysiologic dysfunction, temporal bone fracture on CT, and no evidence of recovery for at least 5 weeks.

Unlike cases of neonatal traumatic paralysis, those associated with developmental causes are unlikely to spontaneously resolve. Surgical exploration is not indicated because the nerve generally tapers to thin fibers that preclude decompression or grafting.

CHRONIC FACIAL PARALYSIS

Children with long-standing paralysis (more than 1 year) despite medical treatment and in whom there is no physical or electrophysiologic evidence of recovery may be candidates for reparative reanimation surgery. The type of surgery depends on the status of the facial musculature and age of the child as well as his or her development. Repair includes nerve transposition, muscular slings, and microneurovascular free muscle grafts. These repairs are usually deferred until the child's facial growth is complete.

■ Conclusion

Pediatric facial paralysis is a challenge for PCCs who need to assess the etiology. Bell palsy is the most common cause of facial paralysis, but the diagnosis is made only after other important etiologies are ruled out. Medical and surgical management of facial paralysis depends on the etiology. Eye care remains a key component of management because corneal desiccation is the most common complication. Appropriate and early referral to an otolaryngologist is warranted for the evaluation of pediatric facial paralysis.

■ Selected References

Adour KK. Otological complications of herpes zoster. *Ann Neurol.* 1994;35 (Suppl): S62–S64

Adour KK, Byl FM, Hilsinger RL Jr, Kahn ZM, Sheldon MI. The true nature of Bell's palsy: analysis of 1,000 consecutive patients. *Laryngoscope.* 1978;88(5):787–801

Adour KK, Ruboyianes JM, Trent CS, et al. Bell's palsy treatment with acyclovir and prednisone compared with prednisone alone: a double-blind, randomized, controlled trial. *Ann Otol Rhinol Laryngol.* 1996;105(5):371–378

Barrs DM. Facial nerve trauma: optimal timing for repair. *Laryngoscope.* 1991;101(8):835–848

Bergman I, May M, Wessel HB, Stool SE. Management of facial palsy caused by birth trauma. *Laryngoscope.* 1986;96(4):381–384

Brodie HA, Thompson TC. Management of complications from 820 temporal bone fractures. *Am J Otol.* 1997;18(2):188–197

Ellefsen B, Bonding P. Facial palsy in acute otitis media. *Clin Otolaryngol Allied Sci.* 1996;21(5):393–395

Fisch U. Surgery for Bell's palsy. *Arch Otolaryngol.* 1981;107(1):1–11

Gallagher PG. Facial nerve paralysis and Kawasaki disease. *Rev Infect Dis.* 1990;12(3): 403–405

Gantz BJ, Rubinstein JT, Gidley P, Woodworth GG. Surgical management of Bell's palsy. *Laryngoscope.* 1999;109(8):1177–1188

Gorlin RJ, Cohen MM, Levin LS. *Syndromes of the Head and Neck.* 3rd ed. New York, NY: Oxford University Press; 1990:641–652

Green JD Jr, Shelton C, Brackmann DE. Iatrogenic facial nerve injury during otologic surgery. *Laryngoscope.* 1994;104(8 Pt 1):922–926

Greene RM, Rogers RS III. Melkersson-Rosenthal syndrome: a review of 36 patients. *J Am Acad Dermatol.* 1989;21(6):1263–1270

House JW, Brackmann DE. Facial nerve grading system. *Otolaryngol Head Neck Surg.* 1985;93(2):146–147

Ishman SL, Friedland DR. Temporal bone fractures: traditional classification and clinical relevance. *Laryngoscope.* 2004;114(10):1734–1741

Lee D, Honrado C, Har-El G, Goldsmith A. Pediatric temporal bone fractures. *Laryngoscope.* 1998;108(6):816–821

Little SC, Kesser BW. Radiographic classification of temporal bone fractures: clinical predictability using a new system. *Arch Otolaryngol Head Neck Surg.* 2006;132(12): 1300–1304

Madhok VB, Gagyor I, Daly F, et al. Corticosteroid for Bell's palsy (idiopathic facial paralysis). *Cochrane Database Syst Rev.* 2016;7:CD001942

May M, Fria TJ, Blumenthal F, Curtin H. Facial paralysis in children: differential diagnosis. *Otolaryngol Head Neck Surg.* 1981;89(5):841–848

McHugh HE, Sowden KA, Levitt MN. Facial paralysis and muscle agenesis in the newborn. *Arch Otolaryngol.* 1969;89(1):131–143

Murakami S, Mizobuchi M, Nakashiro Y, Doi T, Hato N, Yanagihara N. Bell palsy and herpes simplex virus: identification of viral DNA in endoneurial fluid and muscle. *Ann Intern Med.* 1996;124(1 Pt 1):27–30

Peitersen E. Bell's palsy: the spontaneous course of 2,500 peripheral facial nerve palsies of different etiologies. *Acta Otolaryngol Suppl.* 2002;122(7):4–30

Pitts DB, Adour KK, Hilsinger RL Jr. Recurrent Bell's palsy: analysis of 140 patients. *Laryngoscope.* 1988;98(5):535–540

Ramsey MJ, DerSimonian R, Holtel MR, Burgess LP. Corticosteroid treatment for idiopathic facial nerve paralysis: a meta-analysis. *Laryngoscope.* 2000;110(3 Pt 1):335–341

Robillard RB, Hilsinger RL Jr, Adour KK. Ramsay Hunt facial paralysis: clinical analyses of 185 patients. *Otolaryngol Head Neck Surg.* 1986;95(3 Pt 1):292–297

Skogman BH, Croner S, Nordwall M, Eknefelt M, Ernerudh J, Forsberg P. Lyme neuroborreliosis in children: a prospective study of clinical features, prognosis, and outcome. *Pediatr Infect Dis J.* 2008;27(12):1089–1094

Sood AJ, Houlton JJ, Nguyen SA, Gillespie MB. Facial nerve monitoring during parotidectomy: a systematic review and meta-analysis. *Otolaryngol Head Neck Surg.* 2015;152(4):631–637

Sullivan FM, Swan IR, Donnan PT, et al. Early treatment with prednisolone or acyclovir in Bell's palsy. *N Engl J Med.* 2007;357(16):1598–1607

Sunderland S. *Nerves and Nerve Injuries.* 2nd ed. London, England: Churchill Livingstone; 1978:88–89, 96–97, 133

Wiet RJ. Iatrogenic facial paralysis. *Otolaryngol Clin North Am.* 1982;15(4):773–780

CHAPTER 4

Diseases and Anomalies of the Auricle and External Auditory Canal

Stephanie Moody-Antonio, MD

Congenital Malformations
and Deformities
Embryologic Development
of the Auricle and
External Auditory
Canal
Congenital Malformations
of the External Ear
Auricle
Traumatic Injuries to the
Auricle
Infections of the Auricle
Inflammatory Disorders
of the Auricle

External Auditory Canal
Traumatic Injuries to the
Ear Canal
Infectious Disorders of
the Ear Canal
Inflammatory Disorders
of the Ear Canal
Other Disorders Affecting
the Ear Canal
Cerumen Impaction
Keratosis Obturans and
External Auditory
Canal Cholesteatoma
Cysts

■ Congenital Malformations and Deformities

EMBRYOLOGIC DEVELOPMENT OF THE AURICLE AND EXTERNAL AUDITORY CANAL

The external ear develops from the first and second branchial arches starting at about week 4 of gestation. During weeks 5 and 6, 6 small hillocks arise and fuse, becoming adult shape by about month 4 of gestation. The early pinna is initially located high in the neck and moves dorso-cranially with the development of the mandible, reaching the adult location by gestational week 20. The pinna attains 80% of its adult size by age 4 to 5 years.

The external ear canal develops during this same period, starting with extension of the first branchial cleft toward the first pharyngeal pouch during gestational weeks 4 and 5. In the next phase, mesodermal tissue proliferates between the cleft and pouch, and the branchial cleft grows deeper into the mesodermal tissue, forming the primitive cartilaginous portion of the canal. During week 9, ectodermal lining from the first branchial cleft proliferates, temporarily filling the canal with an epidermal plug. This meatal plug begins to resorb during the 21st week starting medially and extending laterally, forming a patent canal by week 28 and leaving a layer of epithelium to line the canal and lateral surface of the tympanic membrane (TM). The ossicles and fibrous layer of the TM arise from mesodermal tissue from the first (incus and malleus) and second (stapes arch) branchial arches. The bony portion of the canal is formed from centers of ossification within the mesodermal tissue, initially forming a u-shaped incomplete ring. Postnatally, maturation of the bony portion of the canal continues as ossification centers fuse to become a complete tympanic ring by about age 2. The tympanic rings grows laterally during childhood, reaching adult size and orientation by about age 9 years. The TM is notably more horizontal at birth and becomes more vertically oriented with the lateral growth of the tympanic ring. Congenital abnormalities of the ear occur with disruption of the branchial structures, generally with more severe abnormalities occurring during gestational weeks 4 and 5 and less severe abnormalities occurring later.

CONGENITAL MALFORMATIONS OF THE EXTERNAL EAR

Congenital malformations of the external ear range from mild deformity and mild stenosis to complete absence of the auricle and ear canal. In some cases, mild deformities of the auricle are inconsequential, while some may be indicative of a genetic syndrome or congenital association. Mild anomalies of the pinna include low-set ears, normally shaped but large or small ears, cupping or folding of the helix, hooding of the helical rim, flattening or absence of the antihelical fold, poor definition of the scaphoid fossa, and protruding or prominent ear. Syndromes commonly associated with minor deformities of the external ear include Turner syndrome (low-set ears with large lobules), Potter syndrome (low-set ears with deficient auricular cartilage and stenotic canal), Trisomy 13 (low-set and malformed auricles, small TM, and abnormal middle ear), and Trisomy 21 (low-set ears).

Many minor deformities require no intervention. Some minor deformities of the auricle can be treated effectively with molding or splinting in the newborn period. During the first 6 weeks after birth, the cartilage is very pliable owing to the effect of circulating maternal estrogen promoting high levels of proteoglycans. Splinting with dental roll or a commercial system for a few weeks has shown a high rate of effectiveness for improving mild-to-moderate deformities. Referral to an otolaryngologist or a plastic surgeon within a few days or weeks after birth is important if nonsurgical correction of minor deformities is desired.

One of the most common mild deformities is the prominent ear, affecting about 5% of the population. A prominent ear projects from the head with a wider-than-normal angle, typically because of deficient antihelical fold or conchal hypertrophy (**Figure 4-1**). Having prominent ears may negatively affect an older child's self-image and referral should be considered if the child shows any sign of social withdrawal or sensitivity regarding his or her appearance. For this and other significant deformities, otoplasty or surgical correction may be considered, typically after age 4, when the auricle is 85% of adult size. Surgical correction of mild/moderate deformities of the pinna generally yields good results, although revision surgery occasionally

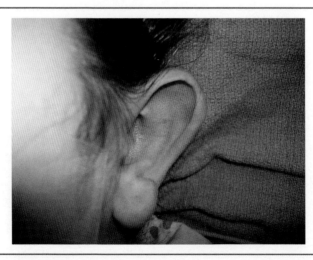

Figure 4-1. Prominent auricle. This congenital anomaly is severe enough to warrant surgical correction.

is needed. Unfortunately, some medical insurance companies consider otoplasty to be a cosmetic procedure and will not pay for the operation.

Microtia and Aural Atresia

Microtia is a deformity of the auricle that ranges from a small but normally formed ear to complete absence of the ear (anotia). Microtia is usually, but not always, associated with congenital aural atresia, absence of the ear canal, and TM. It is more commonly unilateral and right sided and is more common in males. It may occur independently or be associated with a syndrome such as oculoauriculovertebral dysplasia (hemifacial microsomia, Goldenhar syndrome), Crouzon syndrome, Klippel-Feil syndrome, CHARGE syndrome, VATER syndrome, and Kabuki syndrome. When bilateral, the defect is often associated with Treacher Collins or Nager syndrome.

Microtia is categorized by severity. Grade 1 microtia is a slightly small or malformed ear. Often, no surgery is required because the malformation is mild. In some cases, newborn molding is effective in remodeling the ear to a more typical shape. Grade 2 microtia (**Figure 4-2**) is a significant congenital ear deformity, usually consisting of absence of most of the superior half of the auricle, often with a small folded-over "lop ear." Grade 3 microtia (**Figure 4-3**) is a severe auricular deformity in which only a lobule and a small sausage-shaped

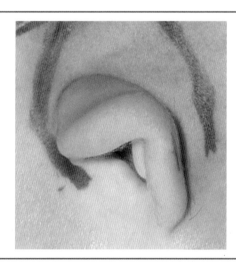

Figure 4-2. Grade 2 microtia. The inferior portion of the auricle is well formed but the superior portion is deficient and folded over. This patient also has a stenotic external auditory canal.

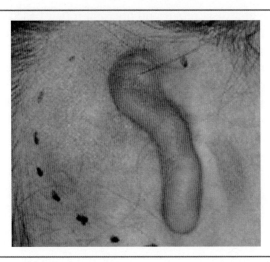

Figure 4-3. Grade 3 microtia with congenital aural atresia. This patient has the cosmetic deformity of absence of the auricle except for a lobule and very small rudimentary auricular remnant. The associated congenital aural atresia results in a handicapping 60-dB conductive hearing loss.

auricular remnant (similar to the shape of a peanut) are present. Grades 2 and 3 microtia and anotia are usually associated with significant hearing loss due to ear canal stenosis or atresia.

Once airway, feeding, renal, and cardiac problems have been addressed or ruled out, the patient should be referred to an otolaryngologist and a plastic surgeon skilled in the evaluation and treatment of microtia and aural atresia. Early evaluation includes hearing evaluation of both the normal and abnormal ears. Bone conduction auditory brainstem evoked responses can detect sensorineural function on the atretic side. Computed tomography (CT) is warranted by age 4 or 5 to rule out a cholesteatoma trapped deep to a partially atretic or severely stenotic ear canal. Speech and language assessment should be ongoing during childhood.

Management of concurrent microtia and atresia should be considered in concert, since corrective techniques are intertwined with respect to timing and surgical procedures. No treatment is absolutely necessary for uncomplicated microtia/atresia. First and foremost, early hearing rehabilitation is critical for infants and children with bilateral hearing loss and is accomplished with a bone conduction device held in place with a soft elastic band or adhesive.

When surgical correction of either the microtic ear or atretic canal is desired, the otolaryngologist and plastic surgeon team will consider the sequence of atresia repair and microtia repair based on their preferred approach, in some cases performing portions of the procedures simultaneously vs performing the atresia repair or microtia repair first and in stages. Surgery for microtia and atresia is usually covered by insurance.

A temporal bone CT scan is required to assess candidacy for surgical opening of the ear canal (aural atresiaplasty). The anatomy is graded based on the presence of middle-ear structures, location of the facial nerve, and size of the middle ear and mastoid. If the anatomy is favorable, atresiaplasty can be considered, but not until age 5 to 6 years when the ear canal is closer to adult size and the child is more likely to tolerate office management of the operated ear. Surgical repair of atresia is extremely difficult, with risk of facial nerve injury, sensorineural hearing loss, and restenosis, and should be performed only by surgeons (typically otologists or pediatric otolaryngologists) with appropriate training and experience. Restoration of long-lasting normal hearing is highly unusual, although significantly improved hearing can be achieved in about 50% of cases. Revision surgeries are common because of restenosis of the ear canal or persistent hearing loss.

When atresia repair is deemed impossible or undesirable, the most effective approach for managing the related hearing loss is a bone conduction device, which can be converted to an osseointegrated surgical implant after about age 5 years, when the skull bone has achieved adequate thickness. These devices include a processor that communicates with the implant, either directly or via magnetic attraction, and stimulates the inner ear through bone conduction (**Figure 4-4**). The decision to undergo bone conduction implantation versus atresiaplasty is made on a case-by-case basis, depending on the child's anatomy, medical comorbidities, and patient and/or family wishes. In the case of unilateral microtia/atresia, there is no harm in waiting until the child reaches the age of consent for atresia repair. There is much less urgency for hearing rehabilitation in a child with unilateral atresia and hearing loss than in a child with bilateral aural atresia. The timing of atresia repair is also influenced by the plan for repair of an associated microtia.

A cosmetically acceptable auricle may be attained in several ways. The simplest method is use of a glue-on prosthetic auricle that has the advantage of no surgery, but may be easily dislodged during play, which can be embarrassing. A second method is surgical placement of osseointegrated implants in the postauricular area to be used

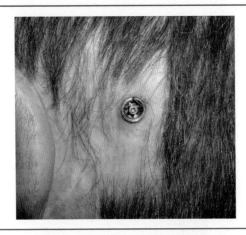

Figure 4-4. Bone-anchored hearing aid (BAHA). This child with Treacher Collins syndrome has bilateral microtia and congenital aural atresia. The BAHA titanium osseointegrated transcutaneous implant is seen here. The external processor is clipped onto the implant.

as anchors for a clip-on or magnetic prosthetic auricle. Prosthetic auricles are modeled after the normal auricle and can be almost impossible to detect on casual visual inspection. A third option is surgical reconstruction with a rib graft or prefabricated synthetic implant (**figures 4-5** and **4-6**). Surgical reconstruction of the pinna is

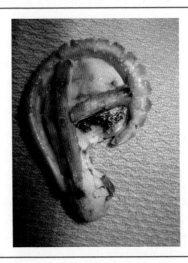

Figure 4-5. Rib cartilage graft for microtia reconstruction. Ribs were harvested and sculpted into this cartilaginous auricle, which was implanted under the scalp in the first stage of the multistage auricular reconstruction.

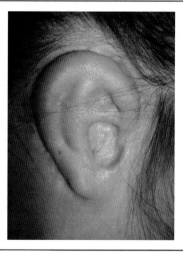

Figure 4-6. Final result of 4-stage auricular reconstruction with rib cartilage for grade 3 microtia. The patient had insufficient anatomical structures to allow congenital aural atresia reconstruction.

performed in 1 or multiple stages interwoven with repair of the aural atresia (if planned). It is also a technically difficult surgery that should be performed by an experienced otolaryngologist or plastic surgeon. The decision regarding each of these options depends on the patient's anatomy, medical comorbidities, and family and surgeon preferences.

Preauricular Sinuses and Cysts

Preauricular pits are thought to arise from abnormal fusion or entrapment of the groove between the first and second hillocks during embryologic fusion, resulting in a closed cyst or a sinus with an opening to the skin between the tragus and the root of the helix or between the antihelix and helix. Anomalous development of or supernumerary hillocks can also result in preauricular tags or appendages. They are more common on the right side, but also can be bilateral. Preauricular pits manifest as an autosomal dominant trait and are rarely associated with hearing loss or renal problems. Further evaluation is warranted if there are other auricular deformities or a cyst or sinus that could indicate branchio-oto-renal syndrome, which is also associated with hearing loss, preauricular tags, and renal deformities.

Preauricular cysts and sinuses may remain asymptomatic and require no treatment. Alternatively, they may drain, be painful, or be a site of recurrent infection (**Figure 4-7**). Infections may be managed with antimicrobial agents, fine-needle aspiration, or incision and drainage as

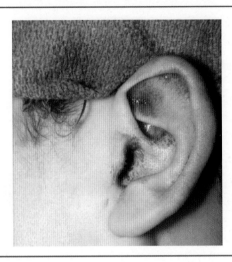

Figure 4-7. First branchial cleft cyst. Note that the cystic structure is just below the lobule, which should alert the primary care clinician to the possibility of a first branchial cleft anomaly.

needed, depending on the patient's response to therapy and the severity of the infection. Recurrent infections, constant drainage, or persistent enlargement of the lesion are indications for referral for surgical excision. Excision of preauricular pits typically includes a small section of related tragal or helical cartilage to reduce the risk of recurrence.

First Branchial Cleft Anomalies

A pit, sinus tract, or cyst located near the lobule, in the postauricular sulcus or within the canal, may be due to duplication of the first branchial groove or incomplete fusion of the first and second branchial arches. Because fusion of the branchial arches occurs concurrent with the development of the parotid gland and facial nerve, first branchial cleft tracts or cysts are often anatomically related to these structures. There are 2 types of first branchial cleft anomalies. A Work type 1 first branchial cleft anomaly contains only ectoderm and is considered to be a duplication of the membranous external auditory canal. It is characterized as a fistula tract opening in the postauricular or preauricular area extending parallel to the ear canal and ending in a bony plate near the middle ear. A Work type 2 branchial cleft anomaly contains ectoderm and mesoderm (often cartilage) (**Figure 4-8**). The tract usually presents at the level of the angle of the mandible and extends through the parotid gland either lateral or medial to the facial nerve, opening into the external canal. These lesions may be difficult to identify because the tract may be hidden in the canal. They may

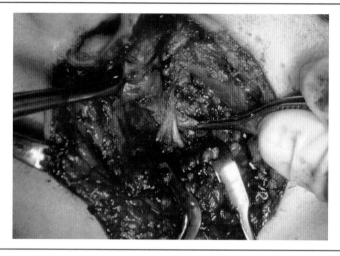

Figure 4-8. Deep portion of the first branchial cleft cyst. The bifurcation of the facial nerve is found to be immediately lateral and juxtaposed to the deep portion of the first branchial cleft anomaly. To avoid nerve injury, facial nerve dissection and preservation are required prior to safe removal of the deep portion of this anomaly.

drain mucus or become infected and present as a neck or periauricular abscess. A CT scan with a fistulogram can be helpful in identifying the path of a tract. When the mass enlarges or becomes infected, surgical excision is the treatment of choice. The deep extension or tract of these lesions may be juxtaposed with the bifurcation or trunk of the facial nerve. Thus, proper technique requires facial monitoring, and dissection is critical (**Figure 4–9**).

■ Auricle

TRAUMATIC INJURIES TO THE AURICLE

Lacerations

Minor lacerations or animal bites of the auricle may be repaired by any competent surgeon. However, patients with more severe injuries should be referred to an experienced auricular surgeon. Whenever cartilage is exposed, prophylactic antimicrobial agents that cover *Staphylococcus aureus* and *Pseudomonas aeruginosa* should be administered.

Auricular Hematoma

Trauma to the auricle may avulse the skin from the cartilage, and hematomas may form in the resultant space. If left untreated, several problems may occur. The hematoma may be replaced by a

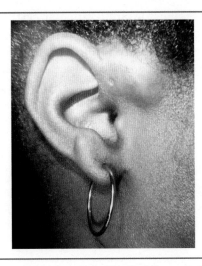

Figure 4-9. Infected preauricular sinus. Note the pit of the preauricular sinus anterior to the root of the helix. The swelling and erythema are caused by infection of the sinus.

scar, and a cosmetic deformity known as cauliflower ear may result. In this condition, a raised scar fills the hematoma site and the auricle is permanently deformed; thickened portions may resemble a cauliflower. An untreated hematoma may also become infected, and cartilage reabsorption of the auricle may result in significant auricular deformity.

The initial treatment of auricular hematoma is fine-needle aspiration or incision and drainage of the blood, followed by placement of sterile dental rolls or gauze packing over the area that is fixed with sutures for 3 to 5 days. The dental rolls act as a bolster or packing that holds the avulsed skin in close proximity to the underlying cartilage. This prevents the reaccumulation of blood or serous fluid and recurrence of the lesion. Alternatively, a quilting stitch through the front and back of the ear cartilage at the hematoma site may prevent re-formation of hematoma. Culture and sensitivity studies are sent and prophylactic antibiotic treatment is considered.

INFECTIONS OF THE AURICLE
Perichondritis and Chondritis
Perichondritis implies an infection limited to the perichondrium, while chondritis implies a deeper infection of the cartilage and is often associated with permanent auricular deformity. Infectious perichondritis and chondritis may be triggered by blunt trauma,

lacerations, and piercings through auricular cartilage. Piercings of the ear cartilage are particularly susceptible to complications because of the avascular nature of the auricular cartilage. The auricle is erythematous, edematous, indurated, and exquisitely tender. *Staphylococcus aureus* and *P aeruginosa* are often involved; therefore, antimicrobial treatment should cover these pathogens. Intravenous antimicrobials are required for severe cases. If an abscess or a seroma forms, fine-needle aspiration or incision and drainage may be required, followed by placement of antibiotic-impregnated cotton or gauze and a gentle mastoid-type pressure dressing to prevent reaccumulation. The ear must be examined regularly and the dressing changed frequently to check for improvement and avoid complications, such as the aforementioned cauliflower ear.

INFLAMMATORY DISORDERS OF THE AURICLE

Relapsing Polychondritis

Relapsing polychondritis is a multisystem autoimmune disease targeting cartilage and connective tissue. Autoantibodies against type II collagen are implicated in this disease, which may affect elastic cartilage of the ear and nose, hyaline cartilage of the peripheral joints, and fibrocartilage of the spine. Additional clinical manifestations include ocular inflammation, vasculitis, myocarditis, sensorineural hearing loss, and peripheral vestibulopathy. The disease often presents with pain, erythema, and swelling of the auricle, sparing the lobule. Peripheral joints and the nose are the next most commonly involved structures. Tracheal cartilage involvement is the most serious manifestation of relapsing polychondritis, affecting 20% to 50% of patients and resulting in cartilage disintegration and increased morbidity due to airway obstruction. Mild episodes of polychondritis are managed with nonsteroidal anti-inflammatory medications. More severe episodes are treated with prednisone (1 mg/kg), with a taper after clinical improvement is observed. Other therapies include administration of immunosuppressive medications such as methotrexate, dapsone, or cyclosporine for more aggressive disease.

Allergic Reactions

Allergic reactions of the auricle to nickel-rimmed eyeglasses or earrings are common in susceptible patients. Only the portion of the ear in direct contact with the implicated material is involved in the reaction.

Treatment involves removal of the causative material and local treatment in the form of mild steroid creams.

Insect Bites

Insect bites may cause an inflammatory reaction of the auricle that may appear at first to be suspicious for relapsing polychondritis. The primary care clinician (PCC) needs to examine the skin carefully to search for any signs of cutaneous puncture, indicating a possible insect bite. Most insect bites heal well with local treatments, including cold compresses, and do not require any medical intervention. Certain insect bites may be more serious, such as brown recluse spider bites, in which the venom may cause tissue necrosis, requiring debridement. If the causative insect can be captured, it should be placed in a closed, clear container and brought in for proper identification.

▓ External Auditory Canal

TRAUMATIC INJURIES TO THE EAR CANAL

Foreign Bodies

Foreign bodies of the external auditory canal may be inert (beads), organic (peas), or biological (insects). Patients with foreign bodies of the external auditory canal must be evaluated for changes in their hearing, for vertigo, and for facial paralysis. Inert, organic, and biological foreign bodies of the ear canal are often removed in the ear, nose, and throat specialist's office using instruments such as curettes, alligator forceps, right-angle hooks, and suction. However, while such instruments are occasionally used by the PCC as well, the rate of successful extraction of globular and other foreign bodies without an edge to grasp is quite low. Care is taken to avoid pushing the object deeper into the canal or traumatizing the surrounding skin to prevent tissue edema, which may complicate foreign body removal. The use of saline irrigation to flush out foreign bodies is discouraged because the status of the TM is often unknown, and if a perforation is present, it may result in further injury or infection. Otologic drops are unnecessary and contraindicated in cases of organic foreign bodies because the solution may cause the object to swell, preventing its removal. In situations in which removal in the office is not possible or when middle-ear injury is suspected, it is appropriate to perform an examination of the ear in the operating room under anesthesia.

INFECTIOUS DISORDERS OF THE EAR CANAL

Acute Otitis Externa

Diffuse acute otitis externa, or swimmer's ear, is diagnosed by the rapid onset of symptoms, including otalgia, aural fullness, otorrhea, and tenderness to manipulation of the auricular cartilage. There may be cervical lymphadenitis and cellulitis of the surrounding skin or pinna. Frequent water exposure and humidity predispose to disruption of the usual cerumen lining, compromise epithelial integrity, and contribute to alkalinization of the canal from its usual slightly acidic pH. Swollen, wet skin is easily traumatized, leading to exposure to bacteria. Accumulation of desquamated skin and wet debris in a neutral pH environment provides an excellent culture medium for bacterial infection. Typical agents include *Pseudomonas, Proteus, Escherichia coli, Staphylococcus epidermidis,* and *Staphylococcus aureus.* The ear will be exquisitely tender to manipulation and the canal will be swollen, erythematous, and filled with purulent and sometimes foul-smelling exudate (**Figure 4-10**). First-line medical therapy for otitis externa not complicated by abscess formation, osteitis, middle-ear disease, or recurrent episodes of infection is gentle cleaning followed by application of topical otic preparations consisting of antibiotic with or without corticosteroid. When external auditory canal edema is severe, it may be necessary to place a wick in the narrowed ear canal to enhance topical drug delivery. Systemic antibiotics and cultures may be required in persistent or severe cases, when there is an associated otitis media or cellulitis, and in immunocompromised patients. Culture and sensitivity studies are important for refractory cases.

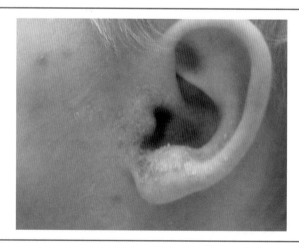

Figure 4-10. Crusting and inflammation caused by otitis externa.

Recurrent Otitis Externa

Recurrent otitis externa may be secondary to predisposing host factors such as diabetes or dermatologic conditions such as atopic dermatitis, psoriasis, or seborrhea. Immunocompromised patients with diabetes, cancer, or HIV may require aggressive management of their systemic illness to effectively control recurrent otitis externa. Overuse of cotton swabs results in traumatic atrophy of cerumen glands, loss of cerumen, abrasion trauma, and contamination of the skin of the ear canal. The protective properties of cerumen include its hydrophobic nature, acidic pH, and lysozyme content, all of which inhibit bacterial and fungal growth. Culture and sensitivity studies are important for recurrent and refractory cases of otitis externa.

Otomycosis

Otomycosis is a superficial fungal infection of the external auditory canal. Symptoms include pruritus and otalgia. The ear canal tends to be occluded by thick debris that is usually fluffy and white, but may also be black, gray, bluish-green, or yellow depending on the causative organism. Cultures are important to identify the pathogens. On otoscopy, black or white conidiophores on white hyphae are often indicative of *Aspergillus*, which causes 90% of cases of otomycosis. Use of strong antibacterial and steroid drops predisposes to otomycosis. Uncomplicated presentations are best treated with local debridement and topical antifungal drops, lotion such as clotrimazole, or acidifying drops such as acetic acid. Restoration of external auditory canal pH, adequate and often-repeated debridement, and moisture reduction are essential for resolution of the infection. Culture and sometimes oral antifungal agents are required for refractory or severe cases.

Necrotizing (Malignant) External Otitis

Necrotizing otitis externa is osteomyelitis of the skull base involving the cancellous bone of the skull, periosteum, dura, blood vessels, and cranial nerves. Individuals with compromised immunity, such as patients with diabetes and those undergoing chemotherapy, are at increased risk of developing this disease. The presence of granulation tissue in the external auditory canal at the bony cartilaginous junction, along with disproportionate pain despite adequate topical treatment, are signs of necrotizing otitis externa. Facial paralysis may result from involvement of the bone surrounding the stylomastoid foramen. Thrombosis of the sigmoid dural sinus also may occur, with resultant septic emboli and cranial nerve palsies.

Treatment of necrotizing otitis externa includes prolonged culture-directed systemic antibiotic therapy in the form of intravenous third-generation cephalosporins or oral fluoroquinolones, along with appropriate management of any correctable metabolic derangements. Adjunctive treatment includes use of hyperbaric oxygen to increase the phagocytic oxidative killing of aerobic organisms and to promote osteoneogenesis.

Furunculosis

Furunculosis may be differentiated from acute otitis externa in that it involves a focal segment of the external auditory canal. A single infected hair follicle in the lateral auditory canal results in pain and possibly drainage. *Staphylococcus aureus* is the usual etiologic pathogen, and treatment involves warm compresses, incision, and drainage along with topical and possibly systemic antibiotics.

INFLAMMATORY DISORDERS OF THE EAR CANAL

Noninfectious Otitis Externa

Dermatologic conditions such as contact dermatitis, psoriasis, seborrhea, and eczema may result in inflammation of the external auditory canal and predispose individuals to secondary infections. Symptoms include aural fullness, itching, clear fluid discharge, and dry flaking skin. Neomycin is the most common otic preparation resulting in sensitization reactions in susceptible individuals; it presents with a red, weepy rash in and around the treated area. Asteatotic dermatitis of the ear canal can result from overuse of cotton swabs, with resulting atrophy of cerumen glands. Otitis externa due to eczema causes severe itching of the ear. It can result in fissuring and weeping of the auricle, particularly of the postauricular crease and ear lobe. There may be crusting, flaking, thickening, oozing, and erythema of the skin of the lateral ear canal, meatus, and conchal bowl. The patient should be counseled to avoid using potentially irritating soaps, shampoos, and sprays around the ear. Otic solutions of 2% acetic acid help to dry an acutely inflamed ear. Steroid-containing creams, lotions, or ointments are useful for long-term control.

Exostoses/Osteomas

Exostoses and osteomas are common lesions of the external auditory canal. Exostoses are bony growths of the external auditory canal arising from the bony cartilaginous junction. They are usually found in individuals with significant exposure to cold water or air, notably surfers and swimmers. These lesions occur bilaterally and, when advanced, may result in recurring otitis externa or conductive hearing loss. Osteomas are generally unilateral, pedunculated growths based on the temporal-squamous suture line in the external auditory canal. They do not have an association with cold water exposure and usually are of no consequence.

▓ Other Disorders Affecting the Ear Canal

CERUMEN IMPACTION

Sebaceous and ceruminous glands of the lateral canal secrete an acidic substance that contains peptides, long-chain fatty acids, alcohols, squalene, pigment, and cholesterol. Cerumen is composed of these secretions mixed with keratin. Cerumen provides a protective coating of the skin lining the canal and aids in clearing of debris and desquamated epithelium. The squamous epithelium of the TM and ear canal follows a medial-to-lateral migration that carries desquamated epithelial cells and debris along with cerumen to the meatus. Cerumen may be wet or dry, depending on composition. This characteristic trait is inherited and tends to follow racial patterns, with dry cerumen common in Asian individuals and wet cerumen common in white and black racial groups.

The cerumen and desquamated epithelium in the external auditory canal are usually self-cleaning owing to epithelial migration and water exposure during swimming and bathing. Excessive production, a narrow ear canal, or disrupted epithelial migration may predispose to cerumen impaction. Some individuals may cause impactions by pushing the cerumen in with cotton-tipped swabs during attempted cleaning. The old saying, "Nothing smaller than your elbow should ever be put in your ear," should be evoked for such patients.

For routine cerumen removal, an otoscope and curettes, alligator forceps, or ear suctions may be used. A variety of sizes of curettes and suctions are required to treat patients with different-sized ear canals. The patient is instructed to "hold still like a statue." Uncooperative patients may be gently restrained by parents or a nurse. A second critical point is that the PCC must rest part of his or her hands that are holding the otoscope and instrument on the head of the child. Bracing is critical to ensure that if the child moves during cerumen removal, the hand and ear-cleaning instrument move with the child to avoid injury to the ear. Cerumen should be removed under direct visualization with a microscope, an otoscope, or a headlight. Gentle manipulation of the cartilaginous portion of the ear is typically well tolerated. Touching the bony portion of the canal with an instrument should be avoided, because it will invariably be painful and may cause a hematoma or bleeding. If a child experiences pain with cerumen management, he or she will likely be more anxious and less cooperative with any future ear examinations. Thus, every attempt should be made to ease anxiety and avoid pain and trauma to the canal. When someone without the requisite skill attempts to remove cerumen, significant complications can result, including perforation of the TM, damage to the ossicles, and otitis externa. If the cerumen is hard or copious and cannot be removed easily with a curette, an alligator forceps, or a 3 French or 5 French ear suction, a course of mineral oil or cerumen-softening drops (sodium bicarbonate, water, saline, docusate sodium, acetic acid, or peroxide) is prescribed for 5 to 7 days prior to a second attempt.

If mechanical removal is not possible, irrigation may be performed in the office using syringes and gentle pressure with warmed saline. It is critical to note that if the PCC is not certain whether the patient's TM is intact, saline irrigation, peroxide, and mineral oil are contraindicated. Irrigation may be complicated by perforation of the TM and perilymphatic fistula if the irrigant is applied under high pressure. The procedure may also lead to otitis externa and malignant otitis externa in predisposed individuals, especially those with diabetes.

For individuals with a history of repeated cerumen impactions and documented intact TMs, 3 drops of mineral oil may be applied to each ear canal at bedtime several times a week. Doing so may help to soften the cerumen and allow spontaneous egress or at least easier cleaning of the softened cerumen.

KERATOSIS OBTURANS AND EXTERNAL AUDITORY CANAL CHOLESTEATOMA

Keratosis obturans is a disease resulting from abnormal epithelial migration from the TM. The resulting collection of desquamated debris develops into a dense obstructive mass in the external auditory canal. There is widening of the bony external auditory canal without erosion of the osseous structures, thereby differentiating these lesions from external auditory canal cholesteatomas. Many patients with this disorder also have a history of sinusitis and bronchiectasis. This problem is best managed by an otolaryngologist, who can clean the ear routinely. Reaccumulation can be prevented with routine application of steroid oil, mineral oil, or acetic acid solution.

External auditory canal cholesteatoma is a disorder that rarely occurs spontaneously in children, but may develop as a result of trauma, radiation therapy, stenosis, or surgical changes in the case of a prior tympanoplasty or atresia repair. As opposed to keratosis obturans, cholesteatoma of the canal is associated with focal periosteitis and osteonecrosis. Superinfection, pain, and otorrhea are common, and the disease progresses if not brought under control. It is managed with frequent debridement and application of antimicrobial drops, followed by surgical canalplasty and a possible skin graft.

CYSTS

Sebaceous cysts may develop in the external auditory canal secondary to the occlusion of a follicular ostium, with the accumulation of sebaceous material. These lesions are prone to superinfection with *S aureus* or other normal skin flora. The pinna may be tender to manipulation, and surgical incision and drainage followed by excision are occasionally required to manage these lesions. Other similar lesions include epidermal inclusion cysts and dermoid cysts. Epidermal inclusion cysts result from the introduction of dermal elements into the subcutaneous tissues by trauma or piercings. Dermoid cysts are congenital lesions in which epidermal tissue becomes trapped under embryologic skin flaps. These lesions are also treated with complete surgical excision.

Acknowledgments

The author wishes to thank Dr Robert F. Yellon and Dr Raymond Maguire for writing the original version of this chapter.

■ Selected References

Baluch N, Nagata S, Park C, et al. Auricular reconstruction for microtia: a review of available methods. *Plast Surg (Oakv)*. 2014;22(1):39–43

Cohen D, Friedman P. The diagnostic criteria of malignant external otitis. *J Laryngol Otol*. 1987;101(3):216–221

Jahrsdoerfer RA. Congenital atresia of the ear. *Laryngoscope*. 1978;88(9 Pt 3 Suppl 13):1–48

Nadaraja GS, Gurgel RK, Kim J, Chang KW. Hearing outcomes of atresia surgery versus osseointegrated bone conduction device in patients with congenital aural atresia: a systematic review. *Otol Neurotol*. 2013;34(8):1394–1399

Rafeq S, Trentham D, Ernst A. Pulmonary manifestations of relapsing polychondritis. *Clin Chest Med*. 2010;31(3):513–518

Rosenfeld RM, Schwartz SR, Cannon CR, et al. Clinical practice guideline: acute otitis externa. *Otolaryngol Head Neck Surg.* 2014;150(1 Suppl):S1–S24

Schwartz SR, Magit AE, Rosenfeld RM, et al. Clinical practice guideline (update): earwax (cerumen impaction). *Otolaryngol Head Neck Surg.* 2017;156(1 Suppl):S1–S29

Takagi D, Nakamaru Y, Maguchi S, Furuta Y, Fukuda S. Otologic manifestations of Wegener's granulomatosis. *Laryngoscope.* 2002;112(9):1684–1690

Triglia JM, Nicollas R, Ducroz V, Koltai PJ, Garabedian EN. First branchial cleft anomalies: a study of 39 cases and a review of the literature. *Arch Otolaryngol Head Neck Surg.* 1998;124(3):291–295

Verhagen CV, Hol MK, Coppens-Schellekens W, Snik AF, Cremers CW. The Baha Softband: a new treatment for young children with bilateral congenital aural atresia. *Int J Pediatr Otorhinolaryngol.* 2008;72(10):1455–1459

Yellon RF. Congenital external auditory canal stenosis and partial atretic plate. *Int J Pediatr Otorhinolaryngol.* 2009;73(11):1545–1549

Complications of Chronic Eustachian Tube Dysfunction: Retractions, Perforations, Cholesteatoma

Christopher R. Grindle, MD

Introduction	**Tympanic membrane**
Tympanostomy tube	**perforation**
concerns	**Cholesteatoma**
Mastoiditis	**Conclusion**

■ Introduction

Otitis media is one of the most common illnesses of childhood, with greater than 2 million visits to primary care clinicians (PCCs) and more than $4 billion in health care costs annually. It is the second most common reason for children to be brought to their PCCs, behind upper respiratory infection. Children between the ages of 6 months and 4 years are particularly susceptible to otitis media owing to several reasons, including anatomical factors in the development of the temporal bone, mastoid, and eustachian tube (ET). During this time, the ET elongates and its angle through the temporal bone changes, becoming more vertically elongated. Most cases of acute otitis media (AOM) or otitis media with effusion (OME) resolve either spontaneously or after medical intervention. Treatment with antibiotics tends to speed the recovery from AOM, but antibiotics are not used to treat OME. Fluid in the middle-ear space (OME) may linger for up to several months after an acute infection, and at least 25% of cases of OME linger for more than 3 months. This may cause a transient conductive hearing loss, but providing the effusion resolves, the hearing loss should resolve. **Figure 5-1** shows the typical appearance of OME.

In some instances, the OME does not resolve and the child may have a persistent conductive hearing loss. This may be an indication for tympanostomy tubes. In other rare instances, other complications of AOM or OME may develop, including perforation of the tympanic membrane, acute coalescent mastoiditis, middle-ear atelectasis, adhesive otitis media, tympanosclerosis, ossicular erosion or fixation, and cholesteatoma formation or chronic otomastoiditis. Other, exceedingly rare, complications include labyrinthitis, facial paralysis, and intracranial infection.

> **Pearl:** Otitis media with effusion is exceedingly common in children 6 months to 4 years of age. Most episodes of otitis media with effusion resolve spontaneously, but up to 25% may last for more than 3 months. Oral antibiotics are not recommended for otitis media with effusion without infection.

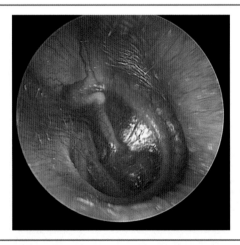

Figure 5-1. Right ear with typical appearance of otitis media with effusion including a slightly retracted tympanic membrane.

■ Tympanostomy Tube Concerns

Tympanostomy tubes are indicated for chronic otitis media lasting longer than 3 months with associated conductive hearing loss. They are also indicated for patients with recurrent AOM with abnormalities of the middle ear noted during evaluation for the surgical procedure. Complication rates from tympanostomy tubes are low but include tympanic membrane perforation (1%–3%) and tube retention (1%). Tube otorrhea is commonly seen after tympanostomy tube insertion (30%–40%) and should not be considered a complication. Although tubes do not specifically drain the middle ear, they allow for the middle-ear contents under pressure—as can be found with AOM or middle-ear effusion—to release out of the external auditory canal. This drainage can be mildly uncomfortable and irritating to the child. It should be gently wicked from the ear, and over-the-counter analgesics can be used for the discomfort. Medical therapy can also include topical antibacterial agents. The most commonly used are the quinolone-containing ear drops, which are not ototoxic. If there is evidence of granulation tissue in the external auditory canal surrounding the tympanostomy tube, a steroid-containing quinolone ear drop is recommended. Advantages to using topical otic drops are that they achieve significantly higher concentrations of antibiotic at the source of the infection, they are well tolerated, and they do not have associated systemic complications such as poor oral tolerance, nausea, and diarrhea. Oral antibiotics are rarely needed. Most otorrhea will resolve in 4 to 7 days with treatment. Persistent drainage (particularly otorrhea that is white and itchy) recalcitrant to standard courses of antibiotic drops should raise suspicion of fungal otorrhea. The topical antifungal 1% clotrimazole solution is an effective treatment. Patients should be told to avoid water exposure to the affected ear.

> **Pearl:** Otorrhea after tympanostomy tube placement is common. Quinolone-containing ototopical drops should be the first-line therapy given their effectiveness and lack of ototoxicity. Oral antibiotics are rarely needed for tube otorrhea.

Mastoiditis

Acute coalescent mastoiditis as a complication of AOM occurs when there is erosion of the bony trabeculae of the mastoid as a result of the infection. It has an annual reported incidence in developed countries of 1 to 6 per 100,00 children aged 0 to 14 years. Symptoms include ear pain, redness, and tenderness in the postauricular area. Postauricular edema often develops, resulting in proptosis of the affected ear. If imaging is performed, acute mastoiditis should be differentiated from fluid within the mastoid (which will be present in AOM or OME as the mastoid and middle ear are contiguous) by the erosion of the bony trabeculae (**Figure 5-2**). The most common complication of mastoiditis is postauricular subperiosteal abscess wherein the infection has spread throughout the mastoid cortex. Management is surgical and medical. Intravenous antibiotics are used and tympanostomy tubes are placed. Incision and drainage of a postauricular subperiosteal abscess is performed if present. Antibiotic ear drops should also be used. Mastoidectomy is reserved for complications of mastoiditis or for patients whose conditions fail to improve with the above management (**Figure 5-3**).

> **Pearl:** Mastoiditis is a rare but serious complication of acute otitis media. Management includes intravenous antibiotics and tympanostomy tube placement and, possibly, mastoidectomy.

Tympanic Membrane Perforation

Tympanic membrane perforations can occur as a result of trauma or infection/inflammation or as a sequela of tympanostomy tubes. Despite warnings to the contrary, people continue to put objects in their ears, such as cotton tip swabs and bobby pins, which are common culprits in traumatic tympanic membrane perforations. Other causes of traumatic tympanic membrane perforation include barotrauma and blast injuries. Perforations often present with acute pain, variable amounts of bleeding, and complaints of ear fullness. The patient should be examined, and attempts should be made to gently remove debris from the external auditory canal. Often with a good examination, the patient can be reassured that, in fact, no

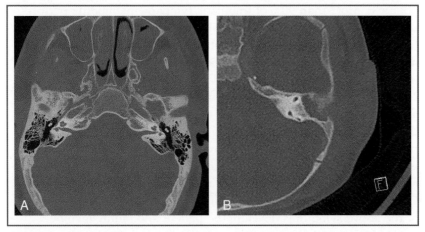

Figure 5-2. A, Normal axial computed tomographic (CT) scan showing well-aerated mastoids with normal trabeculae. B, Axial CT of the left temporal bone with fluid opacification and loss of trabeculae suggestive of coalescent mastoiditis.

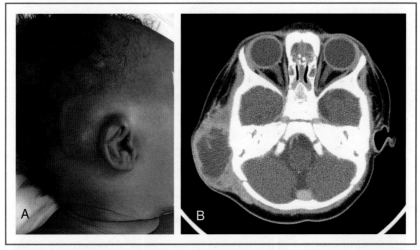

Figure 5-3. A, Right ear with severe postauricular edema, erythema, and proptosis. B, Axial computed tomographic scan with contrast of the same patient showing a large right postauricular subperiosteal abscess.

perforation of the tympanic membrane occurred, but rather a laceration of the skin of the external auditory canal. In cases of tympanic membrane perforation, the patient can be treated with analgesics for any discomfort. Topical ear drops suitable for perforated ears (quinolone) may be used if any infection is present. Additionally, steroid-containing drops may be used if any inflammatory tissue/ granulomas or polyps are present. An audiogram should also be obtained. More than 90% of traumatic tympanic membrane perforations will heal spontaneously and should be followed up to resolution, with a repeat audiogram obtained after closure. Tympanic membrane perforations as a complication of tympanostomy tube insertion are estimated to occur 2% of the time (**Figure 5-4**).

The management of tympanic membrane perforations is variable and depends on symptoms. Often, there are no symptoms related to the perforation, and it can be managed conservatively. The perforation can be observed as long as it remains clean and dry, and there is no significant otalgia, no recurrent drainage, no development of cholesteatoma, and no-to-minimal associated conductive hearing loss. Occasionally, these perforations will heal spontaneously. Should any of the above symptoms develop, the patient and family members should be counseled regarding tympanoplasty to attempt closure of the perforation. There is debate about the optimal timing for tympanoplasty in children, which depends most often on the presence of comorbidities and persistent ET dysfunction rather than on the patient's age. Most otologists wait until the patient is at least 6 years of age before performing surgery to close eardrum perforations.

> **Pearl:** Tympanic membrane perforations have a variety of etiologies. Management is variable, but persistent drainage, infection, significant hearing loss, and/or cholesteatoma would favor surgical management.

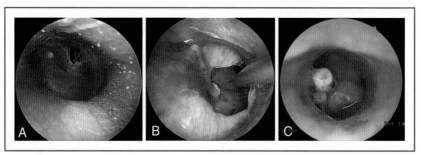

Figure 5-4. A, Clean and dry right tympanic membrane perforation, likely from a previous tympanostomy tube. B, Larger, clean and dry perforation of the right tympanic membrane. Note the extensive plaque of myringosclerosis throughout the tympanic membrane. C, Large, almost total, perforation of the right ear with associated fluid and sclerotic debris in the middle ear.

As discussed earlier, young children are at risk of developing AOM, which is thought to be due, in large part, to underdevelopment of the ET and decreased ventilation of the middle ear. Additionally, it may result in atelectasis of the tympanic membrane secondary to damage to the collagen-containing fibrous layer of the tympanic membrane. The result is a retraction of the tympanic membrane to variable degrees, with partial-to-complete obliteration of the middle-ear space. Several staging systems of tympanic membrane retraction have been described, detailing the range of presentations from focal retractions to obliteration of the middle-ear space and adhesion of the tympanic membrane to the promontory. Management of retractions is based on symptoms. Again, if the ear remains clean and dry and there is minimal conductive hearing loss, the ear can be observed. In earlier stages, tympanostomy tubes may be used to reestablish middle-ear ventilation. However, in later stages, tympanostomy tubes are not beneficial as the tympanic membrane adheres to the floor of the middle ear (**Figure 5-5**).

■ Cholesteatoma

Cholesteatomas are epidermal inclusion cysts of the middle ear and mastoid. The term *cholesteatoma* was first used in 1838 by the German physiologist Müller. However, the lesions contain no cholesterol or bile. The cysts are composed of desquamated debris (primarily keratin) from the keratinizing squamous epithelial lining of the

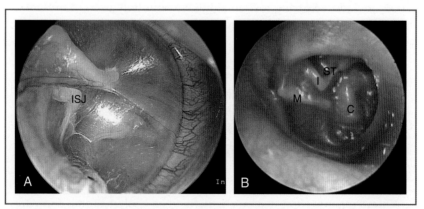

Figure 5-5. A, Retracted right tympanic membrane (TM) showing contact between the TM and the incudostapedial joint (ISJ). B, "Shrink-wrap" retraction of left TM with complete loss of the middle-ear space. Seen clearly are the malleus (M), incus (I), stapes tendon (ST), and basal turn of the cochlea (C).

cyst. They are broadly classified as congenital or acquired and may arise spontaneously or secondarily as a result of trauma. Symptoms of cholesteatoma can vary widely, ranging from no symptoms to chronic otorrhea to conductive hearing loss. Symptoms are related to the size of the cholesteatoma, the location of the lesion within the middle ear/mastoid, and the amount of destruction caused by the lesion. They can be confined within the tympanic membrane (intra-tympanic), involve only the middle ear, or involve the middle ear and the mastoid. Although the lesions themselves are benign, they induce an inflammatory reaction in the middle ear and mastoid mucosa that gives rise to osteoclast activity adjacent to the cholesteatoma. This can lead to the breakdown and destruction of the ossicles and other areas of the mastoid (eg, erosion of the scutum). The endochondral bone of the cochlea, vestibule, and semicircular canals is more resistant than the intramembranous bone of the mastoid, but it can be affected as a late consequence of disease, leading to labyrinthine fistula and sensorineural hearing loss.

The diagnosis of cholesteatoma is made on otoscopic examination. Abnormalities are often noted in the posterior superior aspect of the tympanic membrane in acquired cholesteatoma and in the anterior superior quadrant in congenital cholesteatoma. There also may be chronic, painless otorrhea. In fact, persistent, painless, often foul-smelling otorrhea unresponsive to topical ear drops should raise suspicion of cholesteatoma. Also, persistent unilateral conductive hearing loss in a child older than 4 years should prompt further evaluation. Additional workup of a patient suspected of having cholesteatoma should include a hearing test. Imaging is commonly used to evaluate the extent of the disease and often can guide surgical management.

> **Pearl:** Chronic otorrhea that is unresponsive to treatment or persistent, unilateral conductive hearing loss in a child older than 4 years should raise suspicion of cholesteatoma.

Intratympanic cholesteatoma is defined as cholesteatoma confined to the tympanic membrane. It is rare, with only small case series reported in the literature; however, it is probably underreported. It may occur spontaneously or as a result of perforation of the tympanic

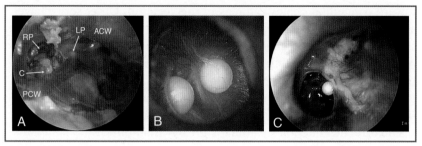

Figure 5-6. Retraction pocket (RP) of right ear with acquired cholesteatoma (C). The lateral process (LP) of the malleus, anterior canal wall (ACW), and posterior canal wall (PCW) are marked for orientation.

membrane (traumatic or after ear tube extrusion) (**Figure 5-6**). Epithelial cells become trapped within the lateral epithelial layer of the tympanic membrane, and the inclusion cyst is formed. If identified early, intratympanic cholesteatoma may resolve spontaneously with the normal migration and sloughing of the tympanic membrane epithelium. If larger or persistent, they should be removed through the ear canal; traditionally, this has been done using an operative microscope, but in recent years, an endoscope has been used. Recurrence is rare.

Congenital cholesteatomas are classically described as round, pearl-like masses located in the anterior superior aspect of the tympanic membrane (anterior to the malleus and superior to an imaginary line perpendicular to the malleus drawn through the umbo) behind an intact tympanic membrane (**Figure 5-7**). They are rare, representing only 5% of cholesteatomas. It has been shown that there is a small area of keratinizing epithelium in the anterior middle ear of the developing fetus that may be responsible for the predilection

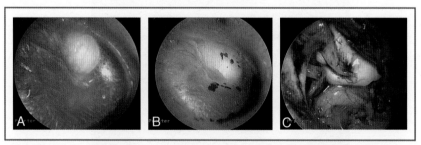

Figure 5-7. A, Congenital cholesteatoma in the right ear with classic, round pearl-like appearance in the anterior superior quadrant. B, Congenital cholesteatoma in the right middle ear. C, Same congenital cholesteatoma with tympanic membrane reflected showing the extent of the mass in the middle ear and association with ossicles.

toward congenital cholesteatomas in this location. Other series have shown that, although most common in the anterior superior quadrant, congenital cholesteatomas may develop anywhere in the middle ear. Additionally, with growth and progression, these lesions expand to involve other aspects of the middle ear and mastoid. Management is surgical. Recurrence is rare, though it increases dramatically with increased extent of disease. If the mastoid is involved, the risk of residual/recurrent cholesteatoma is greater than 60%.

Acquired cholesteatoma is believed to be a consequence of poor middle-ear ventilation and chronic OME. Primary acquired cholesteatoma often forms in the posterior superior aspect of the ear at a retraction pocket in the pars flaccida, a weaker area in the tympanic membrane that does not contain the fibrous middle layer; as such, it is less resistant to the pressure changes with chronic OME and ET dysfunction. As the retraction pocket deepens, the desquamated keratin cannot migrate out normally, and an epithelial inclusion cyst (cholesteatoma) forms (**Figure 5-8**). Secondary acquired cholesteatoma starts as an ingrowth of epithelial tissue through a perforation in the tympanic membrane, with resultant cholesteatoma formation (**Figure 5-9**). As the lesion grows, inflammation increases, triggering osteoclast activity and adjacent bony destruction. Secondary to this inflammation, patients may have painless otorrhea, and, on examination, they often are found to have polyps and granulation tissue in the ear canal. Steroid-containing ear drops may be used to treat this inflammation and aid in the visualization/identification of the underlying causative lesion.

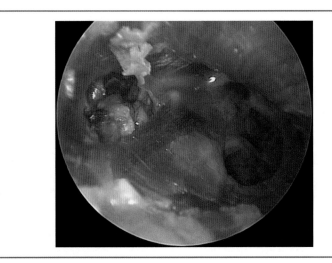

Figure 5-8. Retraction pocket with acquired cholesteatoma of the right ear.

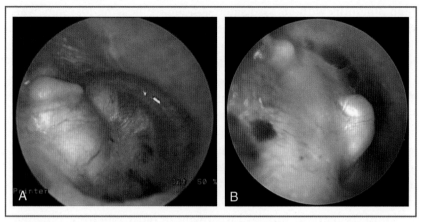

Figure 5-9. Two images of middle-ear masses consistent with cholesteatomas extending through the tympanic membrane.

Management of cholesteatoma is surgical, with several approaches available, all aimed at eradicating the disease, preventing complications, and creating a clean, dry, and stable ear. Secondary goals are to close tympanic membrane perforations and improve hearing. The scope of surgery is dictated by the extent of the disease. If the cholesteatoma is confined to the middle ear, transcanal (either endoscopic or microscopic) surgical approaches can be used. If the mastoid is involved, a postauricular, transmastoid approach is necessary. Recurrence is common, and additional surgical procedures are often required.

> **Pearl:** Cholesteatoma is an epithelial cyst of the middle ear that can develop on the tympanic membrane or in the middle ear, with or without extension into the mastoid air cells. Management is surgical and aimed at restoring a clean, dry, and stable ear and preventing complications. Secondary goals are closing tympanic membrane perforations and improving hearing.

■ Conclusion

Otitis media is a common diagnosis in children. Otitis media with effusion may persist for months, although it typically resolves spontaneously. Otitis media with effusion that persists for more than 3 months with an associated conductive hearing loss may warrant surgery. Fortunately, complications of otitis media are rare. Tympanostomy tubes and intravenous antibiotics are often used to treat mastoiditis, with mastoidectomy reserved for those whose conditions fail to improve or who have additional complications. Tympanic membrane perforations may occur as a result of infection or trauma or they may be iatrogenic. Management depends on symptoms, but surgical management may be considered in patients with significant hearing loss, pain, or infection. Cholesteatoma is an epithelial cyst in the middle ear and/or mastoid. Management is always surgical, and the scope of surgery depends on the extent of disease. Unilateral chronic otorrhea or unilateral conductive hearing loss unresponsive to standard treatment in older children is highly suspicious of cholesteatoma.

■ Selected References

Alzahrani M, Saliba I. Tympanic membrane retraction pocket staging: is it worthwhile? *Eur Arch Otorhinolaryngol.* 2014;271(6):1361–1368

Ching HH, Spinner AG, Ng M. Pediatric tympanic membrane cholesteatoma: systematic review and meta-analysis. *Int J Pediatr Otorhinolaryngol.* 2017;102:21–27

Chole RA, Sudhoff HH. Chronic otitis media, mastoiditis, and petrositis. In: Flint PW, Haughey BH, Lund VJ, et al, eds. *Cummings Otolaryngology—Head and Neck Surgery.* 5th ed. Philadelphia, PA: Mosby Elsevier; 2010:1963–1978

Cohen MS, Basonbul RA, Kozin ED, Lee DJ. Residual cholesteatoma during second-look procedures following primary pediatric endoscopic ear surgery. *Otolaryngol Head Neck Surg.* 2017;157(6):1034–1040

Dornhoffer JL, Friedman AB, Gluth MB. Management of acquired cholesteatoma in the pediatric population. *Curr Opin Otolaryngol Head Neck Surg.* 2013;21(5):440–445

Groth A, Enoksson F, Hultcrantz M, Stalfors J, Stenfeldt K, Hermansson A. Acute mastoiditis in children aged 0-16 years: a national study of 678 cases in Sweden comparing different age groups. *Int J Pediatr Otorhinolaryngol.* 2012;76(10):1494–1500

Hardman J, Muzaffar J, Nankivell P, Coulson C. Tympanoplasty for chronic tympanic membrane perforation in children: systematic review and meta-analysis. *Otol Neurotol.* 2015;36(5):796–804

Hunter JB, Zuniga MG, Sweeney AD, et al. Pediatric endoscopic cholesteatoma surgery. *Otolaryngol Head Neck Surg.* 2016;154(6):1121–1127

James AL, Papsin BC. Ten top considerations in pediatric tympanoplasty. *Otolaryngol Head Neck Surg.* 2012;147(6):992–998

Kay DJ, Nelson M, Rosenfeld RM. Meta-analysis of tympanostomy tube sequelae. *Otolaryngol Head Neck Surg.* 2001;124(4):374–380

Kazahaya K, Potsic WP. Congenital cholesteatoma. *Curr Opin Otolaryngol Head Neck Surg.* 2004;12(5):398–403

Koltai PJ, Nelson M, Castellon RJ, et al. The natural history of congenital cholesteatoma. *Arch Otolaryngol Head Neck Surg.* 2002;128(7):804–809

Lambert E, Roy S. Otitis media and ear tubes. *Pediatr Clin North Am.* 2013;60(4): 809–826

Levi J, Grindle C, O'Reilly R. Pie-slice tympanoplasty for transcanal removal of small congenital cholesteatoma. *Int J Pediatr Otorhinolaryngol.* 2012;76(11):1583–1587

Marchioni D, Alicandri-Ciufelli M, Molteni G, Genovese E, Presutti L. Endoscopic tympanoplasty in patients with attic retraction pockets. *Laryngoscope.* 2010;120(9): 1847–1855

McGuire JK, Wasl H, Harris T, Copley GJ, Fagan JJ. Management of pediatric cholesteatoma based on presentations, complications, and outcomes. *Int J Pediatr Otorhinolaryngol.* 2016;80:69–73

Michaels L. An epidermoid formation in the developing middle ear: possible source of cholesteatoma. *J Otolaryngol.* 1986;15(3):169–174

Nelson M, Roger G, Koltai PJ, et al. Congenital cholesteatoma: classification, management, and outcome. *Arch Otolaryngol Head Neck Surg.* 2002;128(7):810–814

Ramakrishnan Y, Kotecha A, Bowdler DA. A review of retraction pockets: past, present and future management. *J Laryngol Otol.* 2007;121(6):521–525

Rosenfeld RM, Schwartz SR, Pynnonen MA, et al. Clinical practice guideline: tympanostomy tubes in children. *Otolaryngol Head Neck Surg.* 2013;149(1 Suppl):S1–S35

Smith JA, Danner CJ. Complications of chronic otitis media and cholesteatoma. *Otolaryngol Clin North Am.* 2006;39(6):1237–1255

Nose and Sinus

CHAPTER 6

Neonatal Nasal Obstruction

Tulio A. Valdez, MD, MSc, and Kara D. Meister, MD

▓ Introduction

Infants are preferential nasal breathers for at least 6 weeks and up to 6 months. Therefore, nasal airway obstruction is a cause of significant morbidity and must remain high on the differential diagnosis in infants with respiratory compromise.

The etiology of nasal obstruction in a child can often be determined on the basis of a combination of symptoms and physical findings (**Figure 6-1**). Nasal obstruction can be unilateral or bilateral, and intranasal or nasopharyngeal. The spectrum of symptoms and presentations is the result of the degree of obstruction and location. Unilateral or mild symptoms (eg, unilateral rhinorrhea, mild work of breathing) suggest an intranasal or a unilateral level of

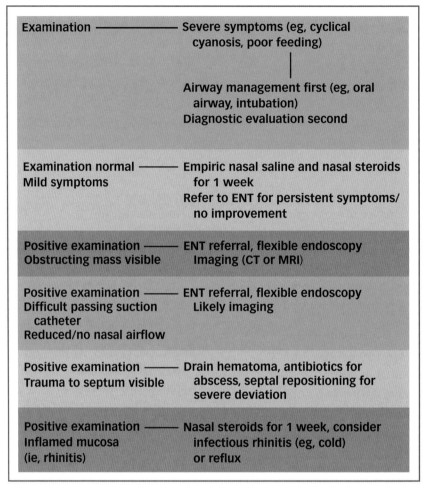

Figure 6-1. Diagnostic approaches to nasal obstruction.

Abbreviations: CT, computed tomography; ENT, ear, nose, and throat; MRI, magnetic resonance imaging

obstruction. Nasopharyngeal obstruction or processes affecting both nostrils will present with significant, even life-threatening, respiratory distress, cyclical cyanosis, and feeding difficulties. Cyclical cyanosis is the process by which infants with nasal obstruction develop increasing work of breathing, culminating in crying, which prompts the infant to breathe through the mouth. Feeding difficulties include fatigue secondary to the inability to breathe while feeding, and poor coordination secondary to the potential mass effect on the palate.

> **Pearl:** Cyclical cyanosis is a key feature of bilateral nasal obstruction.

◼ Physical Examination and Diagnosis

Physical examination of the infant with respiratory distress must focus first on assessing the need for stabilizing the airway. Children with severe respiratory distress may require intubation or placement of an oral airway before undergoing further examination. Placement of a McGovern nipple may also be a temporizing solution. Also, patients with congenital nasal obstruction may have other congenital anomalies such as severe cardiac and neurologic anomalies, which may contribute to cyanosis and poor respiratory effort.

Examination of the infant with nasal obstruction includes anterior rhinoscopy and possible flexible fiberoptic nasopharyngoscopy. Rigid nasal endoscopy often is not feasible in the neonate. A primary care clinician (PCC) may use a mirror or passage of a 5F suction catheter to evaluate for posterior obstruction. A dental mirror that does not fog when placed under a nostril with the opposite nostril occluded denotes a complete obstruction on the tested side. The failure to pass a 5F suction catheter through the nares into the oropharynx when the anterior nasal examination findings are normal suggests an obstruction at the nasopharynx (eg, choanal atresia), while difficulty passing the catheter into the anterior aspect of the nasal cavity suggests a pyriform aperture stenosis. Identifying the level of obstruction with cross-sectional imaging may be required to further investigate the nature of the obstruction. Magnetic resonance imaging (MRI) may provide better soft-tissue detail of an obstructing mass such as encephaloceles or gliomas, while computed tomography (CT) provides the bony detail ideal for diagnosis of choanal atresia and pyriform aperture stenosis. The advent of fetal MRI may provide clinicians with the opportunity to plan for life-threatening respiratory distress in newborns with large obstructing lesions and certain congenital malformations.

Given the complexity of breathing and swallowing, infants with nasal airway obstruction should undergo a swallowing evaluation before the initiation of oral feeds. This may include a clinical swallowing evaluation or instrumented swallowing studies such as a videofluoroscopic swallow study or fiberoptic endoscopic evaluation of swallowing.

◼ Nasal Embryology and Anatomy

Around the fifth week of gestation, paired ectodermal nasal placodes develop on the frontonasal process. These placodes are the beginning of the neonatal nose. Grooves form on the medial and lateral sides of the placodes, and the nose projects forward. By the seventh week, the grooves form blind-ending pits. The medial grooves form the septum and midline nasal structures. The lateral grooves form the lateral nasal sidewall and ala. As the nasal pits deepen, they form the nasal sac. At the posterior portion of the nasal sac, an epithelial membrane separates the nares from the developing oropharynx. By days 42 to 44, the oronasal membrane ruptures to provide a direct communication from the nose to the oropharynx. A cartilaginous capsule encases the developing nasal cavity. This cartilage develops into the turbinates and lateral nasal wall, which eventually will ossify. The lateral nasal wall evaginates to form the paranasal sinuses.

The nasal cavity is divided by the nasal septum, which is composed of bony and cartilaginous structures. Most of the septum in the neonate is cartilage; ossification begins during childhood. Additionally, the mostly cartilaginous septum is thicker in the neonate to support the nasal dorsum. The nasal septum is composed of the quadrilateral cartilage anteriorly with the premaxilla. Posteriorly, the septum is formed by the perpendicular ethmoidal plate and sphenoidal crest. Inferiorly, the vomer articulates with maxillary and palatine bones.

The external nose is composed of paired nasal bones, upper lateral cartilages, and lower lateral cartilages. The internal and external nasal valves are the narrowest portions of the airway. The internal nasal valve is defined by the septum medially, the upper lateral cartilage laterally, and the anterior head of the inferior turbinate posteriorly. The external nasal valve (ie, nasal vestibule) is formed by the lower lateral cartilages and the nasal septum. The internal nasal valve is the narrowest segment of the 2 and is responsible for two-thirds of nasal airway resistance.

> **Pearl:** The internal nasal valve is the narrowest portion of the nasal airway. Borders include the septum, upper lateral cartilages, and inferior turbinate.

■ Differential Diagnosis

There are multiple etiologies of neonatal nasal obstruction, which can be categorized as congenital anatomical deformities, obstructing masses, traumatic obstructions, and inflammatory mucosal changes. Congenital anatomical deformities are aberrations of normal anatomy, present at birth, that alter normal nasal physiology. They can be subdivided into external and internal nasal malformations. External malformations include unilateral nostril agenesis, arhinia, and nostril hypoplasia. External nasal malformations are exceedingly rare and easily diagnosed by visual inspection. Internal nasal cavity malformations include choanal atresia and pyriform aperture stenosis. Obstructing nasal masses include vascular malformations (eg, lymphatic malformation, arteriovenous malformation, venous malformation, capillary malformation), dermoid cysts, encephaloceles, gliomas, dacryocystoceles, and teratomas. Of the obstructing lesions, glioma, dermoid, and encephalocele are the most common. Malignant neoplasms of the nasal cavity and nasopharynx are most commonly lymphoma and rhabdomyosarcoma. However, these lesions are exceptionally uncommon in neonates. Traumatic neonatal causes of obstruction are septal deviation and septal hematoma, which may be secondary to birth trauma.

Inflammatory etiologies, while rarely a cause of complete obstruction, may worsen a fixed obstruction. Neonatal rhinitis and rhinitis medicamentosa are examples of inflammatory etiologies. Neonatal syphilis, termed *snuffles*, can present as copious rhinorrhea. This mucoid discharge is highly infectious, harboring a high concentration of spirochetes. Adenoid hypertrophy is a rare cause of neonatal obstruction. It is significantly more common in children. As a child grows, inflammatory etiologies (eg, allergic rhinitis) become the most common cause of obstruction.

■ Congenital Anatomical Deformities

CHOANAL ATRESIA

Choanal atresia is a congenital obstruction of the posterior nasal aperture on 1 or both sides. The incidence is approximately 1 in 5,000 to 1 in 8,000 live births. Syndromic association with congenital anomalies is linked to unilateral choanal atresia 50% of the time, and there is a syndromic association 75% of the time if the atresia is bilateral. The female-to-male ratio is 2:1. The right side is affected more often than the left. Sixty percent of cases are a mixed bony-membranous obstruction, 30% are only bony, and 10% are only membranous.

Associated syndromes include CHARGE (Colobomas, Heart defects, choanal Atresia, Retarded growth, Genital and Ear anomalies) syndrome, Treacher Collins, Crouzon, Apert, velocardiofacial, Trisomy 18, and Trisomy 21. Nonsyndromic associations with other congenital anomalies, such as auricular abnormalities, palatal deformities, and polydactyly, have been reported. CHARGE is the most commonly associated syndrome, and neonates with choanal atresia should be evaluated for this syndrome. The exact point of disruption in embryologic development that leads to choanal atresia is not known. Theories include failure of the oronasal membrane to rupture or abnormal migration of neural crest cells.

Signs and symptoms of choanal atresia can vary depending on the presence of unilateral or bilateral disease. In unilateral choanal atresia, patients can present later in life with unilateral rhinorrhea and obstruction (**Figure 6-2**). In bilateral disease, infants present as early as neonates (often within 48 hours of birth) with complete nasal obstruction and cyclic cyanosis. Diagnosis is suspected with the inability to pass a 5F suction catheter through the nose into the nasopharynx. Endoscopic evaluation further validates a fixed obstruction suggested by the failed passage of a suction catheter (**Figure 6-2**). Fine-cut craniofacial CT confirms the diagnosis and, more importantly, provides anatomical information about the thickness of the atresia, the character of the stenosis, and other associated craniofacial anomalies.

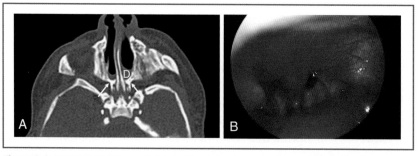

Figure 6-2. Choanal atresia. A, Computed tomography scan demonstrating atretic choanae bilaterally (arrows). Inspissated mucus in the nasal cavity creates the "delta sign" (D). B, Endoscopic view of bilateral choanal atresia affecting the nasopharynx.

Pearl: Failure to pass a 5F suction catheter can signify anterior or posterior levels of obstruction.

Treatment of choanal atresia is surgical. Two surgical approaches are available for repair. The first is the more classically described transpalatal approach. In this approach, incisions are made to gain access to the hard palate. Portions of the posterior hard palate are removed to allow resection of the membranous or bony atresia plate. While the exposure is superior in this approach, it entails a greater risk of dental and facial growth abnormalities. The transnasal approach uses nasal dilators and rigid instrumentation to penetrate and resect the membranous or bony atresia plate while using endoscopic visualization. Because this technique does not involve the palate, there is no risk to palatal and dental growth. Recent literature examining surgical approaches in 73 patients noted comparable restenosis rates in the transpalatal and endoscopic transnasal approaches (12.5% and 17%, respectively). Endoscopic transnasal approaches are becoming the standard of care in most urban settings. Classically, nasal stenting of the choana was used to prevent restenosis. However, more recently, no increased risk of restenosis with stentless endoscopic approaches has been noted in various studies. Oral and nasal steroids are also used to help prevent restenosis. Patients with bilateral atresia and those with syndromes (eg, CHARGE) have a greater risk of developing restenosis.

The timing of surgical repair and airway management in the interim are areas of controversy. Unilateral atresia treatment is delayed to allow for growth to decrease operative risk and potential restenosis as long as the child is able to feed and grow without difficulty. Most children with unilateral atresia undergo surgical repair by age 4 or 5 years. In patients with bilateral atresia, airway and management concerns necessitate an earlier repair. Establishing a secure airway may necessitate a tracheotomy or prolonged intubation in these patients while they await further nasal growth and a definitive repair. Most of these children undergo definitive surgical repair as young as 1 week old and nearly always by 12 months of age.

Pearl: Neonates with syndromic disorders (eg, CHARGE) are at greater risk of developing restenosis after choanal atresia repair.

CONGENITAL PYRIFORM APERTURE STENOSIS

Congenital pyriform aperture stenosis (CPAS) is an anterior nasal obstruction of the nasal valve area. It is caused by excessive bony growth of the nasal process of the maxilla into the nasal cavity (**Figure 6-3**). Congenital pyriform aperture stenosis is associated with holoprosencephaly (ie, forebrain abnormality) and other congenital midline anomalies (eg, hypertelorism, flat nasal bridge, a central incisor, pituitary disorders).

Congenital pyriform aperture stenosis generally presents in the neonatal period. Like choanal atresia, CPAS presents with cyclical cyanosis. This is more pronounced during feeding as the infant tries to increase nasal airflow against a fixed obstruction. In older infants and children, a respiratory infection may trigger exacerbation of milder obstructive symptoms and, therefore, come to the attention of the PCC.

Diagnosis is made on physical examination and by performing nasal endoscopy or CT. Although a suction catheter may or may not be

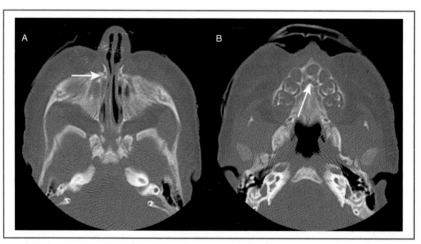

Figure 6-3. Congenital pyriform aperture stenosis. A, Pyriform aperture width of <11 mm between the medial processes of the maxillae (arrow) is diagnostic of pyriform aperture stenosis. B, Single central megaincisor (arrow) is present in over 75% of patients with pyriform aperture stenosis.

passable through the nares in a patient with CPAS, the site of obstruction in CPAS is directly visible on physical examination, whereas the anterior nares seem patent in choanal atresia. Radiographic diagnosis requires less than 11 mm of space between the medial aspects of the maxilla at the level of the inferior meatus, as measured on axial CT cuts. Further imaging (ie, MRI), endocrine and neurologic consultations, and laboratory analysis for pituitary function should be considered given the association with holoprosencephaly and pituitary disorders.

Management and treatment of CPAS are guided by the degree of stenosis and symptoms. Mild cases can be managed with topical vasoconstrictive drops, nasal steroids, and humidification until further growth increases the size of the nasal airway. Indications for surgical correction include sleep apnea, repeated intubation, frequent difficulties feeding, persistent or frequent respiratory distress, and failure of medical management.

> **Pearl:** Congenital pyriform aperture stenosis is associated with holoprosencephaly and a central incisor as well as with pituitary disorders.

Surgical management includes a sublabial approach to expose the pyriform aperture. Typically, an endoscopic drill or a microdebrider is used to widen the lateral and inferior margin. Care is taken to prevent damage to tooth buds. Nasal stents are commonly placed postoperatively to prevent restenosis.

ARHINIA

Congenital nasal absence (arhinia; absence of the external nose, nasal cavities, and olfactory apparatus) is a rare malformation, occurring most often with other anomalies of the eyes, palate, or ears. Approximately 50 cases are documented in the literature; therefore, the etiology is not completely elucidated. Cases of familial arhinia have been reported, and there is a suspicion that the malformation may be a sequela of maternal medication use. Arhinia is life threatening because of the resultant severe airway obstruction and feeding difficulties. Placement of a tracheostomy tube and gastrostomy tube may be needed. Reconstruction is complex and often delayed until preschool age.

▓ Obstructing Masses

NASOLACRIMAL DUCT CYST

The most common obstructing mass causing neonatal airway obstruction is arguably a nasolacrimal duct cyst, or dacryocystocele. Lesions can be unilateral or rarely bilateral and are characterized by a blue-gray or blue-purple cystic mass just inferior and lateral to the inferior turbinate at the location of the valve of Hasner. Lesions also may present elsewhere on the course of the nasolacrimal duct, such as near the medial canthus, but it is the intranasal lesions that are implicated in nasal airway obstruction. Obstruction with resultant inflammation and infection can lead to marked erythema and edema of the affected eye, face, and naris. Surgical intervention by an otolaryngologist and ophthalmologist is often carried out in a multidisciplinary manner to address the nasolacrimal duct and its associated nasolacrimal duct cyst.

DERMOID CYST OR SINUS

A dermoid cyst or sinus is derived from ectoderm and mesoderm. The sinus tract or cyst cavity is lined by squamous epithelium and contains adnexal structures (eg, hair follicles, sebaceous glands, sweat glands). Nasal dermoids are responsible for 10% to 12% of all head and neck dermoids. Nasal dermoids occur as a midline pit or mass on the nasal dorsum and may be associated with a widened nasal bridge. When presenting as a dorsal nasal mass, they are firm, often lobulated, noncompressible, and nonpulsatile. If associated with a sinus opening, keratin-like discharge is common. A protruding hair from the sinus is pathognomonic for nasal dermoid. A dermoid may extend into the nasal septum.

> **Pearl:** The most common obstructing lesions in a neonate are encephalocele, glioma, and dermoid.

A dermoid cyst or sinus is thought to occur as a persistent connection between the prenasal space and intracranium during fetal development. The prenasal space is located posterior to the nasal bones and anterior to the nasal and septal cartilages. This space has a connection with the intracranium through a defect between the developing frontal bones. During development, the dura extends through this defect in the prenasal space and attaches to ectoderm on the dorsal nose. As the defect closes, the dural attachment to the ectoderm releases and the dura retracts into the cranium. A nasal dermoid cyst or sinus represents a failure of separation and obliteration of the connection between the ectoderm and cranium through the prenasal space. As a result, a nasal dermoid may be found anywhere along this connection, including intracranially. A dural connection is reported in approximately 30% of these lesions.

> **Pearl:** Brain magnetic resonance imaging is necessary in nasal dermoids to rule out intracranial extension.

Computed tomography and MRI are used to evaluate these lesions. Thin-slice CT with contrast is used to examine for potential skull-base defects. In particular, a bifid crista galli or an enlarged foramen cecum are suggestive of possible intracranial extension. Contrast-enhanced MRI provides information about intracranial extension in addition to delineating normal soft tissue from dermoid. Nasal dermoid is hyperintense on T1-weighted imaging.

Management of nasal dermoids consists of surgical excision. If intracranial extension is present, a combined intracranial-extracranial approach is pursued by the otolaryngologist and neurosurgeon in collaboration. If a sinus is present, the skin surrounding the sinus is excised with the tract. Complete excision of the cyst is required to prevent recurrence.

TERATOMA

Teratomas are typically benign lesions that include tissue from all 3 germ layers (ie, ectoderm, mesoderm, and endoderm). Less than 5% of all teratomas occur in the head and neck, and among those that do, a frequent location includes the nasopharynx. Nasopharyngeal teratomas typically protrude into the oropharynx (**Figure 6-4**). As a result of the mass effect on surrounding development, nasopharyngeal teratomas are associated with palatal defects.

Presentation in the prenatal period is common. Polyhydramnios secondary to impaired swallowing and elevated α-fetoprotein levels can lead to a diagnosis of large lesions via ultrasonography. If not diagnosed

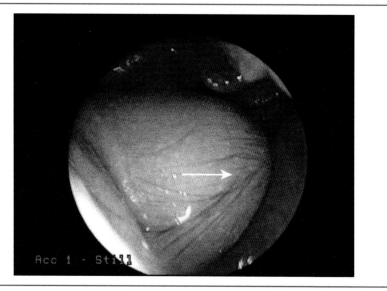

Figure 6-4. Nasopharyngeal teratoma extending into the oropharynx almost to the level of the epiglottis. Notice the hairs on the lesion (arrow).

prenatally, presentation in the early neonatal period is common. Acute severe respiratory distress is common. Typically, the degree of respiratory distress necessitates endotracheal intubation or tracheotomy. If diagnosed prenatally, an ex-utero intrapartum treatment (EXIT) procedure may be performed that uses maternal-fetal circulation to provide oxygenation to the neonate while the airway is secured. However, if the teratoma is small, feeding difficulties may be the only presenting symptom.

After adequate airway control is achieved, management of these lesions is surgical excision. The approach to these lesions is dictated by their size. Alpha-fetoprotein can be used to monitor for recurrence.

> **Pearl:** Teratomas include tissue from all 3 germ layers (ie, ectoderm, mesoderm, and endoderm).

ENCEPHALOCELE

Encephaloceles are intracranial contents displaced through a bony defect in the skull. A meningocele is an encephalocele that includes only meninges without any actual brain tissue. A meningoencephalocele contains brain and meninges. Given that a skull-base defect is present, encephaloceles may present with meningitis or cerebrospinal fluid leak. Encephaloceles can present as glabellar or dorsal nasal masses. As masses, they appear bluish, soft, pulsatile, and compressible. Owing to the intracranial connection, there is pulsation, expansion, and discoloration of the mass with increases in intrathoracic pressure (crying, straining) or manual compression of the jugular vein (Furstenberg sign). Encephaloceles that herniate through a defect in the cribriform plate or through the junction of the posterior ethmoid air cells and sphenoid sinus present as a unilateral intranasal mass. Computed tomography and MRI help to make the diagnosis. Thin-cut CT characterizes the bony defect, while MRI distinguishes a meningocele from meningoencephalocele. Management is surgical repair of the bony defect with reduction of herniated contents. Typically, surgical intervention is performed early to eliminate the risk of meningitis and cosmetic deformities with large external encephaloceles.

GLIOMA

Gliomas are masses of heterotopic glial tissue that lack a patent cerebrospinal fluid intracranial connection. As a result, these masses are firm, noncompressible, nonpulsatile, and lobular. When found on the external aspect of the nasal dorsum, they have cutaneous telangiectasias. Intranasal gliomas often arise from the lateral nasal wall or skull base. Performing CT to assess for a skull-base defect is recommended. Magnetic resonance imaging and nasal endoscopy better delineate the location in relation to surrounding structures. Management is via surgical excision, often with a combined otolaryngological and neurosurgical approach. Surgical intervention often is performed early to relieve obstruction, promote feeding, obtain a pathological diagnosis, and avoid midface growth distortion.

> **Pearl:** Intranasal gliomas most often arise from the lateral nasal wall.

▪ Traumatic Obstructions

SEPTAL DEVIATION AND EXTERNAL NASAL DEVIATION

The incidence of septal deviation in neonates is approximately 1%. It has been postulated to be attributable to forceps trauma and passage through the birth canal during delivery. Anterior quadrilateral cartilage deviation is more common in newborns delivered vaginally than via cesarean. However, internal rotation of the head toward the pelvic wall during cesarean delivery can also lead to septal deviation. Management of septal deviation is guided by symptoms. If there is significant septal deviation and severe obstruction, the septum can be repositioned. For milder cases of deviation, surgical correction via septoplasty at an older age may be helpful in increasing the size of the nasal airway. Although most minor deformities often normalize during the first few months after birth, indications for surgical correction have been advocated at any age if deformity causes significant obstruction and nasal stenosis.

> **Pearl:** Neonatal septal deviation has an incidence of 1%.

SEPTAL HEMATOMA AND ABSCESS

Septal hematomas form most often as a result of minor nasal trauma. While septal hematomas are far more common in toddlers and children, minor birth trauma can lead to septal injury and hematomas in neonates. The trauma to the septum leads to rupture of blood vessels. As blood collects between septal cartilage and mucoperichondrium, ischemia and pressure necrosis begin to damage septal cartilage. As the cartilage necroses, bacteria can colonize and the developing infection can form an abscess. Cartilage necrosis can lead to significant septal and nasal deformities. The primary presenting symptom of a septal hematoma is nasal obstruction. The resulting deformity leads to a fixed anatomical obstruction. Management of a septal hematoma and an abscess involves urgent drainage and placement of nasal packing to prevent recollection. Depending on the type of packing or splints used, antibiotics may be prescribed to prevent a sinus infection while the drainage ostia are obstructed. In a recent study of patients who experienced recollection, all had recollection within 3 days of packing removal.

■ Inflammatory Etiologies

NEONATAL RHINITIS

Rhinitis of infancy, or neonatal rhinitis, tends to be self-limited and symptoms frequently resolve within weeks. Diagnosis is made by clinical history and examination, including nasal endoscopy, and is often a diagnosis of exclusion. Findings include pale, boggy nasal mucosa, watery rhinorrhea, and obstructing rhinoliths. Conservative management includes use of nasal saline drops, gentle nasal suctioning to avoid inflammation, humidification of ambient air, and use of topical decongestants. Treatment with topical steroid drops (or steroid-containing drops such as ciprofloxacin-dexamethasone) is recommended in cases of severe respiratory distress. While treatment is highly effective, the PCC should be mindful of potential adverse effects, including epistaxis, mucosal ulceration, and rebound inflammation. The use of intranasal steroid drops for nasal obstruction in infants has also been linked to iatrogenic Cushing syndrome and adrenal insufficiency.

MEDICATION-INDUCED RHINITIS

Rhinitis secondary to placental transfer of maternal medications can result in sinonasal inflammation in newborns. The most frequently implicated substances include β-blockers, hormonal therapies, antidepressants, and cocaine. Treatment is generally supportive and conservative.

■ Selected References

April MM, Ward RF, Garelick JM. Diagnosis, management, and follow-up of congenital head and neck teratomas. *Laryngoscope*. 1998;108(9):1398–1401

Belden CJ, Mancuso AA, Schmalfuss IM. CT features of congenital nasal piriform aperture stenosis: initial experience. *Radiology*. 1999;213(2):495–501

Brown OE, Myer CM III, Manning SC. Congenital nasal pyriform aperture stenosis. *Laryngoscope*. 1989;99(1):86–91

Canty PA, Berkowitz RG. Hematoma and abscess of the nasal septum in children. *Arch Otolaryngol Head Neck Surg*. 1996;122(12):1373–1376

Cedin AC, Peixoto Rocha JF Jr, Deppermann MB, Moraes Manzano PA, Murao M, Shimuta AS. Transnasal endoscopic surgery of choanal atresia without the use of stents. *Laryngoscope*. 2002;112(4):750–752

Dispenza F, Saraniti C, Sciandra D, Kulamarva G, Dispenza C. Management of naso-septal deformity in childhood: long-term results. *Auris Nasus Larynx.* 2009;36(6): 665–670

Hengerer AS, Strome M. Choanal atresia: a new embryologic theory and its influence on surgical management. *Laryngoscope.* 1982;92(8 Pt 1):913–921

Joshi RR, Maresh A. Iatrogenic Cushing's syndrome and adrenal insufficiency in infants on intranasal dexamethasone drops for nasal obstruction: case series and literature review. *Int J Pediatr Otorhinolaryngol.* 2018;105:123–126

Korantzis A, Cardamakis E, Chelidonis E, Papamihalis T. Nasal septum deformity in the newborn infant during labour. *Eur J Obstet Gynecol Reprod Biol.* 1992;44(1):41–46

Losee JE, Kirschner RE, Whitaker LA, Bartlett SP. Congenital nasal anomalies: a classification scheme. *Plast Reconstr Surg.* 2004;113(2):676–689

Losken A, Burstein FD, Williams JK. Congenital nasal pyriform aperture stenosis: diagnosis and treatment. *Plast Reconstr Surg.* 2002;109(5):1506–1511

Min YG. The pathophysiology, diagnosis and treatment of allergic rhinitis. *Allergy Asthma Immunol Res.* 2010;2(2):65–76

Myer CM III, Cotton RT. Nasal obstruction in the pediatric patient. *Pediatrics.* 1983; 72(6):766–777

Neskey D, Eloy JA, Casiano RR. Nasal, septal, and turbinate anatomy and embryology. *Otolaryngol Clin North Am.* 2009;42(2):193–205, vii

Osguthorpe JD, Shirley R. Neonatal respiratory distress from rhinitis medicamentosa. *Laryngoscope.* 1987;97(7 Pt 1):829–831

Otteson TD, Hackam DJ, Mandell DL. The Ex Utero Intrapartum Treatment (EXIT) procedure: new challenges. *Arch Otolaryngol Head Neck Surg.* 2006;132(6):686–689

Rahbar R, Shah P, Mulliken JB, et al. The presentation and management of nasal dermoid: a 30-year experience. *Arch Otolaryngol Head Neck Surg.* 2003;129(4):464–471

Schoem SR. Transnasal endoscopic repair of choanal atresia: why stent? *Otolaryngol Head Neck Surg.* 2004;131(4):362–366

Sohal M, Schoem SR. Disorders of the neonatal nasal cavity: fundamentals for practice. *Semin Fetal Neonatal Med.* 2016;21(4):263–269

Stankiewicz JA. The endoscopic repair of choanal atresia. *Otolaryngol Head Neck Surg.* 1990;103(6):931–937

Tewfik TL, Mazer B. The links between allergy and otitis media with effusion. *Curr Opin Otolaryngol Head Neck Surg.* 2006;14(3):187–190

Van Den Abbeele T, Triglia JM, François M, Narcy P. Congenital nasal pyriform aperture stenosis: diagnosis and management of 20 cases. *Ann Otol Rhinol Laryngol.* 2001;110(1):70–75

Zhang MM, Hu YH, He W, Hu KK. Congenital arhinia: a rare case. *Am J Case Rep.* 2014;15:115–118

CHAPTER 7

Rhinosinusitis

Alexandra G. Espinel, MD, and Maria T. Peña, MD

Background	**Evaluation**
Definitions	**Microbiology**
Anatomy	**Medical Management**
Pathophysiology	**Surgical Management**
Contributing Factors	**Complications**

▤ Background

Pediatric rhinosinusitis (RS) is one of the most prevalent diseases that can significantly affect a child's quality of life, especially if it is recurrent or chronic. Persistent RS symptoms, including rhinorrhea, cough, headache, and fatigue, are likely to interfere with a child's sleep and concentration at school, which can affect emotional well-being. Caregivers and families of children with recurrent acute RS (ARS), chronic RS (CRS), or both experience considerable disruption in daily routines. Indeed, sinusitis creates a substantial health care burden, with 20 million pediatric cases of ARS occurring annually in the United States (US). Between 6% and 18% of children in primary care settings with upper respiratory tract infections (URTIs) may have acute bacterial sinusitis. The economic cost is high because of the direct and indirect costs, including lost caregiver workdays, additional child care expenses for the patient and siblings, and other related expenses. Additional economic burdens are created by this disease because the prevalence of pediatric RS is increasing, and it is known to exacerbate other airway pathologies such as reactive airway disease.

Children develop, on average, between 6 and 8 URTIs per year, with 0.5% to 5% progressing to acute sinusitis. Symptoms of viral URTIs and acute bacterial RS are similar, which makes it challenging to differentiate between them. The immaturity of the pediatric immune system, the various clinical presentations of RS, and the symptoms from associated medical conditions also add to the difficulties in making a correct diagnosis.

> **Pearl:** Children develop, on average, between 6 and 8 upper respiratory tract infections per year, with 0.5% to 5% progressing to acute sinusitis.

■ Definitions

The International Rhinosinusitis Advisory Board, the Sinus and Allergy Health Partnership, the European Academy of Allergology and Clinical Immunology, the European Rhinologic Society, and the American Academy of Pediatrics (AAP) Subcommittee on Management of Sinusitis and Committee on Quality Improvement divided RS into clinical categories based on the duration and frequency of symptoms (**Table 7-1**). Rhinosinusitis presenting for less than 12 weeks is classified as ARS. The 2012 European position paper on Rhinosinusitis and Nasal Polyps further subdivides pediatric ARS into acute viral, acute postviral, and acute bacterial RS. Acute bacterial RS is an infection of the nose and paranasal sinuses that presents with the key signs and symptoms of rhinorrhea and cough. The quality of the nasal discharge varies (eg, clear, mucoid, purulent, thick, thin). Other manifestations include nasal congestion, low-grade fever, otitis media, halitosis, irritability, and, rarely, headache. Sore throat may develop as a result of chronic mouth breathing secondary to nasal congestion. Acute bacterial RS should be suspected when symptoms of nasal discharge, daytime cough, or both persist beyond 10 days. Severe ARS is classified as purulent rhinorrhea for 3 to 4 consecutive days, temperature above 39.0°C, and periorbital edema. The 2013 updated AAP clinical practice guideline for the diagnosis and management of acute bacterial sinusitis in children also recommends that a diagnosis of ARS be made for a worsening clinical course (increased pain or headache, persistent fever, increasing nasal secretions, or ocular symptoms) after initial improvement of symptoms or for severe onset, defined as concurrent fever higher than 39.0°C and purulent nasal discharge for at least 3 consecutive days.

Table 7-1. Rhinosinusitis Definitions

Term	Definition
Acute rhinosinusitis	Sudden onset of 2 or more of the following symptoms for <12 weeks: mucopurulent drainage (anterior, posterior, or both), nasal obstruction/congestion, facial pain/pressure, or cough
Acute viral rhinosinusitis	Suspected viral etiology; duration of sinonasal symptoms <10 days
Acute postviral rhinosinusitis	An increase in sinonasal symptoms after 5 days, or persistent symptoms after 10 days, but lasting <12 weeks
Acute bacterial rhinosinusitis	Persistent upper respiratory tract symptoms lasting >10 days (cough or nasal discharge or both) OR Recurrence of symptoms (fever, worsening cough, worsening or new purulent rhinorrhea) after initial improvement (double worsening) OR Severe onset of symptoms such as fever or purulent nasal discharge lasting at least 3 consecutive days
Chronic rhinosinusitis	At least 90 continuous days of 2 or more of the following symptoms: mucopurulent rhinorrhea (anterior, posterior, or both), nasal obstruction/congestion, facial pain/pressure, or cough AND endoscopic signs of mucosal edema, purulent drainage, or nasal polyps and/or Computed tomographic scan evidence of mucosal changes in the ostiomeatal complex and/or the paranasal sinuses
Recurrent acute rhinosinusitis	Four or more episodes of acute bacterial rhinosinusitis per year without signs or symptoms of rhinosinusitis between episodes

From Wald ER, Applegate KE, Bordley C, et al. Clinical practice guideline for the diagnosis and management of acute bacterial sinusitis in children aged 1 to 18 years. *Pediatrics*. 2013;132(1):262–280; Brietzke SE, Shin JJ, Choi S, Lee JT, Peña M, Prager JD. Clinical consensus statement: pediatric chronic rhinosinusitis. *Otolaryngol Head Neck Surg*. 2014;151(4):542–553; Fokkens WJ, Lund VJ, Mulliol J, et al. European Position Paper on rhinosinusitis and nasal polyps 2012. *Rhinol Suppl*. 2012;23:1–298.

An indolent infection lasting more than 12 consecutive weeks without improvement is defined as CRS. During this time, the respiratory symptoms of purulent rhinorrhea, nasal obstruction, facial pain or pressure, and cough are persistent. Headache and fever are uncommon. The 2014 American Academy of Otolaryngology-Head and Neck Surgery (AAO-HNS) Clinical Consensus Statement on Pediatric Chronic Rhinosinusitis supports the use of both subjective symptoms and objective elements when defining CRS. The consensus statement defines pediatric CRS as 90 continuous days of 2 or more of the following symptoms: facial pain/pressure, nasal obstruction/congestion, nasal discharge, hyposmia/anosmia, or cough and either endoscopic signs of mucosal edema, purulent drainage, or nasal polyposis or computed tomographic (CT) evidence of mucosal changes within the ostiomeatal complex and/or sinuses. Individuals with CRS may experience an abrupt worsening of their symptoms, defined as acute exacerbation of CRS, which resolves with antimicrobial therapy.

> **Pearl:** Pediatric rhinosinusitis is divided into clinical categories based on the duration and frequency of symptoms.

▌ Anatomy

The paranasal sinuses consist of 4 paired cavities or collections of air cells—maxillary, ethmoid, frontal, and sphenoid sinuses (**Figure 7-1**)—that ultimately drain into the nasal cavity via channels called *ostia*. The ostiomeatal complex is the space between the middle and inferior turbinates where there is a confluence of sinus drainage from the frontal, anterior ethmoid, and maxillary sinuses. The paranasal sinuses are lined with pseudostratified ciliated epithelium that contains goblet cells and submucosal glands that produce seromucinous secretions and innate immune mediators.

The maxillary and ethmoid sinuses are present, albeit small, at birth. In neonatal life, the maxillary sinuses begin as a small slit-like cavity inferior to the orbits. They slowly enlarge laterally and vertically. Between ages 8 and 12 years, the floor of the maxillary sinuses reaches the floor of the nose. By age 15 years, the maxillary sinuses are adult size and have an inverted pyramidal shape. The natural opening of the maxillary sinus is positioned superiorly on the medial maxillary sinus wall and beneath the middle turbinate into the middle meatus.

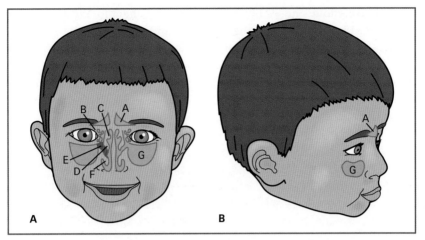

Figure 7-1. Coronal and sagittal depictions of the nose and paranasal sinuses. A, Frontal sinus. B, Ethmoid sinus. C, Superior turbinate. D, Middle turbinate. E, Ostiomeatal complex. F, Inferior turbinate. G, Maxillary sinus.

The ethmoid sinuses consist of a honeycomb of air cells that are divided by thin, bony partitions and lie medial to the orbits. They reach their final form when children are between 12 and 14 years of age. The ethmoid sinuses are divided into anterior and posterior. The anterior ethmoids drain into the middle meatus, and the posterior ethmoids drain into the superior meatus, which is between the middle and superior turbinates. The orbit is separated from the ethmoid sinuses by a thin bone, the lamina papyracea. Infection of the ethmoids can spread easily to the orbit, directly through small congenital bony dehiscences of the lamina or by traversing neurovascular foramina.

The frontal sinuses arise from an anterior ethmoid air cell and move above the superior orbital rim by age 5 to 6 years. They continue to develop throughout late adolescence and drain into the middle meatus. The walls of the frontal sinuses are shared with the orbit and intracranial cavity. Therefore, frontal sinus infections are capable of spreading directly to these adjacent structures. The diploic veins, a valveless venous system that extends through the posterior wall of the frontal sinus to connect the vasculature of the sinus mucosa with the intracranial sinuses and veins, also provide a potential route of infectious spread. Septic thrombi can easily produce intracranial complications via this venous drainage system.

The sphenoid sinuses begin to develop by age 3 to 5 years. They are located just posterior to the ethmoids and anterior to the pituitary fossa. The optic nerve and carotid artery are often located on the lateral wall of the sphenoid sinuses. The sphenoid sinuses represent another direct route for infections to spread into the central nervous system. Their strategic position anterior to the pituitary fossa also can be used to access tumors of the pituitary gland intranasally.

> **Pearl:** The paranasal sinuses consist of 4 paired cavities or collections of air cells—maxillary, ethmoid, frontal, and sphenoid sinuses—that ultimately drain into the nasal cavity via channels called *ostia*. The paranasal sinuses are in close proximity to the orbits and intracranial cavity.

■ Pathophysiology

The normal functioning of the paranasal sinuses depends on 3 factors: patency of the sinus ostia, mucociliary function, and character of sinus secretions. The diameter of the sinus ostia ranges from 1 mm to a few millimeters. Consequently, they are easily occluded by systemic illnesses that cause mucosal inflammation or structural abnormalities of the sinonasal cavities. Allergic rhinitis, immune disorders, extra-esophageal reflux disease, and viral infections are commonly encountered pathologies that contribute to mucosal inflammation characteristic of RS, with subsequent ostial obstruction. Trauma, intranasal growths such as nasal polyps and tumors, or obstructive sinonasal anatomical abnormalities such as a deviated nasal septum are common causes of mechanical obstruction of the sinus ostia. Viral URTIs and allergic rhinitis are the most common causes of pediatric RS.

Prolonged sinus ostial obstruction creates conditions that support unchecked bacterial growth. The secretions produced by the goblet cells and submucosal glands in the sinus mucosa stagnate as sinus outflow tracts are closed off. Over time, sinus oxygenation becomes significantly reduced, which increases the acidity of sinus secretions, creating a nutrient-rich medium for bacteria to thrive. Complete ostial obstruction also creates a negative intrasinus pressure and impairs bacterial export to the nasal cavity. Alterations in intranasal pressure from sneezing, sniffing, and nose blowing may allow the heavily colonized intranasal contents to enter the usually sterile sinus cavity.

The mucociliary apparatus of the sinonasal cavities is an essential defense mechanism against bacterial and viral pathogens as well as environmental irritants. It consists of a mucous layer that is moved by cilia located beneath the mucus. The mucous layer itself is subdivided into 2 compartments. The deep compartment is thin and serous, permitting normal cilia motility, while the superficial layer's increased viscosity captures particulate matter and pathogens. The mucous layer and cilia play a pivotal role in normal sinonasal function. Alterations in the quality of mucus or in cilia morphology and number, as seen with diseases such as cystic fibrosis (CF) and primary ciliary dyskinesias (PCD), respectively, interrupt the normal physiology of the paranasal sinuses.

> **Pearl:** The normal functioning of the paranasal sinuses depends on 3 factors: patency of the sinus ostia, mucociliary function, and character of sinus secretions.

CONTRIBUTING FACTORS

Viral URTIs are the most common contributing factor that predisposes children to acute bacterial sinusitis. On average, children develop between 6 and 8 viral URTIs each year, and this number may increase by a factor of 3 in those who regularly attend child care. Through the production of various inflammatory and immune mediators, viral infections cause obstructive inflammation of the sinonasal outflow tracts and inhibition of normal ciliary function, predisposing factors for increased bacterial overgrowth. Other than supportive measures, no standard treatment exists for viral URTIs. Frequent handwashing is recommended. In severe cases, removing the child from the child care setting for a prolonged period may be necessary.

Second to viral URTIs, allergy is the most common comorbidity associated with bacterial sinusitis, especially in older children. Sixty percent of children with refractory sinusitis were found to have positive results on allergy testing. These children frequently have a history of sneezing, copious watery nasal secretions, pruritus of the eyes and throat, and nighttime cough. On physical examination, clear rhinorrhea or pale, boggy, inferior turbinates may be identified. These clinical symptoms and signs are thought to be related to the release of major basic protein and histamine by eosinophils and mast cells, respectively. Both substances disrupt mucociliary clearance by causing inflammatory obstruction of the sinus ostia. Major basic protein is thought to be toxic to the sinonasal mucosa. Other environmental pollutants, such as cigarette smoke, may contribute to an increased risk of pediatric RS by directly irritating the sinonasal mucosa. Secondhand smoke exposure has recently been linked with a higher likelihood of sinonasal symptoms and CRS.

> **Pearl:** Second to viral upper respiratory tract infections, allergy is the most common comorbidity associated with bacterial sinusitis.

Immunodeficiency is present in 0.5% of the general population. Up to a third of refractory RS cases may involve immune deficiencies, especially in patients with a history of frequent bacterial infections or illnesses soon after discontinuing antibiotic treatment. Children with immune deficiencies will likely have a history of multiple upper and lower respiratory infections, including otitis media, RS, bronchitis, and pneumonia. Immunology evaluation should be considered in patients who have manifestations of a specific immune disorder, in those with recurrent and/or chronic sinus infections that have an atypical presentation (ie, particularly virulent or prolonged), and in patients in whom an unusual organism has been isolated as the cause of the sinus infection.

Anatomical variations in the nasal and sinus cavities have been postulated to predispose patients to sinus disease by narrowing sinus outflow tracts. However, studies in children have not found a relationship between intranasal anatomical variations and sinus disease. Consequently, contributing factors other than anatomical abnormalities likely play a more integral role in the development of pediatric ARS and CRS.

Gastroesophageal reflux (GER) has been implicated in many aerodigestive disorders, including RS. Nasopharyngeal reflux has been documented in children with symptoms of CRS and is associated with coughing paroxysms. Acid-induced injury of the sinus lining is suspected of initiating and sustaining an inflammatory response that leads to sinonasal edema and impaired mucociliary clearance. Although the medical treatment of GER in children with CRS has shown improvement in nasopharyngeal reflux, hoarseness, and asthma, the relationship between GER and CRS is unclear. In the 2014 AAO-HNS Clinical Consensus Statement on pediatric CRS, no consensus could be reached with respect to the contribution of GER to pediatric CRS or the management of GER in these patients.

> **Pearl:** Immunology evaluation should be considered in patients with manifestations of a specific immune disorder; in those who have recurrent and/or chronic infections with an atypical presentation; and in those in whom an unusual pathogen has been isolated as the cause of the sinus infection.

The primary care clinician (PCC) must consider chronic medical diseases that affect the function of the sinonasal mucosa, such as CF and PCD. In the US, CF has a prevalence of 1 in 3,200 white newborns. The disease manifests as chronic upper and lower respiratory tract infections, malnutrition, intestinal obstruction, and pancreatic insufficiency. The presentation and manifestations of CF are variable, and many children with the disease have nasal obstruction and CRS with nasal polyps. Primary ciliary dyskinesia, such as Kartagener syndrome, is a rare disorder of ciliary structure or function. Children with PCD also have recurrent upper and lower respiratory infections.

> **Pearl:** The presentation and manifestations of cystic fibrosis are variable, and many children with the disease have chronic rhinosinusitis with nasal polyps.

■ Evaluation

The diagnosis of RS is made by means of a thorough clinical history and supported by findings on physical examination. In infants or young children, irritability and decreased energy may be the only signs. In older children, the diagnosis of acute bacterial RS is strongly suggested by the presence of 2 major symptoms or 1 major and 2 minor symptoms (**Table 7-2**). Self-limiting viral URTIs may be indistinguishable from acute bacterial RS. Viral etiology is suggested by rhinitis preceded by fever. Lack of improvement or worsening of symptoms at 7 to 10 days is highly suggestive of acute bacterial RS. A careful head and neck examination, while often difficult in children, may corroborate a suspected diagnosis of RS. Turbinate erythema and induration with pooled purulent secretions on the nasal floor may be seen on anterior rhinoscopy. The PCC should examine the posterior oropharynx for erythema and purulent secretions coming from the nasopharynx. Transillumination of the paranasal sinuses correlates poorly with sinus disease. Nasal endoscopy may be helpful to evaluate for purulence in the middle meatus, intranasal polyps, and adenoid size or adenoid pad inflammation/ infection. Mucopurulent secretions in the region of the middle meatus are highly suggestive of bacterial RS. Nasal polyps (**Figure 7-2**) are uncommon in children and constitute a different subtype of CRS; they should prompt an evaluation for CF and other comorbidities, such as allergic fungal sinusitis or antrochoanal polyps.

> **Pearl:** Identification of sinonasal polyps in any child is an indication for cystic fibrosis testing.

Plain radiographs are considered of low utility in cases of pediatric RS because of high false-positive rates. Positive signs of ARS on radiographs are complete opacification of the sinus, thickening (>4 mm) of the sinus mucoperiosteum, and air-fluid levels within

| Table 7-2. Diagnosis of Rhinosinusitis ||
Major Symptoms	Minor Symptoms
Facial pain/pressure	Nasal obstruction/congestion
Nasal discharge	Hyposmia/anosmia
Cough	Headache
Fever	Halitosis
Fatigue	Dental pain Ear fullness/pain

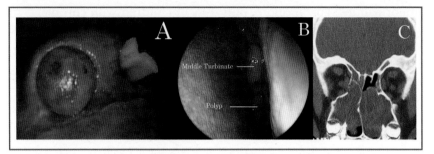

Figure 7-2. Nasal polyposis. A, Patient with large nasal polyp. B, Nasal endoscopic view of a small nasal polyp. C, Computed tomographic scan of a patient with bilateral extensive nasal polyposis.

the sinus. Correlation of abnormal sinus findings on radiographs with positive culture results (>104 colony-forming units/mL) is reported to range from 70% to 75%. A thorough history identifying symptoms of more than 10 days' duration has been shown to significantly correlate with abnormal radiographic findings and positive cultures, thereby obviating the need for imaging.

Based on the 2012 AAO-HNS Clinical Consensus Statement on appropriate use of CT for paranasal sinus disease, CT imaging is indicated in pediatric patients for CRS when medical management and/or adenoidectomy have failed to control symptoms, in cases of suspected tumor and/or complications from sinusitis, and before surgery. It is not indicated in patients with symptoms of less than 10 days' duration or in those with uncomplicated acute sinusitis who have not received proper medical management. Magnetic resonance imaging is considered in the assessment of immunocompromised pediatric patients when invasive fungal sinusitis is suspected.

While CT is considered the gold standard in imaging, a positive scan alone is not diagnostic of bacterial RS. Roughly 70% of the CT scans of children with purulent rhinorrhea lasting from 2 to 9 days demonstrated sinus opacification or air-fluid levels. Despite treatment with antibiotics or placebo, 60% of the scans were normal and 40% showed improvement on follow-up imaging at 3 weeks.

Radiologic evidence of paranasal mucosal thickening or other sinonasal abnormalities on CT scans is common, occurring in 27% to 45% of asymptomatic adults. These findings also can be seen in adults with headache, but no association has been found between sinus opacification and headache. Similarly, 50% of CT scans of asymptomatic children younger than 13 years showed sinonasal abnormalities. Furthermore, only 10% of children with chronic, nonprogressive headache had radiographic evidence of sinus pathology, which responded to medical management.

> **Pearl:** Computed tomography should be reserved for patients with suspected complications of rhinosinusitis, patients who are unresponsive to medical therapy, and patients who are under consideration for surgical intervention.

The gold standard for the diagnosis of bacterial RS is maxillary sinus puncture with aspiration and culture. However, this procedure is unnecessary in uncomplicated cases of ARS, as diagnosis is based on a thorough clinical history. Furthermore, maxillary sinus puncture and aspiration is a painful, invasive procedure that typically requires general anesthesia in the pediatric population. In addition, it has potential complications, such as facial numbness and injury to the tooth roots, especially in young children in whom the floor of the maxillary sinus is above the floor of the nose. Therefore, sinus aspiration for culture should be reserved for patients in whom appropriate medical therapy has failed and in patients with immunodeficiency or toxemia. Nasal cavity bacterial cultures correlate poorly with cultures from the maxillary sinus. However, an 83% to 94% correlation has been demonstrated between endoscopically guided middle meatal cultures and aspiration-obtained maxillary sinus cultures. This procedure has few risks and is less painful than maxillary sinus puncture and aspiration.

> **Pearl:** Sinus aspiration for culture should be reserved for patients in whom appropriate medical therapy has failed and in patients with immunodeficiency or toxemia.

Because many factors contribute to RS, testing for associated medical conditions may be indicated. Allergy testing is recommended in all children whose symptoms are unresponsive to medical therapy, especially those with recurrent ARS, those with a strong family history of allergy, or those with a history of urticaria. The PCC should perform an evaluation for immunodeficiency in children with recurrent RS, severe symptoms, or an inadequate response to appropriate medical management. Initial immunologic testing includes an assessment of total serum immunoglobulin (Ig) and IgG subclass levels, as well as antibody responses to diphtheria, tetanus, and pneumococcal vaccines. In cases of suspected GER, a 24-hour pH probe is considered the gold standard for diagnosis. Children with nasal polyps should be evaluated for CF. While an elevated sweat chloride concentration is often found in patients with CF, genetic testing is more accurate and reliable. Primary ciliary dyskinesia is diagnosed via biopsy of the nasal or tracheal mucosa.

> **Pearl:** Evaluation for associated medical conditions such as allergy, gastroesophageal reflux, cystic fibrosis, primary ciliary dyskinesias, and immune disorders may be indicated in patients with recurrent or chronic rhinosinusitis.

■ Microbiology

The most common pathogens in acute bacterial RS isolated from maxillary sinus taps over 35 years ago were *Streptococcus pneumoniae,* nontypeable *Haemophilus influenzae,* and *Moraxella catarrhalis.* *Streptococcus pneumoniae* was isolated from 30% to 40% of specimens. *Haemophilus influenzae* and *M catarrhalis* each accounted for approximately 15% to 20% of cases. Recent data on the bacteriology of pediatric acute bacterial RS showed that *S pneumoniae, H influenzae, M catarrhalis, Streptococcus pyogenes,* and anaerobes are the most common pathogens currently isolated. Widespread use of the heptavalent pneumococcal conjugate vaccine (PCV7) has resulted in a decrease in the incidence of *S pneumoniae* and an increase in *H influenzae.*

Chronic RS does not have a well-defined bacterial population but is often polymicrobial. The most frequently cultured bacteria include α-hemolytic streptococci, *Staphylococcus aureus,* coagulase-negative staphylococci, *S pneumoniae,* nontypeable *H influenzae, M catarrhalis,* anaerobic bacteria, and *Pseudomonas.* Positive *Pseudomonas* cultures are frequently encountered after multiple courses of antibiotic treatment. This bacteriology has remained stable in multiple studies over the last 30 years.

■ Medical Management

Antibiotics should be reserved for children with respiratory symptoms that persist beyond 10 to 14 days or those with significant purulent rhinorrhea lasting for at least 3 to 4 consecutive days and a temperature of 39.0°C. In children with mild-to-moderate symptoms of uncomplicated acute bacterial RS who have not been treated with antibiotics for at least 90 days prior to the infection and who do not attend child care, first-line therapy is amoxicillin. The recommended dosage is 45 mg/kg/day divided into 2 doses. In communities with a high prevalence of *S pneumoniae*, the dosage should be increased to 90 mg/kg/day divided into 2 doses. For children with penicillin allergy, cefdinir (14 mg/kg/day in 1 or 2 doses), cefuroxime (30 mg/kg/day in 2 doses), or cefpodoxime (10 mg/kg/day once daily) is recommended. Clarithromycin (15 mg/kg/day divided into 2 doses) or azithromycin (10 mg/kg/day on day 1, then 5 mg/kg/day once daily for 4 days) is suggested for patients with serious allergic reactions to penicillin. If a patient's culture reveals penicillin-resistant *S pneumoniae*, clindamycin at 30 to 40 mg/kg/day in 3 divided doses is indicated. The duration of antibiotic treatment varies, but at least 14 days is recommended for patients with acute bacterial RS. The 2013 AAP clinical practice guideline for the diagnosis and management of acute bacterial sinusitis permits an additional 3 days of outpatient observation for children with symptoms lasting more than 10 days without improvement. Factors that may influence this decision include symptom severity, the child's quality of life, recent use of antibiotics, previous experience with sinusitis, or caregiver concerns regarding antibiotics. Primary care clinicians must reassess the initial management if there is a report of worsening symptoms or failure to improve within 72 hours. Should this occur, antibiotic regimens should be changed or initiated.

For children whose symptoms do not improve after 48 to 72 hours of treatment with the usual dosage of amoxicillin; those who have been treated with antibiotics within 90 days prior to an infection; those who attend child care; or those with moderately severe symptoms, initial therapy should be high-dose amoxicillin-clavulanate (80–90 mg/kg/day of amoxicillin, 6.4 mg/kg/day of clavulanate, in 2 divided doses). Other therapeutic alternatives include cefdinir, cefuroxime, or cefpodoxime. In patients with vomiting that prevents administration of oral antibiotics, a single dose of intravenous (IV) or intramuscular ceftriaxone (50 mg/kg/day) may be administered. An oral antibiotic should be initiated 24 hours later to complete therapy. Children whose conditions do not improve with a second course of antibiotics or who are acutely ill should be treated with IV cefotaxime or ceftriaxone. Consultation with an otolaryngologist may be necessary to obtain sinus cultures for culture-directed therapy.

> **Pearl:** Children whose symptoms do not improve after 48 to 72 hours of treatment with the usual dose of amoxicillin; those who have been treated with antibiotics in the last 90 days; those who attend child care; or those with moderately severe symptoms should receive high-dose amoxicillin-clavulanate as the initial therapy.

Children with CRS should be treated with antibiotics and adjunctive medical therapies. The 2014 AAO-HNS Clinical Consensus Statement on Pediatric Chronic Rhinosinusitis suggests that a 20-day course of antibiotics may produce a superior response compared with a 10-day course of antibiotics, and that daily use of topical nasal saline and nasal steroids is beneficial. Antibiotics directed at resistant pneumococci, *S aureus,* and anaerobic bacteria have been advocated as part of initial medical treatment in CRS. Since the emergence of community-acquired methicillin-resistant *S aureus* (MRSA), much attention has been directed toward the management of sinonasal MRSA. In patients with heavy growth of MRSA in the setting of acute sinonasal inflammation, a 1- to 2-week course of culture-directed oral antibiotics and topical mupirocin is advocated.

Nasal saline rinses in children are a common supplemental therapy, especially in those with CRS. Recent studies have demonstrated improvement in patients' quality of life and in CT findings after 6 weeks of daily nasal rinses in patients with CRS. Daily nasal rinses are also particularly helpful in patients with CF and PCD, particularly after functional endoscopic sinus surgery (FESS) because the sinus ostia have been enlarged. Mechanical flushing with nasal saline rinses assists in clearing the nose and paranasal sinuses of stagnant secretions and biofilms—thus reducing bacterial counts—which improves sinus ventilation, drainage, and mucociliary transport. Saline may also aid in reducing nasal edema because of its mild vasoconstrictive properties.

Intranasal steroids may be helpful as they can reduce the swelling around the sinus ostia and encourage drainage. In patients with ARS, intranasal steroids have been shown to be beneficial as an adjunct to antibiotics in reducing the time until symptom improvement. For patients with CRS, 2 trials conducted exclusively in children showed that inhaled nasal steroids resulted in a greater reduction in symptoms and hastened the rate of complete resolution. Benefit has also been shown in improvement of quality of life scores among patients with CRS. Patients with CRS may need to use intranasal steroids for years. Short-term studies (4–6 weeks) have shown that intermittent use in patients with allergic rhinitis is helpful. This may be attempted to limit exposure to the medications.

Local side effects of intranasal steroids, which include dryness or a burning sensation of the nasal mucosa and epistaxis, are related to the corticosteroid vasoconstrictive activity. Septal perforations are rare and occur most commonly in the first year of use. Patients treated with these medications should undergo an annual examination of the nasal mucosa to check for injury. These complications are minimized when the spray is directed at the lateral nasal wall, away from the nasal septum. Doing this also directs the medication laterally, where it is most effective. Studies have demonstrated elevated intraocular pressure (IOP) with long-term use of the first-generation intranasal steroid dexamethasone and betamethasone. A recent study of fluticasone and mometasone did not show increased IOP during a 6-month follow-up. While there is little concern regarding increased IOP in healthy individuals, caution should be exercised in those with IOP risk factors such as open angle glaucoma, diabetes, high myopia, connective tissue disorders, or a first-degree relative with primary open angle glaucoma.

Systemic absorption via the nasal mucosa occurs but is low (<1%) with both fluticasone and mometasone. Neither of these medications has been shown to affect children's growth. Fluticasone has been approved by the US Food and Drug Administration for use in children older than 4 years, and mometasone has been approved for children older than 2 years. Disruption of the hypothalamic axis has not been reported with fluticasone and mometasone. However, the older first-generation intranasal steroids, dexamethasone and betamethasone (not currently available in the US), with higher systemic absorption have some effect. To date, no studies have evaluated side effects of concurrent use of intranasal steroids with other topical steroids or parenteral forms.

> **Pearl:** Local side effects of intranasal steroids include dryness or a burning sensation of the nasal mucosa, epistaxis, and, rarely, nasal septal perforation. These side effects are mitigated by directing the administration of the intranasal steroid spray at the lateral nasal wall, away from the nasal septum.

Oral steroids may be considered in patients with ARS who do not respond to initial therapy, in those with nasal polyposis, and in those with severe nasal mucosal edema. Caution should be exercised when prescribing these medications owing to potential significant side effects, such as osteoporosis, diarrhea, hypertension, increased appetite, weight gain, and stomach irritation among others. Nasal decongestants, except intranasal steroids, and mucolytics may provide some short-term symptomatic relief, but have limited efficacy. Topical nasal decongestants may improve symptomatic nasal congestion but should be limited to the first 4 to 5 days of medical treatment to avoid rebound vasodilatation.

Correcting or ameliorating associated comorbidities is essential to the treatment of pediatric RS. In patients with specific environmental allergies, optimizing the home environment to decrease or avoid allergens is vital. Antihistamines are indicated in cases of suspected or documented allergy. Also, secondhand smoke exposure should be avoided. Patients with diagnosed immunodeficiencies should be referred to an immunologist and may require immunoglobulin therapy. In patients with CRS and suspected GER, further testing for GER may be warranted. Empirical GER treatment is not a beneficial adjunct and is not recommended in the 2014 AAO-HNS Clinical Consensus Statement on Pediatric Chronic Rhinosinusitis. Patients with CF or PCD should be managed with the assistance of a pulmonologist.

■ Surgical Management

Surgery is indicated in cases of failed maximal medical management. Adenoidectomy is usually first-line surgical management. In children 12 years and younger, adenoiditis is an important contributing factor to CRS. The beneficial effect of adenoidectomy is independent of endoscopic sinus surgery. Culture of the middle meatus or maxillary sinus may also be performed at the time of adenoidectomy. The adenoid pad can contribute to recurrent acute bacterial RS and CRS because it acts as a bacterial reservoir that is a nidus for infection. Adenoidectomy, regardless of adenoid size, has been shown to decrease nasopharyngeal pathogens implicated in CRS. Studies have shown that adenoidectomy alone improves the symptoms of recurrent RS and CRS in 50% to 60% of children. However, children with asthma or those exposed to secondhand smoke did not respond as well to adenoidectomy.

Indications for other surgical interventions remain controversial. Although FESS has been performed safely in children for more than 20 years, pediatric otolaryngologists are performing it less often and with a much more conservative dissection than in previous years. Pediatric FESS is currently indicated in patients with persistent sinonasal disease despite maximal medical therapy, adenoidectomy, and culture-directed systemic antibiotic treatment; sinonasal tumors, obstructing nasal polyps, or CF; and intraorbital or intracranial complications of RS. Success rates of 82% to 100%, with an overall complication rate of only 1.4%, were reported in a 22-year review of the Cochrane and PubMed databases.

Functional endoscopic sinus surgery for recurrent acute sinusitis is considered when disease is persistent after maximum medical therapy, and it continues to have a significant impact on the patient's quality of life. No studies suggest the number of recurrent infections necessary for FESS to be of benefit. Before recommending FESS for recurrent disease, the PCC should ensure that there are no undiagnosed contributing factors and that each episode of acute sinusitis is appropriately managed.

Balloon sinuplasty has recently emerged for the treatment of sinusitis. This procedure uses endoscopic techniques and intraoperative radiographic guidance to dilate the sinus ostia with a balloon instead of a sharp instrument. It is a potentially less traumatic and safer procedure than FESS; however, more research is needed. As it is a novel technique, its use in children is limited, and the indications and long-term outcomes have not yet been studied.

> **Pearl:** The indications for sinus surgery are persistent sinonasal disease despite maximal medical therapy, adenoidectomy, and culture-directed systemic antibiotic treatment; sinonasal tumors or obstructing nasal polyposis; and intraorbital or intracranial complications.

■ Complications

Children are more susceptible to orbital complications of RS because of the thinness of their sinus walls and bony septa, greater bony porosity, open suture lines, and larger vascular foramina. Pediatric patients with orbital infections caused by sinusitis can have decreased visual acuity, gaze restriction, diminished pupillary reflex, and proptosis. These infections can range in severity from eyelid edema, to abscess of the orbital soft tissues (**Figure 7-3**), to cavernous sinus thrombosis. Cavernous sinus thrombosis occurs because of retrograde spread of orbital infection through the valveless orbital veins and is a life-threatening condition. Urgent consultation with an otolaryngologist and ophthalmologist is indicated in any patient with ophthalmologic findings and sinusitis.

> **Pearl:** Urgent consultation with an otolaryngologist and ophthalmologist is indicated in any patient with ophthalmologic findings and sinusitis.

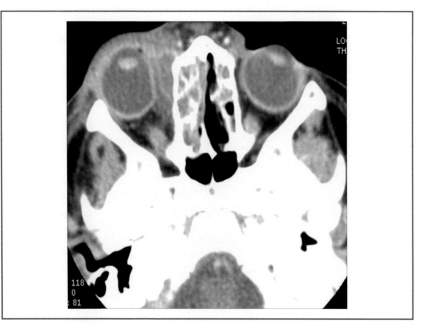

Figure 7-3. Orbital complications of sinusitis. Computed tomographic scan of a patient with a right orbital abscess.

Intracranial complications can also be associated with acute sinusitis and include meningitis, epidural and subdural abscesses, cavernous and sagittal sinus thromboses, and intraparenchymal brain abscesses (**figures 7-4** and **7-5**). The most common presenting symptoms of intracranial complications are fever and headache. Lethargy, seizures, and neurologic deficits are ominous signs associated with increased morbidity and mortality. Extension of frontal sinusitis through the valveless diploic veins or direct extension of an infection through osteitic bone are the most common anatomical routes for infections to access the central nervous system. However, the remaining sinuses may be sources of intracranial infection. In cases of potentially life-threatening intracranial complications of RS, prompt neurosurgical and otolaryngological evaluation is necessary.

> **Pearl:** Patients with fever, mental status changes, and sinusitis need emergent otolaryngological and neurosurgical intervention.

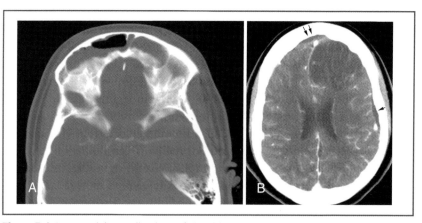

Figure 7-4. Intracranial complications of sinusitis. A, Computed tomographic (CT) scan showing frontal sinusitis with an air-fluid level. B, CT scan showing left frontal cerebritis, left subdural abscess (single arrow), and midline epidural empyema (double arrows) in a 15-year-old with acute mental status changes.

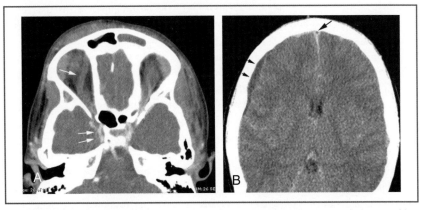

Figure 7-5. Intracranial complications of sinusitis. A, Axial contrast computed tomographic (CT) scan revealing thrombosis of the superior ophthalmic vein (single arrow) and right cavernous sinus (double arrows) in an 11-year-old with right orbital pain and periorbital edema. B, Contrast CT scan of the brain demonstrates thrombosis of the superior sagittal sinus (single arrow) and a right subdural abscess (double arrows) in the same patient.

■ Selected References

Barlan IB, Erkan E, Bakir M, Berrak S, Başaran MM. Intranasal budesonide spray as an adjunct to oral antibiotic therapy for acute sinusitis in children. *Ann Allergy Asthma Immunol.* 1997;78(6):598–601

Becker SS, Russell PT, Duncavage JA, Creech CB. Current issues in the management of sinonasal methicillin-resistant *Staphylococcus aureus. Curr Opin Otolaryngol Head Neck Surg.* 2009;17(1):2–5

Brietzke SE, Shin JJ, Choi S, et al. Clinical consensus statement: pediatric chronic rhinosinusitis. *Otolaryngol Head Neck Surg.* 2014;151(4):542–553

Brook I. Microbiology and antimicrobial treatment of orbital and intracranial complications of sinusitis in children and their management. *Int J Pediatr Otorhinolaryngol.* 2009;73(9):1183–1186

Chan R, Astor FC, Younis RT. Embryology and anatomy of the nose and paranasal sinuses. In: Younis RT, ed. *Pediatric Sinusitis and Sinus Surgery.* New York, NY: Taylor & Francis Group; 2006:1–14

Chur V, Small CB, Stryszak P, Teper A. Safety of mometasone furoate nasal spray in the treatment of nasal polyps in children. *Pediatr Allergy Immunol.* 2013;24(1):33–38

Clayman GL, Adams GL, Paugh DR, Koopmann CF Jr. Intracranial complications of paranasal sinusitis: a combined institutional review. *Laryngoscope.* 1991;101(3):234–239

Cunningham MJ, Chiu EJ, Landgraf JM, Gliklich RE. The health impact of chronic recurrent rhinosinusitis in children. *Arch Otolaryngol Head Neck Surg.* 2000;126(11):1363–1368

Dykewicz MS, Kaiser HB, Nathan RA, et al. Fluticasone propionate aqueous nasal spray improves nasal symptoms of seasonal allergic rhinitis when used as needed (prn). *Ann Allergy Asthma Immunol.* 2003;91(1):44–48

Fiocchi A, Sarratud T, Bouygue GR, Ghiglioni D, Bernardo L, Terracciano L. Topical treatment of rhinosinusitis. *Pediatr Allergy Immunol.* 2007;18(Suppl 18):62–67

Fokkens WJ, Lund VJ, Mullol J, et al. EPOS 2012: European position paper on rhinosinusitis and nasal polyps 2012. A summary for otorhinolaryngologists. *Rhinology.* 2012;50(1):1–12

Goldsmith AJ, Rosenfeld RM. Treatment of pediatric sinusitis. *Pediatr Clin North Am.* 2003;50(2):413–426

Hansen AG, Stovner LJ, Hagen K, et al. Paranasal sinus opacification in headache sufferers: a population-based imaging study (the HUNT study-MRI). *Cephalalgia.* 2017;37(6):509–516

Havas TE, Motbey JA, Gullane PJ. Prevalence of incidental abnormalities on computed tomographic scans of the paranasal sinuses. *Arch Otolaryngol Head Neck Surg.* 1988; 114(8):856–859

Herrmann BW, Forsen JW Jr. Simultaneous intracranial and orbital complications of acute rhinosinusitis in children. *Int J Pediatr Otorhinolaryngol.* 2004;68(5):619–625

International Rhinosinusitis Advisory Board. Infectious rhinosinusitis in adults: classification, etiology and management. *Ear Nose Throat J.* 1997;76(12 Suppl):1–22

Juniper EF, Guyatt GH, Archer B, Ferrie PJ. Aqueous beclomethasone dipropionate in the treatment of ragweed pollen-induced rhinitis: further exploration of "as needed" use. *J Allergy Clin Immunol.* 1993;92(1 Pt 1):66–72

Leo G, Mori F, Incorvaia C, Barni S, Novembre E. Diagnosis and management of acute rhinosinusitis in children. *Curr Allergy Asthma Rep.* 2009;9(3):232–237

Levine HL, Setzen M, Cady RK, et al. An otolaryngology, neurology, allergy, and primary care consensus on diagnosis and treatment of sinus headache. *Otolaryngol Head Neck Surg.* 2006;134(3):516–523

Lippincott LL, Brown KR. Medical management of pediatric chronic sinusitis. *J La State Med Soc.* 2000;152(10):470–474

Lund VJ, Kennedy DW; The Staging and Therapy Group. Quantification for staging sinusitis. *Ann Otol Rhinol Laryngol Suppl.* 1995;167:17–21

Lusk R. Pediatric chronic rhinosinusitis. *Curr Opin Otolaryngol Head Neck Surg.* 2006;14(6):393–396

Lusk RP, Stankiewicz JA. Pediatric rhinosinusitis. *Otolaryngol Head Neck Surg.* 1997; 117(3 Pt 2):S53–S57

Muntz HR, Lusk RP. Bacteriology of the ethmoid bullae in children with chronic sinusitis. *Arch Otolaryngol Head Neck Surg.* 1991;117(2):179–181

Pasha R, Soleja RQ, Ijaz MN. Imaging for headache: what the otolaryngologist looks for. *Otolaryngol Clin North Am.* 2014;47(2):187–195

Passalacqua G, Canonica GW, Baiardini I. Rhinitis, rhinosinusitis and quality of life in children. *Pediatr Allergy Immunol.* 2007;18(suppl 18):40–45

Phipps CD, Wood WE, Gibson WS, Cochran WJ. Gastroesophageal reflux contributing to chronic sinus disease in children: a prospective analysis. *Arch Otolaryngol Head Neck Surg.* 2000;126(7):831–836

Pien LC. Q: How long can my patient use intranasal steroid sprays? *Cleve Clin J Med.* 2005;72(12):1079–1080, 1082

Rahmati MB, Mohebi S, Shahmohammadi S, Rezai MS. Fluticasone nasal spray as an adjunct to Amoxicillin for acute sinusitis in children: a randomized controlled trial. *Eur Rev Med Pharmacol Sci.* 2013;17(22):3068–3072

Ramadan HH. Surgical management of chronic sinusitis in children. *Laryngoscope.* 2004; 114(12):2103–2109

Ray NF, Baraniuk JN, Thamer M, et al. Healthcare expenditures for sinusitis in 1996: contributions of asthma, rhinitis, and other airway disorders. *J Allergy Clin Immunol.* 1999;103(3 Pt 1):408–414

Reh DD, Lin SY, Clipp SL, Irani L, Alberg AJ, Navas-Acien A. Secondhand tobacco smoke exposure and chronic rhinosinusitis: a population-based case-control study. *Am J Rhinol Allergy.* 2009;23(6):562–567

Rosenfeld RM. Pilot study of outcomes in pediatric rhinosinusitis. *Arch Otolaryngol Head Neck Surg.* 1995;121(7):729–736

Rosenstein BJ, Cutting GR; Cystic Fibrosis Foundation Consensus Panel. The diagnosis of cystic fibrosis: a consensus statement. *J Pediatr.* 1998;132(4):589–595

Schwartz RH, Pitkaranta A, Winther B. Computed tomography imaging of the maxillary and ethmoid sinuses in children with short-duration purulent rhinorrhea. *Otolaryngol Head Neck Surg.* 2001;124(2):160–163

Setzen G, Ferguson BJ, Han JK, et al. Clinical consensus statement: appropriate use of computed tomography for paranasal sinus disease. *Otolaryngol Head Neck Surg.* 2012;147(5):808–816

Shapiro GG, Virant FS, Furukawa CT, Pierson WE, Bierman CW. Immunologic defects in patients with refractory sinusitis. *Pediatrics.* 1991;87(3):311–316

Silberstein SD. Headaches due to nasal and paranasal sinus disease. *Neurol Clin.* 2004;22(1):1–19, v

Şimşek A, Bayraktar C, Doğan S, Karataş M, Sarıkaya Y. The effect of long-term use of intranasal steroids on intraocular pressure. *Clin Ophthalmol.* 2016;10:1079–1082

Sinus and Allergy Health Partnership. Antimicrobial treatment guidelines for acute bacterial rhinosinusitis. Executive summary. *Otolaryngol Head Neck Surg.* 2000; 123(1 Pt 2):1–4

Sobol SE, Samadi DS, Kazahaya K, Tom LW. Trends in the management of pediatric chronic sinusitis: survey of the American Society of Pediatric Otolaryngology. *Laryngoscope.* 2005;115(1):78–80

Vogan JC, Bolger WE, Keyes AS. Endoscopically guided sinonasal cultures: a direct comparison with maxillary sinus aspirate cultures. *Otolaryngol Head Neck Surg.* 2000;122(3):370–373

Wald ER. Microbiology of acute and chronic sinusitis in children. *J Allergy Clin Immunol.* 1992;90(3 Pt 2):452–456

Wald ER. Sinusitis. *Pediatr Ann.* 1998;27(12):811–818

Wald ER. Sinusitis in children. *N Engl J Med.* 1992;326(5):319–323

Wald ER, Applegate KE, Bordley C, et al. Clinical practice guideline for the diagnosis and management of acute bacterial sinusitis in children aged 1 to 18 years. *Pediatrics.* 2013;132(1):e262–e280

Wang DY, Wardani RS, Singh K, et al. A survey on the management of acute rhinosinusitis among Asian physicians. *Rhinology.* 2011;49(3):264–271

Willner A, Choi SS, Vezina LG, Lazar RH. Intranasal anatomic variations in pediatric sinusitis. *Am J Rhinol.* 1997;11(5):355–360

Yilmaz G, Varan B, Yilmaz T, Gürakan B. Intranasal budesonide spray as an adjunct to oral antibiotic therapy for acute sinusitis in children. *Eur Arch Otorhinolaryngol.* 2000;257(5):256–259

Younis RT, Anand VK, Davidson B. The role of computed tomography and magnetic resonance imaging in patients with sinusitis with complications. *Laryngoscope.* 2002; 112(2):224–229

Epistaxis

Mark S. Volk, MD, DMD

▨ Introduction

Epistaxis is a common, usually benign condition of childhood. Although simple epistaxis can be an inconvenience, chronic or excessive bleeding requires proper diagnosis and management, as nasal bleeding may be a source of morbidity or an indication of serious underlying pathology. Because epistaxis is so common, decisions regarding the extensiveness of the workup as well as treatment of a child with nasal bleeding can be difficult.

▨ Epidemiology

Epistaxis is most common in pediatric and geriatric populations. In the United States, it accounts for 0.5% of all emergency department (ED) visits. More than 50% of children between 6 and 10 years of age have nosebleeds. The peak age is between 8 and 9 years. While epistaxis is no doubt common, not many studies have reported its actual incidences. In 1 study, 30% of children between the ages of 0 and 5 years, 56% of those aged 6 to 10 years, and 64% of those aged 11 to 15 years reported having epistaxis. However, in an Italian study of 1,281 children between 11 and 14 years of age, 8.5% reported having episodes of epistaxis. In addition to the increased incidence of epistaxis during childhood, nosebleeds occur more frequently in cold, dry conditions. In a review of ED visits in a tertiary care general hospital in Boston, MA, researchers reported that nosebleeds accounted for 0.50% of ED visits between the months of December and February. The percentage decreased to 0.34% of ED visits during all other times of the year. Studies show a predisposition to epistaxis after upper respiratory tract infections and in males compared with females.

In most (>90%) patients, the site of the bleeding is the anterior nasal septum. This area is prone to bleeding secondary to a network of small blood vessels known as Kiesselbach plexus (**Figure 8-1**). These vessels are located in a superficial portion of the septal mucosa, which makes them prone to injury from the slightest mechanical or chemical insult.

▦ Presenting Symptoms

The presenting symptom of epistaxis is, of course, bleeding from the nose. Parents bring their children to the primary care clinician (PCC) for varying degrees of nose bleeding, which can range from 1 or 2 episodes every other month to several per day. The quantity of bleeding also can vary from a trace amount that stops spontaneously to copious bleeding that continues for 30 minutes or more and results in significant blood

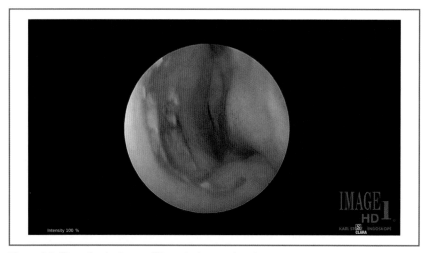

Figure 8-1. Kiesselbach plexus of the anterior nasal septum.

loss. Bleeding episodes can occur in 1 or both nostrils or in alternating nostrils. Recording the location is critical to tailor any needed cauterization in the future. One of the challenges in dealing with this condition is trying to gauge the severity of the bleeding. Katsanis et al developed a grading system that can be a useful guide (**Table 8-1**). Documenting the frequency and severity of episodes is vital to gauge the needed aggressiveness of the workup and therapy, as well as to determine progress

| Table 8-1. Epistaxis Scoring System ||
Component	Score[a]
Frequency	
5–15/y	0
16–25/y	1
>25/y	2
Duration	
<5 min	0
5–10 min	1
>10 min	2
Amount[b]	
<15 mL	0
15–30 mL	1
>30 mL	2
Epistaxis History/Age[c]	
<33%	0
33%–67%	1
>67%	2
Site	
Unilateral	0
Bilateral	2

[a] Mild = 0–6, severe = 7–10.

[b] Estimation of average blood loss per episode: based on fractions or multiples of teaspoons (5 mL), tablespoons (15 mL), or cups (240 mL).

[c] Proportion of the child's life during which nosebleeds have been recurrent (>5 episodes/y).

From Katsanis E, Luke K-H, Hsu E, Li M, Lillicrap D. Prevalence and significance of mild bleeding disorders in children with recurrent epistaxis. *J Pediatr.* 1988;113(1 Pt 1):73-76, with permission from Elsevier.

during treatment. Any use of medicines that increase the chance of bleeding (eg, ibuprofen, salicylates) should be noted. The PCC also should determine if there is a history of any systemic diseases, bleeding, or easy bruising or a family history of bleeding problems.

Physical Examination Findings

A thorough head and neck examination is important in evaluating any patient with epistaxis. The oral cavity has the largest surface area of mucous membrane that can be examined without an endoscope, so it is important to examine the mouth to look for any petechiae or other generalized mucosal lesions that may be more difficult to see in the nose. Anterior rhinoscopy can be performed using an otoscope. This instrument is well known to children and is usually nonthreatening. On examination of the nose, the PCC should pay special attention to the nasal septum. The anterior septum is the location of a network of vessels known as Kiesselbach plexus (see **Figure 8-1**). These vessels can be superficial and fragile and are the origin of most episodes of epistaxis. Although distended vessels sometimes can be seen in this area, this occurs in only about 40% to 50% of children who have nasal bleeding. Often, minimal old blood is seen in the area, even shortly after a nosebleed episode.

> **Pearl:** After nasal trauma, a septal hematoma may form. This bulge in the nasal septum can be differentiated from a septal deviation by palpating for fluctuance using a cerumen loop or the wooden end of a cotton swab. A hematoma of the septum requires referral to an otolaryngologist for incision and drainage.

Differential Diagnosis

Two-thirds of epistaxis episodes occur spontaneously and without apparent trauma. If trauma is involved, it is usually secondary to nose blowing, sneezing, nose picking, or application of preparations such as intranasal steroids. Parents often report a history of discovering their child awakening at night or in the morning with blood on the pillow-case or sheets. These incidents are thought to be secondary to occult trauma such as contact with the pillow or nose picking (intentional or unintentional). Only about 2% of nosebleeds occur secondary to an obvious blow to the nose, such as being struck by a ball or an elbow. Upper respiratory tract infections, dehydration of the nasal mucosa, carriage of *Staphylococcus aureus* in the nasal vestibule, and nose picking all seem to play a part in nasal bleeding. Although some recent data suggest that nose picking may have less of a role than once was thought, the previously mentioned factors frequently have a synergistic effect. Thus, a URTI, dry nasal mucosa, and low-grade *S aureus* infection make it more likely that a child will manipulate or pick the nose. Likewise, frequent nose picking increases the probability that the nose will carry or recolonize with *S aureus.*

Epistaxis can be the first sign of a hematologic disorder. In adult studies, the incidence of hematologic disorders in patients with nosebleeds is between 0.7% and 3.5%. However, determining which patients would benefit from a hematologic workup has been difficult. In 1 study, a total of 36 children with epistaxis were tested, and the results showed no abnormality in the prothrombin time (PT)/partial thromboplastin time (PTT), fibrinogen level, or platelet aggregation. Two of the 12 patients in the severe nose-bleeding group had abnormal von Willebrand factors and were found to have von Willebrand disease (vWd). Another patient in the severe epistaxis group had a factor VIII:c deficiency. A similar study of 20 children with recurrent epistaxis noted that 4 patients had hematologic abnormalities consistent with vWd. Two of the 4 patients had normal PT/PTT, and the other 2 had only a sight elevation of these values. Given that the prevalence of vWd in the general population is approximately 0.82%, it appears that patients who experience recurrent nosebleeds are at a significantly higher risk of having this hematologic disorder.

> **Pearl:** Because of the finding of normal prothrombin time/partial thromboplastin time values despite the diagnosis of von Willebrand disease (vWd) in this population, it is recommended that all patients undergoing blood work for coagulation studies have a vWd panel drawn at the same time.

Other causes of nosebleeds include allergies, vascular abnormalities (eg, hereditary hemorrhagic telangiectasia), and nasal or nasopharyngeal tumors (**Box 8-1**).

Box 8-1. Etiology of Epistaxis

Local Causes of Epistaxis

♦ Inflammatory
  - Allergy
  - Rhinitis sicca
  - Vasomotor rhinitis
♦ Infectious
  - Viral (URTI)
  - Bacterial (vestibulitis, sinusitis)
♦ Trauma
  - Nose picking
  - External trauma (nasal/facial trauma)
  - Foreign body
  - Postoperative: sinus surgery, septoplasty, turbinate reduction
♦ Anatomical
  - Acquired
    ■ Nasal septal deviation
  - Congenital
    ■ Choanal atresia
    ■ Meningocele, encephalocele, glioma

♦ Medications (topical)
  - Decongestants (rhinitis medicamentosa)
  - Cocaine
♦ Inhalants
  - Tobacco
  - Toxic fumes
  - Cannabis
♦ Neoplasms
  - Malignant
    ■ Squamous cell carcinoma
  - Benign
    ■ Angiofibroma
    ■ Inverting papilloma
    ■ Polyp

Systemic Causes of Epistaxis

♦ Medications
  - Aspirin
  - Anticoagulants
  - Antibiotics (chloramphenicol)
  - Antineoplastics (methotrexate)
♦ Bleeding disorders
  - Coagulopathies
    ■ Inherited (factor deficiencies)
    ■ Acquired (vitamin K deficit)

♦ Neoplasms
  - Leukemia
  - Lymphoma
♦ Inflammatory disorders
  - Wegener granulomatosis
  - Lethal midline granuloma
♦ Hypertension
♦ Other
  - Sepsis
  - Liver or bone marrow failure
    ■ Biliary atresia
    ■ Aplastic anemia
♦ Hereditary hemorrhagic telangiectasia (Osler-Weber-Rendu disease)

Abbreviation: URTI, upper respiratory tract infection.

Pearl: Any significant history of epistaxis in a male between the ages of 10 and 24 years requires referral to an otolaryngologist for examination of the nasopharynx to rule out the presence of juvenile nasopharyngeal angiofibroma (Figure 8-2).

■ Treatment

Management of most nosebleeds primarily revolves around educating the parent and patient about the need for treatment at the time of the bleed, as well as ways to prevent bleeding. In general, more than 65% of nosebleeds stop with conservative maneuvers such as applying pressure and occasionally using a vasoconstricting agent. A number of common misconceptions exist as to the best way to stop a nosebleed. In a 1993 study, only 33% of personnel in a Glasgow ED knew the proper anatomical site to which pressure should be applied. This finding is consistent with the many ineffective techniques suggested by PCCs and laypeople to stop a nosebleed. These include lying down, extending the head, pinching the bridge of the nose, putting a tissue under the upper lip, and applying ice (to the nose or back of the neck). These techniques are not useful because they do not address the common site of bleeding, namely the anterior nasal septum.

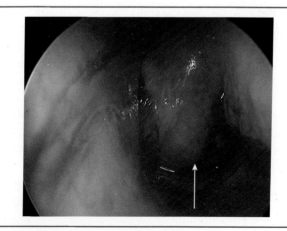

Figure 8-2. Intranasal juvenile nasopharyngeal angiofibroma.

Courtesy of Christopher Grindle, MD.

> **Pearl:** To control a nosebleed at home, patients should place constant pressure on the anterior septum by pinching the caudal (soft) portion of the nose with the fingers for 5 to 10 minutes. Blood clots are a source of fibrinolytic enzymes, so if bleeding persists after 5 to 10 minutes, the nose should be gently blown to evacuate any clots. If available, a vasoconstrictor such as oxymetazoline can be sprayed up the nose and pressure reapplied. These measures are usually effective. However, if bleeding is copious or persists for more than 30 minutes, medical attention at an emergency department is recommended.

Patients who have persistent nosebleeds may benefit from otolaryngological consultation. However, if an otolaryngologist is not readily available, the PCC can perform several maneuvers in the office to stop or reduce the bleeding. First, the patient or parent should continue to squeeze the caudal portion of the nose for 5 minutes. Leaning back will cause blood to enter the pharynx and pool, so the patient should sit straight up or lean slightly forward during these maneuvers. In this acute setting, optimum treatment is localization and cauterization of the bleeding area, which is best accomplished by using a headlight, nasal speculum, and silver nitrate sticks. If this equipment and supplies are not available, the PCC can place a rolled-up piece of absorbable hemostatic agent up against the nasal septum. If bleeding is brisk or unremitting and the patient is showing signs of airway distress or hypovolemia, transfer to an ED. Because small blood vessels in the septal mucosa are the source of most nosebleeds, this is relatively uncommon in children and suggests an arterial source of the bleeding or a systemic cause. Patients brought to the ED in this condition require fluid resuscitation, a workup, and definitive management. The first step in this situation is reassessment and, if necessary, placement of an anterior or posterior nasal pack, which is usually left in place for 24 to 48 hours. If bleeding resumes after pack removal, more definitive therapy is indicated. This treatment can take the form of endoscopic visualization and cautery, angiography with embolization, or surgical clipping of the arteries supplying the bleeding area. All of these treatments require general anesthesia. Depending on the site of the bleeding source, surgical clipping involves ligation of the anterior or posterior ethmoid arteries or clipping of offending branches of the internal maxillary artery. Ligation of the ethmoid vessels is done through a Lynch incision made just medial and superior to the eye. The alternative surgical option involves accessing the internal maxillary artery through the maxillary sinus via an incision under the upper lip (Caldwell-Luc approach).

> **Pearl:** Patients who have continued severe epistaxis may need placement of an anterior nasal pack. If the bleeding area is located posteriorly, placement of anterior and posterior packs may be indicated. This type of packing is often quite uncomfortable and frequently requires hospital admission, intravenous hydration, antibiotics, and sedation or pain control.

As stated earlier, severe nasal bleeding is rare. The most common presentation of epistaxis is frequent, easily controlled episodes. In this setting, there are 2 initial management options. One way to control bleeding is to perform a chemical cauterization of the nasal septum. This can be done in the office by an otolaryngologist. It involves spraying lidocaine or placing a lidocaine-soaked pledget against the nasal septum, followed by application of silver nitrate to any identifiable ectatic vessels or to the vascular plexus. This technique has the advantage of possibly preventing further bleeding episodes. Unfortunately, it has some disadvantages. It can be difficult to reliably pinpoint the offending vessels; there can be associated discomfort; the silver nitrate can stain skin and clothing; and it can be difficult to perform with less-than-cooperative pediatric patients. The second technique is the use of nasal saline followed by application of antibiotic (ie, bacitracin or mupirocin) ointment. Saline is instilled in the form of nose drops or spray, and ointment is applied with cotton applicators to the anterior nasal septum. The saline and ointment combination should be used twice a day, which serves to hydrate the nasal mucosa as well as reduce the population of *S aureus* and other bacteria that may be causing inflammation in the nose. This regimen has the advantage of not requiring intervention by a specialist and is usually well tolerated by the patient. The disadvantage of the saline/ointment regimen is that it can take as long as 10 to 14 days to have an effect, and it must be followed twice daily for at least a month.

Several studies have shown that the efficacy of these techniques (silver nitrate cautery alone, cautery and saline/ointment, and saline/ ointment alone) is similar. Interestingly, saline paired with petroleum jelly, a nonantibiotic ointment, showed no reduction in nosebleeds. This finding supports the theory that nasal vestibulitis may be a cause of epistaxis in some individuals. A surgical intervention to control recurrent epistaxis has also been described. The procedure, a "mini" septodermoplasty, consists of resection of the vascular anterior septal mucosa and replacement with a tiny skin graft.

IF REFERRAL TO A SPECIALIST IS RECOMMENDED, WHAT IS THE OPTIMAL TIME FRAME?

Referral to an otolaryngologist should be done in the presence of severe or unremitting bleeding or when conservative measures, such as application of saline and antibiotic ointment, fail.

NATURAL HISTORY AND PROGNOSIS

Adults often report that they had episodes of nose bleeding as children and that these episodes resolved as they grew older. This frequent remark correlates with observations that nosebleeds exhibit a bimodal peak in incidence. The short-term resolution rate is unknown but has been estimated at approximately 30%. Virtually all children who have uncomplicated epistaxis will experience resolution of their nosebleeds as they mature.

■ Long-term Prognosis and Potential Complications Into Adulthood

Epistaxis in childhood rarely leads to long-standing complications. Individuals with developmental delays can pick their noses obsessively as a response to the crusting after epistaxis episodes. The resulting continued trauma to the septum may result in septal perforation. Cocaine users also run the risk of developing a septal perforation. In such cases, the etiology is vasoconstriction of the septal mucoperichondrium that results in ischemia and loss of the underlying cartilage. A septal perforation, no matter the cause, often leads to chronic crusting and epistaxis.

PROJECTED TIME TO RETURN TO ACTIVITIES OF DAILY LIVING

Most individuals with epistaxis can resume their normal activities shortly after treatment. Those who are being treated conservatively with saline and antibiotic ointment often can continue their normal activities during treatment. Recommendations for children who have been treated for severe epistaxis need to be made on an individual basis.

■ Selected References

Evans J. The aetiology and treatment of epistaxis: based on a review of 200 cases. *J Laryngol Otol.* 1962;76(3):185–191

Glad H, Vainer B, Buchwald C, et al. Juvenile nasopharyngeal angiofibromas in Denmark 1981-2003: diagnosis, incidence, and treatment. *Acta Otolaryngol.* 2007;127(3):292–299

Guarisco JL, Graham HD III. Epistaxis in children: causes, diagnosis, and treatment. *Ear Nose Throat J.* 1989;68(7):522, 528–530, 532 passim

Joice P, Ross P, Robertson G, White P. The effect of hand dominance on recurrent idiopathic paediatric epistaxis. *Clin Otolaryngol.* 2008;33(6):570–574

Juselius H. Epistaxis. A clinical study of 1,724 patients. *J Laryngol Otol.* 1974;88(4): 317–327

Katsanis E, Luke K-H, Hsu E, Li M, Lillicrap D. Prevalence and significance of mild bleeding disorders in children with recurrent epistaxis. *J Pediatr.* 1988;113(1 Pt 1): 73–76

Kiley V, Stuart JJ, Johnson CA. Coagulation studies in children with isolated recurrent epistaxis. *J Pediatr.* 1982;100(4):579–581

Loughran S, Spinou E, Clement WA, Cathcart R, Kubba H, Geddes NK. A prospective, single-blind, randomized controlled trial of petroleum jelly/Vaseline for recurrent paediatric epistaxis. *Clin Otolaryngol Allied Sci.* 2004;29(3):266–269

McGarry GW, Moulton C. The first aid management of epistaxis by accident and emergency department staff. *Arch Emerg Med.* 1993;10(4):298–300

Pallin DJ, Chng YM, McKay MP, Emond JA, Pelletier AJ, Camargo CA Jr. Epidemiology of epistaxis in US emergency departments, 1992 to 2001. *Ann Emerg Med.* 2005;46(1): 77–81

Petruson B. Epistaxis in childhood. *Rhinology.* 1979;17(2):83–90

Qureishi A, Burton MJ. Interventions for recurrent idiopathic epistaxis (nosebleeds) in children. *Cochrane Database Syst Rev.* 2012;(9):CD004661

Rodeghiero F, Castaman G, Dini E. Epidemiological investigation of the prevalence of von Willebrand's disease. *Blood.* 1987;69(2):454–459

Ruddy J, Proops DW, Pearman K, Ruddy H. Management of epistaxis in children. *Int J Pediatr Otorhinolaryngol.* 1991;21(2):139–142

Somers EH, Bhatt K, Dobratz EJ, Darrow DH. Mini septodermoplasty for recurrent epistaxis in children. Presented at: annual meeting of the American Society of Pediatric Otolaryngology; April 2018; Washington, DC

Wertheim HFL, van Kleef M, Vos MC, Ott A, Verbrugh HA, Fokkens W. Nose picking and nasal carriage of *Staphylococcus aureus. Infect Control Hosp Epidemiol.* 2006; 27(8):863–867

CHAPTER 9

Pediatric Nasal and Facial Fractures

T.J. O-Lee, MD

Introduction

Despite advances in child protective measures, trauma remains the leading cause of death of children in the United States. Medical care rendered for all traumatic injuries is valued at greater than $15 billion annually. Pediatric ear, nose, and throat (ENT) trauma accounts for only a small share of this total. Most head and neck injuries consist of soft-tissue trauma, such as laceration, contusion, or abrasion. Bony injuries occur even less frequently. Pediatric maxillofacial injuries account for approximately 5% of all facial fractures, with a reported incidence ranging between 1.5% and 15%. Children younger than 5 years are at a significantly lower risk, ranging from 1% to 1.5%. With increasing age, the incidence of facial fracture increases, ultimately reaching the pattern and frequency of that in adults at around late adolescence.

Diagnosis

In the evaluation of all patients with trauma, airway, breathing, and circulation must first be assessed and restored before treatment is initiated. Following this algorithm is especially important in cases of ENT trauma because injuries of the head and neck can produce dramatic bleeding and distract the treatment team from the most important task: securing the airway.

Once the patient's condition is stabilized, a systematic evaluation should be performed. The ear, nose, and throat should be evaluated separately. Organ functions, such as hearing, nasal patency, and voice, can be important predictors of injury site, but they should not be relied on exclusively because injuries can have subtle or delayed onset of deficits. Evaluating facial symmetry with the patient at rest and in motion is important to assess facial nerve integrity. Progressive breathing or swallowing difficulty can indicate expanding hematoma of the neck or throat.

When suspicion is high for bony or deep-tissue trauma, radiologic imaging often is indicated. A plain radiograph has limited accuracy in the evaluation of the complex bony structures of the face and, therefore, limited applicability. Even in cases of suspected nasal fracture, plain radiographs are infrequently helpful to the treating primary care clinician (PCC). Even though a plain radiograph may show fractures of the nasal bone, such visualization does not affect treatment.

A panoramic radiograph of the mandible, panorex, is obtained with a rotating x-ray source. The result is a linear picture of an otherwise curved mandible. This is likely the most helpful type of plain radiograph in traumatic evaluation of the face and neck. It is sensitive for fractures and often demonstrates the position of the fracture line relative to the teeth and teeth buds.

Computed tomography (CT) is often the study of choice for evaluation of pediatric trauma because of its high resolution and relatively quick procedure time. Compared with magnetic resonance imaging (MRI), CT has better bony resolution and may be performed more quickly than MRI, thereby eliminating the need for general anesthesia. Computed tomographic evaluation of trauma is usually performed without contrast unless deep-tissue bleeding is suspected.

■ Soft-Tissue Injuries

Soft-tissue injury to the face is perhaps the most commonly encountered ENT trauma in pediatric patients. Some general treatment guidelines are as follows:

1. Clean laceration wounds thoroughly, and carefully remove all foreign bodies embedded in the tissue. This process should take place after the wound is adequately anesthetized to minimize secondary trauma to the child and ensure thorough exploration of the wound.

2. Realign the tissue carefully prior to starting repair. Meticulous preservation of tissue will often improve the accuracy of realignment.

3. Close the tissue in layers when possible. This increases the strength of the repair as well as the accuracy of skin approximation. Absorbable sutures should be used whenever possible to avoid the trauma of suture removal for the child.

BITES

Animal and human bites often result in large avulsions of soft tissue. Wounds should be irrigated thoroughly with sterile saline before closure to decrease the bacterial load. Prophylactic antibiotic treatment is indicated, and amoxicillin-clavulanate often is used as a first-line drug to cover oral flora. In children with penicillin allergy, clindamycin or azithromycin often are substituted.

TISSUE LOSS

Any significant tissue loss in a wound presents a challenge to the treating PCC. In the immediate period after the injury, it may not be possible to distinguish viable from nonviable tissue. After a thorough cleaning of the wound, a moist dressing to preserve tissue viability is a reasonable course of action in wounds in which tissue loss prohibits immediate closure. Once the margins of viable tissue are declared, usually within 24 to 48 hours, the use of advancement or other local tissue rotation methods can be considered. Also, skin grafting is an option, although the limited tissue thickness, poor color match, and donor site morbidities diminish the desirability of grafting. Vacuum-assisted wound dressing has shown remarkable results in many instances and should be considered for large wounds.

> **Pearl:** In any trauma assessment, evaluation of the airway, breathing, and circulation must take precedence. Do not become distracted by obvious deformities.

■ Bony Injuries

Great advances have been made in recent decades in treating pediatric facial fractures. Specific techniques used for reconstruction must accommodate a child's developing anatomy, rapid healing, psychological development, and potential for deformity as a consequence of altered facial growth. The prevalence of CT scans enables accurate diagnosis of facial fractures in most instances. Rigid internal fixation has been successfully adapted from adults to pediatric patients with careful modification. Open reduction and rigid internal fixation are indicated for severely displaced fractures. Primary bone grafting is preferred over secondary reconstruction. Alloplastic materials should be avoided when possible.

Associated injuries are a common feature of childhood maxillo-facial trauma. Neurologic and orthopedic injuries are seen in 30% of children with facial fractures, which reinforces the impor-tance of a complete initial assessment of a child with facial trauma and highlights the dilemma with regard to the timing of the reconstruction because of the rapid healing of bony injuries in children.

> **Pearl:** Assessment via computed tomography is preferred over magnetic resonance imaging in cases of trauma because of its higher bony resolution and quicker procedure time. Contrast is not needed to evaluate fractures.

NOSE

Nasal fractures are by far the most common facial bone injuries in chil-dren, followed by dentoalveolar injuries. Nose fractures usually are treated in the outpatient setting and do not require surgical inter-vention. The need for treatment is not dictated by the presence of fracture but by the presence of functional or cosmetic deficits. A nasal obstruction or an external nasal deformity that persists after 3 to 5 days requires a referral to pediatric otolaryngology. Assessment within the first 3 to 5 days is likely to be confounded by tissue swelling and ecchymosis.

The initial examination of a child with nasal fracture may be limited owing to midfacial swelling. The swelling subsides after several days, at which time the true extent of the deformity can be appreciated. On the other hand, immediate intranasal examination is necessary to detect the presence of septal hematoma (**Figure 9-1**). Although rarely seen, septal hematoma can be observed on anterior

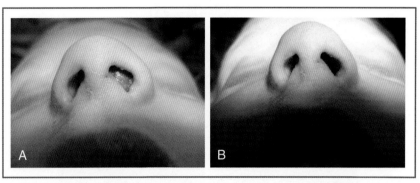

Figure 9-1. A, Nasal septal hematoma visible inside the left nostril. B, Nasal septum after drainage of the hematoma in the same patient.

rhinoscopy as an obvious purple bulge on 1 side of the nose. The bulge is compressible with a cotton tip applicator and does not shrink with topical vasoconstriction. A septal hematoma requires immediate evacuation on detection. An untreated hematoma can become a thick, fibrotic, and obstructive septum. If the hematoma becomes infected, the resulting loss of cartilage can cause a saddle nose deformity.

For isolated nasal fractures, plain radiographs are rarely helpful. A nondisplaced fracture on a radiograph requires no treatment. In addition, a displaced fracture for which closed reduction is warranted is obvious on physical examination. Therefore, plain radiographs rarely change the management of nasal injuries.

In cases of nasal fracture without septal hematoma, the patient should be seen by a specialist within 3 to 4 days after the injury. This delay allows swelling and ecchymosis to dissipate, facilitating a more accurate and thorough evaluation while respecting the 10-day window within which cosmetically or functionally significant fractures can be reduced. Closed reduction of the bony fracture can be performed with intranasal instrumentation and bimanual external manipulation (**Figure 9-2**). If significant dislocations are present or if the injury is more than 2 weeks old, open reduction may be necessary.

> **Pearl:** Evaluation of nasal fractures should be conducted primarily via physical examination. Plain radiography is rarely helpful.

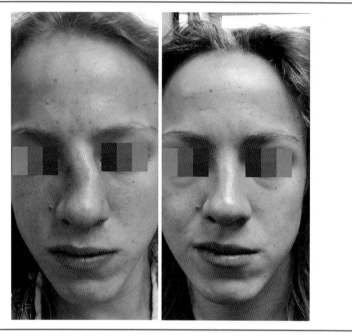

Figure 9-2. Nasal fracture with right nasal depression and shifting of the nasal dorsum. Left, preintervention. Right, 2 weeks after a closed nasal reduction.

MANDIBLE

Fractures of the mandible are the most common facial fractures requiring hospitalization. They account for 30% to 50% of all pediatric facial fractures after nasal fractures are excluded. Because pediatric condyles are highly vascularized, and thin necks are poorly resistant to impact forces, the most vulnerable part of the pediatric mandible is the condyle. More than 50% of pediatric mandibular fractures involve 1 of the condyles, whereas only 30% of mandibular fractures in adults involve the condyles. As patients mature, the frequency of symphyseal, body, and ramus fractures increases.

Clinical signs of mandibular fractures may include displacement of the fragments, mobility, swelling, mucosal tears, limited mouth opening, malocclusion, and pain. Clinical suspicion of a fracture is confirmed by panoramic radiography, a complete mandibular series of plain radiographs, or CT scan. Computed tomography is especially helpful in determining 3-dimensional displacement of the condyles.

Immobilization is difficult in patients younger than 2 years because of incomplete eruption of the primary teeth; however, later growth and remodeling frequently compensate for less-than-ideal postinjury alignment. The primary teeth, which develop firm roots at ages 2 to 5 years, can be used for splints and arch bars. Roots of primary teeth are resorbed at ages 6 to 12 years. Therefore, arch bars may need extra support from circummandibular wiring and pyriform aperture suspension. Permanent teeth are safe anchors for fixation after 13 years of age.

The central consideration when treating pediatric condylar fractures is whether the patient needs immobilization. Although minimally invasive endoscopic open reduction with internal fixation (ORIF) is gaining popularity in treating adult condylar fractures, most authors still advocate conservative measures in pediatric patients. If the patient has normal occlusion and normal mandibular movement, only a soft diet and movement exercises are necessary. However, if open bite deformities with retrusion of the mandible and movement limitation are present, immobilization lasting 2 to 3 weeks followed by use of guiding elastics can yield normal function.

Displaced symphysis fractures can be treated by ORIF through an intraoral incision in children older than 6 years, after the permanent incisors have erupted. Open reduction with internal fixation in para-symphyseal fractures is possible once buds of the canines have moved up from the mandibular border after age 9 years. In body fractures, the inferior mandibular border can be plated when buds of the permanent premolar and molar have migrated superiorly toward the alveolus.

Frequent postoperative follow-up visits are necessary to detect and treat early complications, such as infection, malocclusion, malunion, and nonunion. Late complications such as damage to permanent teeth, temporomandibular joint dysfunction, or midface deformity with facial asymmetry also need attention and possible treatment.

ORBITS

Because of the very thin bones of the orbital walls, fractures are not infrequent, accounting for 20% to 25% of pediatric facial fractures. Medial orbital wall and orbital floor fractures are more common than other facial fractures for the same reason. The mechanism of injury is often direct trauma to the eye or a surrounding structure. Such pressure causes the orbital contents to explode beyond the normal boundary, thus fracturing the bones.

In assessing orbital injuries, the PCC needs to document visual acuity, ocular pressure, and extraocular movements. Diplopia is a sensitive measure of extraocular movement deficit in a cooperative patient. All visual fields need to be inspected before diagnosing diplopia.

The treatment of isolated blowout fractures is symptom dependent. In an asymptomatic patient, no intervention is necessary because fractures will heal spontaneously. If persistent enophthalmos, extraocular muscle restriction, or pain on eye movement is present, surgical exploration is indicated. Large fractures also are routinely explored, as are fractures that on CT entail obvious muscle entrapment (**Figure 9-3**). Absorbable gelatin film usually is sufficient for reconstructing small defects of the orbital floor, while large disruptions are best repaired with calvarial bone grafts.

Orbital roof fractures occur in very young children whose frontal sinuses are underdeveloped. These fractures are often associated with skull injuries.

Orbital roof fractures in children are different from those in adults. They occur more frequently because of the lack of frontal sinus pneumatization. Children have a craniofacial ratio of 8:1 at birth, compared with 2:1 in adults, thus exposing more of their

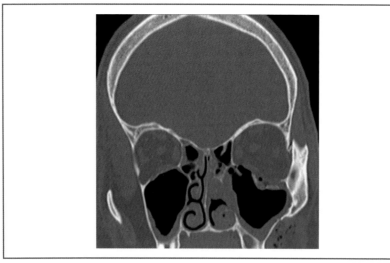

Figure 9-3. Coronal computed tomographic scan demonstrating multiple fractures of the left orbit, including a large orbital floor fracture with herniation of soft tissue into the maxillary sinus.

cranium and skull base to potential injuries. Most orbital roof fractures, particularly those that are nondisplaced or with fragments displaced superiorly (blowout fractures), can be safely observed in the acute setting. Treatment should be directed by the presence of symptoms, such as extraocular muscle entrapment, enophthalmos, exophthalmos, diplopia, vision changes, or dystopia. Large blow-in fractures have a higher chance of resulting in late-onset complications; therefore, surgical thresholds should be lower. Depending on the extent and location of the orbital roof fracture, various approaches are available. Cooperation among neurosurgery, ophthalmology, and head and neck surgery is essential to ensure optimal care for patients.

MIDFACE

Midfacial fractures are rare in children and usually result from high-impact, high-velocity forces such as motor vehicle crashes. Zygomaticomalar complex (ZMC) fractures are seen in 10% to 15% of midfacial fractures, and Le Fort maxillary fractures are seen in 5% to 10% of cases. A free-floating nasal base is a rare injury and indicates a nasoethmoidal fracture.

Zygomaticomalar complex fractures parallel the pneumatization of the maxillary sinus and are uncommon before the age of 5 years. Surgical correction of ZMC fractures is indicated when bony displacement is present. Adequate exposure is essential, and such correction is achieved by a process called *triangulation*. Three key sites need to be directly visualized: the frontozygomatic suture, infraorbital rim, and anterior zygomaticomaxillary buttress. Access can be achieved via the lateral upper eyelid incision, lower eyelid infraciliary or transconjunctival incision, or transoral buccal sulcus incision. Unlike in adults, 1-point fixation at the frontozygomatic suture may suffice in children because of shorter lever arm forces from the frontozygomatic suture to the infraorbital rim.

In ethmonasal fractures, medial canthal ligament integrity must be assessed by inserting a hemostat into the nose toward the medial orbital rim. The child should be anesthetized for this examination. Mobility of the underlying fragments suggests that the bone with its canthal attachment has been displaced and that reconstruction of the nasal maxillary buttress and possible transnasal wiring are necessary. Measurement of soft-tissue intercanthal distance is difficult because ethnic, racial, and gender variations can significantly affect the results. Nevertheless, the average intercanthal distance at 4 years of age is approximately 25 mm; by age 12 years, 28 mm; and by adulthood, 30 mm. Thus, a near-adult intercanthal distance is achieved at a very young age; hence, an easy mistake is to set the intercanthal distance too wide. Intercanthal distances that are 5 mm greater than the average values tend to be indicative of—and 10 mm confirms the diagnosis of—displaced fractures of the ethmonasal complex. Attempts should be made to narrow the excessive distance between the eyes and protect the nose of the child.

■ Conclusion

Children of all ages can experience ENT trauma, often resulting in functional and cosmetic deficits. A thorough understanding of pediatric skull and facial growth enables PCCs to focus the search for subtle fractures on the most age-appropriate locations. Soft-tissue injuries often can point to possible locations of fracture and should be carefully treated. Anticipation of mandibular growth facilitates repair because most injuries can be treated with intermaxillary fixation. Unerupted dentition requires careful selection of fixation methods and cautious screw placement if rigid fixation is ultimately required. Modern rigid plating systems have greatly enhanced surgeons' ability to reconstruct facial fractures in a 3-dimensional fashion. Depending on the site of injury, a multidisciplinary team approach can ensure that injuries to organ systems around the face are cared for in an optimal manner.

■ Selected References

Caldicott WJ, North JB, Simpson DA. Traumatic cerebrospinal fluid fistulas in children. *J Neurosurg*. 1973;38(1):1–9

Gussack GS, Luterman A, Powell RW, Rodgers K, Ramenofsky ML. Pediatric maxillofacial trauma: unique features in diagnosis and treatment. *Laryngoscope*. 1987;97(8 Pt 1):925–930

Hardt N, Gottsauner A. The treatment of mandibular fractures in children. *J Cranio-maxillofac Surg*. 1993;21(5):214–219

Hogg NJ, Horswell BB. Soft tissue pediatric facial trauma: a review. *J Can Dent Assoc*. 2006;72(6):549–552

Holland AJ, Broome C, Steinberg A, Cass DT. Facial fractures in children. *Pediatr Emerg Care*. 2001;17(3):157–160

Kaban LB. Diagnosis and treatment of fractures of the facial bones in children 1943-1993. *J Oral Maxillofac Surg*. 1993;51(7):722–729

Kaban LB, Mulliken JB, Murray JE. Facial fractures in children: an analysis of 122 fractures in 109 patients. *Plast Reconstr Surg.* 1977;59(1):15–20

Koltai PJ. Maxillofacial injuries in children. In: Smith JD, Bumstead RM, eds. *Pediatric Facial Plastic and Reconstructive Surgery.* New York, NY: Raven Press; 1993

Koltai PJ, Rabkin D. Management of facial trauma in children. *Pediatr Clin North Am.* 1996;43(6):1253–1275

Koltai PJ, Rabkin D, Hoehn J. Rigid fixation of facial fractures in children. *J Craniomaxillofac Trauma.* 1995;1(2):32–42

Law RC, Fouque CA, Waddell A, Cusick E. Lesson of the week. Penetrating intra-oral trauma in children. *BMJ.* 1997;314(7073):50–51

Lee D, Honrado C, Har-El G, Goldsmith A. Pediatric temporal bone fractures. *Laryngoscope.* 1998;108(6):816–821

Liu-Shindo M, Hawkins DB. Basilar skull fractures in children. *Int J Pediatr Otorhinolaryngol.* 1989;17(2):109–117

Marom T, Russo E, Ben-Yehuda Y, Roth Y. Oropharyngeal injuries in children. *Pediatr Emerg Care.* 2007;23(12):914–918

McGraw BL, Cole RR. Pediatric maxillofacial trauma: age-related variations in injury. *Arch Otolaryngol Head Neck Surg.* 1990;116(1):41–45

McGuirt WF Jr, Stool SE. Cerebrospinal fluid fistula: the identification and management in pediatric temporal bone fractures. *Laryngoscope.* 1995;105(4 Pt 1):359–364

McGuirt WF Jr, Stool SE. Temporal bone fractures in children: a review with emphasis on long-term sequelae. *Clin Pediatr (Phila).* 1992;31(1):12–18

Nicol JW, Johnstone AJ. Temporal bone fractures in children: a review of 34 cases. *J Accid Emerg Med.* 1994;11(4):218–222

Pierrot S, Bernardeschi D, Morrisseau-Durand MP, Manach Y, Couloigner V. Dissection of the internal carotid artery following trauma of the soft palate in children. *Ann Otol Rhinol Laryngol.* 2006;115(5):323–329

Posnick JC, Wells M, Pron GE. Pediatric facial fractures: evolving patterns of treatment. *J Oral Maxillofac Surg.* 1993;51(8):836–844

Rowe NL. Fractures of the facial skeleton in children. *J Oral Surg.* 1968;26(8):505–515

Shapiro RS. Temporal bone fractures in children. *Otolaryngol Head Neck Surg.* 1979; 87(3):323–329

Stefanopoulos PK, Tarantzopoulou AD. Facial bite wounds: management update. *Int J Oral Maxillofac Surg.* 2005;34(5):464–472

Thorén H, Iizuka T, Hallikainen D, Lindqvist C. Different patterns of mandibular fractures in children: an analysis of 220 fractures in 157 patients. *J Craniomaxillofac Surg.* 1992;20(7):292–296

Troulis MJ, Kaban LB. Endoscopic approach to the ramus/condyle unit: clinical applications. *J Oral Maxillofac Surg.* 2001;59(5):503–509

von Domarus H, Poeschel W. Impalement injuries of the palate. *Plast Reconstr Surg.* 1983;72(5):656–658

Williams WT, Ghorayeb BY, Yeakley JW. Pediatric temporal bone fractures. *Laryngoscope.* 1992;102(6):600–603

Oropharynx

CHAPTER 10

Disorders of the Tonsils and Adenoid

David H. Darrow, MD, DDS, and Cristina M. Baldassari, MD

▦ Introduction

Adenotonsillar disorders in children occur as a result of hyperplasia, infection, inflammation, or malignancy. Hyperplasia is a natural consequence of immune activity within these tissues but may become problematic when tissue size becomes excessive for the pharyngeal space they occupy. Infection of the tonsils and adenoid is common in children because of their participation in immune processes and continuous exposure to inhaled and ingested antigens. Malignancy of the tonsils and adenoid, in contrast, is exceedingly rare. This chapter will review the functions of the tonsils and adenoid, diagnosis and management of diseases of these tissues, and appropriate indications for their surgical removal.

▦ Functions of Tonsils and Adenoid

The palatine tonsils and adenoid are tissues of Waldeyer ring, a group of lymphoepithelial tissues that also includes tubal tonsils in the nasopharynx and the lingual tonsil. Collectively, these tissues participate in the mucosal immune system of the pharynx. Positioned strategically at the entrance of the gastrointestinal and respiratory tracts, the tonsils and adenoid serve as secondary lymphoid organs, initiating immune responses against antigens entering the body through the mouth or nose. The size of the tonsils appears to correlate with their level of immunologic activity, peaking between the ages of 3 and 10 years and demonstrating age-dependent involution. Some evidence also shows that their size increases with bacterial load.

Tonsils are covered by a nonkeratinizing, stratified, squamous epithelium featuring some 10 to 30 deep crypts that effectively increase the surface area exposed to incoming antigens. The crypts occasionally harbor degenerated cells and debris that give rise to so-called tonsilloliths, in which the presence of biofilms has also been implicated. Although tonsils lack afferent lymphatics, the epithelium contains a system of specialized channels lined by M cells that take up antigens into vesicles and transport them to the intraepithelial and subepithelial spaces where they are presented to lymphoid cells. The transport function of M cells serves as a portal for mucosal infections and immunizations. M cells also can initiate immunologic responses within the epithelium, introducing foreign antigens to lymphocytes and antigen-presenting cells (APCs).

After passing through the crypt epithelium, inhaled or ingested antigens reach the extrafollicular region or lymphoid follicles. In the extrafollicular region, APCs process antigens and present them to helper T lymphocytes that stimulate proliferation of follicular B lymphocytes. B lymphocytes ultimately develop into 1 of 2 types of cell—antibody-expressing B memory cells capable of migration to the nasopharynx and other sites, or plasma cells that produce antibodies and release them into crypt lumen. Tonsillar plasma cells can produce all 5 immunoglobulin (Ig) classes helping to combat and prevent infection. In addition, contact of memory B cells in the lymphoid follicles with antigen is an essential part of the generation of a secondary immune response.

Among immunoglobulin isotypes, IgA may be considered the most important product of the adenotonsillar immune system. In its dimeric form, IgA can attach to the transmembrane secretory component (SC) to form secretory IgA (SIgA), a critical component of the mucosal immune system of the upper airway. This component is necessary for binding of IgA monomers to each other and to the SC and is an important product of B-cell activity in tonsil follicles. While tonsils produce immunocytes bearing the J (joining) chain carbohydrate, SC is produced only in the adenoid and extratonsillar epithelium, and, therefore, only the adenoid possesses a local secretory immune system.

> **Pearl:** The tonsils and adenoid are secondary sources of circulating B lymphocytes, but only the adenoid and extratonsillar lymphoid tissues, not the tonsils, possess a local secretory immune system.

■ Infectious and Inflammatory Diseases of Tonsils and Adenoid

Pharyngotonsillitis is a general term used to describe diffuse inflammation of structures of the oropharynx, including the tonsils. The disorder presents with the symptom of sore throat; however, objective signs of inflammation must be present to make the diagnosis. Pharyngotonsillitis may be classified as acute, subacute, or chronic based on the duration of symptoms, with most patients presenting acutely. Alternatively, inflammatory disease of the nasopharynx may be considered *nasopharyngitis,* in which common symptoms include rhinorrhea, nasal congestion, sneezing, and cough. Inflammation limited to the adenoid pad (adenoiditis) is difficult to diagnose in the primary care setting because of inaccessibility of this tissue to direct visualization.

COMMON VIRAL INFECTION

Nasopharyngitis typically occurs in cold weather months among young children during their early exposures to respiratory viruses. Adenoviruses, influenza viruses, parainfluenza viruses, and enteroviruses are the most common etiologic agents. Rhinovirus and respiratory syncytial virus occur almost exclusively in preschool-age children and are rarely associated with overt signs of pharyngeal inflammation. Adenoviruses are more common among older children and adolescents. Nasopharyngitis of viral etiology may also cause a concomitant pharyngotonsillitis. The infection is most commonly acute and self-limited, with symptoms resolving within 10 days. Nonviral agents are associated less frequently with nasopharyngitis but may include *Corynebacterium diphtheriae, Neisseria meningitidis, Haemophilus influenzae,* and *Coxiella burnetii.*

Viruses responsible for pharyngotonsillitis are more diverse than those in nasopharyngitis; adenoviruses, influenza viruses, parainfluenza viruses, enteroviruses, Epstein-Barr virus (EBV), and *Mycoplasma* account for about 70% of these infections. As in nasopharyngitis, most viral pharyngotonsillitis requires no specific therapy.

GROUP A β-HEMOLYTIC STREPTOCOCCAL INFECTION

Group A β-hemolytic streptococcus (GABHS) is the most common bacterium associated with pharyngotonsillitis in children. In the 8 decades since the advent of antibiotics, most pharyngeal infections by GABHS have been benign, self-limited, and uncomplicated processes. In fact, most patients improve symptomatically without any medical intervention whatsoever. However, a small number of affected children continue to develop renal and cardiac complications following GABHS infection, and some authors have implicated GABHS in the development of common childhood neuropsychiatric disorders (PANDAS; see page 201). In addition, there is evidence that early antibiotic therapy may be useful in treating symptoms of GABHS. As a result, appropriate diagnosis and treatment of these infections are imperative. Some critical yet underrecognized concepts in the management of GABHS are listed in **Box 10-1**.

> ## Box 10-1. Key Concepts in the Management of GABHS
>
> 1. Symptoms of group A β-hemolytic streptococcus (GABHS) infection resolve without treatment; the purpose of antimicrobial therapy is prevention of suppurative and nonsuppurative sequelae.
> 2. No naturally occurring penicillin-resistant strains of GABHS have been identified.
> 3. Patients with recurrent sore throat need not be cultured if associated symptoms are suggestive of a viral illness.
> 4. Carriers rarely spread GABHS to close contacts, and there is no evidence that the disease is spread by pets or toothbrushes.
> 5. The importance of identifying GABHS carriers is in determining whether their sore throats associated with positive cultures may be due to viral infection rather than acute streptococcal infection.
> 6. Asymptomatic patients with positive culture results following treatment need not undergo retreatment.

The incidence of GABHS pharyngitis has not been estimated on the basis of population-based data. Nevertheless, "strep throat" is well recognized as a common disease among children and adolescents. The incidence peaks during winter and spring and is more common in cooler, temperate climates. Close contact in schools, military quarters, dormitories, and families with several children appears to be a risk factor for the disease.

Transmission of GABHS is believed to occur through droplet spread. Individuals are most infectious early in the course of the disease, and risk of contagion depends on the inoculum size and virulence of the infecting strain. The incubation period is usually between 1 and 4 days. After antimicrobial therapy is begun, most primary care clinicians (PCCs) will allow affected children to return to school within 36 to 48 hours. The role of individuals colonized with GABHS in the spread of the disease is uncertain, although data suggest that carriers rarely spread the disease to close contacts.

Streptococci are gram-positive catalase-negative cocci characterized by their growth in long chains or pairs in culture. These organisms are traditionally classified into 18 groups with letter designations (Lancefield groups) based on the antigenic carbohydrate component of their cell walls. While GABHS is isolated from most patients with streptococcal pharyngitis, group C, G, and B streptococci also occasionally cause this disorder. Further subclassification of streptococci is made based on their ability to lyse sheep red blood cells in culture;

β-hemolytic strains cause hemolysis associated with a clear zone surrounding their colonies, while α-hemolytic strains cause partial hemolysis, and gamma-hemolytic strains cause no hemolysis. Alpha-hemolytic strains are normal flora of the oral cavity and pharynx and should not be confused with the more pathogenic β-hemolytic strains.

The primary determinant of streptococcal pathogenicity is an antigenically distinct protein known as the *M protein*. This molecule is found within the fimbriae, which are fingerlike projections from the cell wall of the organism that facilitate adherence to pharyngeal and tonsillar epithelium. More than 120 M serotypes are known. The M protein allows *Streptococcus* to resist phagocytosis in the absence of type-specific antibody. In the immunocompetent host, synthesis of type-specific anti-M and other antibodies confers long-term serotype-specific immunity to the particular strain in question. In laboratory-produced penicillin-resistant strains of GABHS, M protein is absent, thereby rendering these strains more vulnerable to phagocytosis. This finding may help to explain why there have been no naturally occur-ring penicillin-resistant GABHS isolated in more than 70 years of penicillin use.

Group A β-hemolytic streptococci are capable of elaborating at least 20 extracellular substances that affect host tissue. Among the most important are streptolysin O, an oxygen-labile hemolysin, and streptolysin S, an oxygen-stable hemolysin, which lyse erythrocytes and damage other cells such as myocardial cells. Streptolysin O is anti-genic, while streptolysin S is not. Group A β-hemolytic streptococci also produce 3 erythrogenic or pyrogenic toxins (A, B, and C) whose activity is similar to that of bacterial endotoxin. Other agents of signifi-cance include exotoxin A, which may be associated with toxic shock syndrome, and bacteriocins, which destroy other gram-positive organ-isms. Spread of infection may be facilitated by a variety of enzymes elaborated by GABHS that attack fibrin and hyaluronic acid.

Signs and symptoms of GABHS pharyngotonsillitis are acute in onset, usually characterized by high fever, odynophagia, headache, and abdominal pain. However, presentation may vary from mild sore throat and malaise (30%–50% of cases) to high fever, nausea and vomiting, and dehydration (10%). Pharyngeal and tonsillar mucosa are typically erythematous and occasionally edematous, with exudate present in 50% to 90% of cases. Cervical adenopathy is also common and is seen in 30% to 60% of cases. Most patients improve sponta-neously in 3 to 5 days, unless otitis media, sinusitis, or peritonsillar abscess occurs secondarily.

The risk of developing rheumatic fever following GABHS infection of the pharynx is approximately 0.3% in endemic situations and 3% under epidemic circumstances. A single episode of rheumatic fever places an individual at high risk for recurrence following additional episodes of GABHS pharyngitis. Acute glomerulonephritis occurs as a sequela in 10% to 15% of patients infected with nephritogenic strains. In patients who develop these sequelae, there is usually a latent period of 1 to 3 weeks.

Pediatric autoimmune neuropsychiatric disorder associated with group A streptococcal infection (PANDAS) has been described as a selective immunopathy similar to Sydenham chorea in which the response to streptococcal infection leads to dysfunction in the basal ganglia, resulting in tic, obsessive-compulsive, and affective disorders. Classically, behaviors are abrupt in onset and must have some temporal relationship to infection by GABHS. Clinical improvement has been reported among some patients treated with antibiotics, particularly as prophylaxis against recurrence. However, a cause-and-effect association of PANDAS with GABHS infection has yet to be established. Many experts believe that infection of any kind may provoke the neuropsychiatric phenomena, as has been observed with other stressors.

Early diagnosis of streptococcal pharyngitis has been a priority in management of the disease, primarily because of the risk of renal and cardiac sequelae. A number of authors have studied the predictive value of various combinations of signs and symptoms in an effort to distinguish streptococcal from nonstreptococcal pharyngitis; however, none of these has been particularly reliable. Taken together, these studies demonstrate a false-negative rate of about 50% and a false-positive rate of 75%. Adenopathy, fever, and pharyngeal exudate have the highest predictive value for a positive culture and rise in anti-streptolysin O (ASO) titer, and absence of these findings in the presence of cough, rhinorrhea, hoarseness, or conjunctivitis most reliably predicts a negative culture or a positive culture without rise in ASO.

Most PCCs advocate throat culture as the gold standard to determine the appropriate treatment of GABHS. For greatest accuracy, the tonsils, tonsillar crypts, or posterior pharyngeal wall must be swabbed. Tests for rapid detection of group-specific carbohydrate simplify the decision to treat at the time of the office visit and often eliminate the need for additional postvisit communication. However, while these tests have demonstrated a specificity of greater than 95%, most studies suggest a sensitivity in the 70% to 90% range. As a result, many PCCs advocate throat culture for children with suspected streptococcal disease and negative findings on traditional rapid strep tests. Several nucleic acid amplification tests and polymerase chain reaction recently received approval by the US Food and Drug Administration, and the sensitivity of these tests has been found to be similar to that of throat culture, obviating the need for follow-up cultures. Rapid antigen detection is usually more expensive than throat culture, and this technique still must be interpreted with care given the high incidence of posttreatment carriers. Studies also suggest possible bias in interpretation of the test results.

Carriage of GABHS may be defined as a positive culture for the organism in the absence of a rise in ASO convalescent titer or absence of symptoms. The prevalence of GABHS carriers has been estimated at anywhere from 5% to 50% depending on the time of year and location; however, the percentage is sometimes overestimated because of the use of antibiotics that occasionally interfere with a rise in ASO titer. Carriers are at low risk of transmitting GABHS or of developing symptoms or sequelae of the disease. The importance of this condition is in distinguishing true acute streptococcal pharyngitis from nonstreptococcal sore throat in a carrier. When this distinction is important, a baseline convalescent ASO titer should be drawn. A subsequent positive test result may be defined as a 2-fold dilution increase in titer between acute and convalescent serum, or any single value above 333 Todd units in children. However, a low titer does not rule out acute infection, and a high titer may represent infection in the distant past. As a result, the American Academy of Pediatrics (AAP) and Infectious Diseases Society of America currently recommend that testing for GABHS should not be performed in children with conjunctivitis, cough, hoarseness, coryza, diarrhea, oral ulcerations, or other clinical manifestations highly suggestive of viral infection. Furthermore, patients referred for potential tonsillectomy for "recurrent strep" must be ruled out as carriers before they are considered candidates for surgery.

Although most upper respiratory infections caused by GABHS resolve without treatment, studies suggest that antimicrobial therapy prevents suppurative and nonsuppurative sequelae, including rheumatic fever, and may also hasten clinical improvement. Therefore, treatment is indicated for most patients with positive rapid test results for the group A antigen. When the test result is negative or not available, one may treat for a few days while formal throat cultures are incubating.

Group A β-hemolytic streptococcus is sensitive to several classes of antibiotics, including penicillins, cephalosporins, macrolides, and clindamycin. Expert panels have designated penicillin the drug of choice in managing GABHS because of its track record of safety, efficacy, and narrow spectrum. To date, no strains of GABHS acquired in vivo have demonstrated penicillin resistance or increased minimum inhibitory concentrations in vitro. Beginning in the 1980s, several studies reported a decrease in bacteriologic control rates, attributed primarily to inoculum effects and increased tolerance to penicillin. Whether cephalosporins may achieve greater eradication of GABHS than penicillin remains controversial.

Depot benzathine penicillin G is still advocated by the American Heart Association for primary treatment of GABHS pharyngitis; however, a 10-day course of oral penicillin is the most widely prescribed regimen. Twice-daily dosing by the enteral route yields similar results to those obtained with 4-times-per-day dosing. Courses of shorter duration are associated with bacteriologic relapse and are less efficacious in preventing rheumatic fever. The efficacy of amoxicillin appears to be equal to that of penicillin. In poorly compliant or penicillin-allergic patients, azithromycin dosed once daily for 5 days may be a reasonable alternative. Erythromycin is now used less commonly than in the past because of its gastrointestinal side effects.

Most patients with positive cultures after treatment are GABHS carriers; these individuals need not undergo retreatment if their symptoms have resolved. For patients in whom complete bacteriologic clearance is desirable, such as those with a family member with a history of rheumatic fever, a course of clindamycin or a second course of penicillin combined with rifampin may yield increased success. In patients with recurrent symptoms, serotyping may aid in distinguishing bacterial persistence from recurrence. No data are available regarding the use of antibiotic prophylaxis in these patients, and in such cases, tonsillectomy may sometimes be advantageous.

During antimicrobial therapy, patients must be monitored carefully for fluid intake, pain control, and impending suppurative complications such as peritonsillar abscess. Small children may become dehydrated rapidly and may require hospitalization for intravenous administration of fluids.

INFECTIOUS MONONUCLEOSIS, EPSTEIN-BARR VIRAL INFECTION, AND POSTTRANSPLANTATION LYMPHOPROLIFERATIVE DISORDER

Pharyngitis is one of the hallmarks of infectious mononucleosis, a disorder associated with primary infection by EBV. The universality of exposure to EBV is demonstrated by studies in populations around the world in which 80% to 95% of adults exhibited serologic reactivity to EBV antigens. However, while primary infection by EBV occurs during the second and third decade in developed nations and regions of high socioeconomic status, young children may still be exposed, especially in developing countries and regions with low socioeconomic status. When the virus is acquired at a younger age, symptoms are generally less severe.

The incidence of infectious mononucleosis in the United States is approximately 1 per 50,000 to 100,000 per year, but the incidence increases to about 100 per 100,000 among adolescents and young adults. Infected individuals transmit EBV by way of saliva exchanged during kissing or other close contact.

Epstein-Barr virus is a member of the herpesvirus family that preferentially infects and transforms human B lymphocytes. The virus enters the cell by attaching to a receptor designed for proteins of the complement chain, and its genetic material is transported by vesicles to the nucleus, where it dwells as a plasmid and maintains a latent state of replication. An incubation period of 2 to 7 weeks follows the initial exposure, during which EBV induces a proliferation of infected B cells. This process is subsequently countered by a potent cellular immune response, characterized by the appearance of atypical lymphocytes (most likely T lymphocytes responding to the B-cell infection) in the blood. The number of infected circulating B cells is reduced during this 4- to 6-week period.

Infectious mononucleosis is characterized by a prodrome of malaise and fatigue, followed by acute onset of fever and sore throat. The physical examination typically reveals enlarged, erythematous palatine tonsils, in most cases with yellow-white exudate on the surface and within the crypts. Cervical adenopathy is present in nearly all patients, and involvement of the posterior cervical nodes often helps distinguish EBV infection from infection by streptococcus or other organisms. Between the second and fourth weeks of illness, approximately 50% of patients develop splenomegaly, and 30% to 50% develop hepatomegaly. Rash, palatal petechiae, and abdominal pain also may be present in some cases. Fever and pharyngitis generally subside within about 2 weeks, while adenopathy, organomegaly, and malaise may last as long as 6 weeks.

A diagnosis of infectious mononucleosis can usually be made on the basis of clinical presentation, absolute lymphocytosis, presence of atypical lymphocytes in the peripheral smear, and detection of Paul-Bunnell heterophil antibodies. The latter is the basis of monospot assays, which screen for agglutination of horse erythrocytes. Children younger than 5 years may not develop a detectable heterophil antibody titer; in these patients, it is possible to determine titers of IgG antibodies to the viral capsid antigen, as well as antibodies to the early antigen complex. Antibodies to EBV nuclear antigen appear late in the course of disease (**Table 10-1**). In most cases, rest, fluids, and analgesics are adequate to manage symptoms of infectious mononucleosis. In more symptomatic patients, particularly those with respiratory compromise caused by severe tonsillar enlargement and those with hematologic or neurologic complications, a course of systemic steroids may hasten resolution of acute symptoms. Placement of a nasopharyngeal trumpet or endotracheal intubation may be necessary on rare occasions when complete airway obstruction is imminent. Antibiotics may be useful in cases of concomitant group A β-hemolytic pharyngotonsillitis; however, ampicillin is known to induce a rash in this setting.

> **Pearl:** Children younger than 5 years may not develop a detectable heterophil antibody titer and should undergo serologic testing for Epstein-Barr viral capsid antigen and early antigen.

The use of antiviral agents in infectious mononucleosis has yielded disappointing results. In clinical trials, acyclovir reduced viral shedding in the pharynx but demonstrated little efficacy in the

Table 10-1. Expected Results of Serologic Testing for Epstein-Barr Virus (EBV)			
	Never Been Infected With EBV	**Infected With EBV Now**	**Infected With EBV in Past**
Antiviral capsid antigen	Negative	Positive	Positive
Anti–Epstein-Barr nuclear antigen	Negative	Negative	Positive

treatment of symptoms. Other agents have exhibited greater in vitro effect than acyclovir but have yet to be tested clinically.

Exposure to EBV has been implicated in the development of post-transplantation lymphoproliferative disorder (PTLD). Children who have received bone marrow and solid organ transplants may develop abnormal proliferation of lymphoid cells in the setting of immunosuppression; approximately 80% of affected individuals have a history of EBV infection. Epstein-Barr virus seronegative transplant recipients may develop acute EBV infection from environmental exposure or from the EBV-seropositive donor once they become immunosuppressed. Clinical presentation is variable and can mimic graft-versus-host disease, graft rejection, or more conventional infections. Signs and symptoms may resemble an infectious mononucleosis–like illness or an extranodal tumor, commonly involving the gut, brain, or transplanted organ. Mononucleosis-like presentations typically occur in children within the first year after transplantation and are often associated with primary EBV infection after transfer of donor virus from the grafted organ. Extranodal tumors are more common among EBV-seropositive recipients several years after transplantation. Studies have shown that young age at the time of transplantation and EBV seronegativity conferred an increased risk of adenotonsillar hyperplasia, which may be a precursor to PTLD. A higher incidence of PTLD has also been demonstrated with use of more potent immunosuppressive agents.

Initial management involves reduction of immunosuppression with care to preserve the transplanted organ. Patients who do not tolerate or respond to reduction of immunosuppression require more aggressive therapy and often have a poorer prognosis. Additional treatments include antivirals such as acyclovir and ganciclovir, antibody therapy, interferon, chemotherapy, and radiation therapy, with varying results. Prognosis is poor, with mortality rates as high as 50% to 90%. Novel forms of immunotherapy have been tested in PTLD, including antibody and cell-mediated approaches.

Pearl: Patients with a history of organ transplantation who develop tonsil enlargement should be evaluated for posttransplantation lymphoproliferative disorder, a condition linked to Epstein-Barr virus infection.

PERITONSILLAR INFECTION

Peritonsillar infection may present as cellulitis or abscess (PTA). Most cases are thought to represent a suppurative complication of tonsil infection. Peritonsillar infection occurs more commonly in adolescents and young adults than in young children. Affected individuals have symptoms of sore throat, odynophagia, fever, voice change, and otalgia. Common physical findings include fever, drooling, trismus, muffled "hot potato" voice, and pharyngeal asymmetry, with inferior and medial displacement of the tonsil. Radiographic evaluation is usually not necessary but may be useful in young or uncooperative children or in equivocal cases. Although some authors have found intraoral ultrasound to be useful in adults, computed tomography with contrast remains the imaging modality of choice in children.

While patients with peritonsillar cellulitis may be treated with antibiotics alone, most abscesses require removal of the pus as definitive therapy. Evacuation of PTA can be managed by needle aspiration, incision and drainage, or immediate (quinsy) tonsillectomy, with nearly equivalent efficacy. In very young or poorly cooperative patients, or in those in whom an abscess has been inadequately drained, tonsillectomy is curative and essentially eliminates any chance of recurrence.

Abscess cultures usually reveal a polymicrobial infection, often containing gram-positive organisms and anaerobes. Appropriate antimicrobial therapy in the emergency department or office setting includes initial parenteral administration of penicillin, with or without metronidazole, clindamycin, or ampicillin-sulbactam. Options for oral therapy include amoxicillin-clavulanate, penicillin, and clindamycin, although children may resist taking the latter due to its taste. Intravenous hydration also should be considered for those individuals who have not been able to take liquids orally.

The efficacy of tonsillectomy in the prevention of recurrent PTA has not been compared with that of watchful waiting in a prospective, controlled trial. In the only large retrospective cohort investigation on the subject, Kronenberg et al studied 290 patients and demonstrated an increased rate of recurrent PTA among those who also had recurrent tonsillitis. A later study by the same group showed no difference in recurrent PTA based on a history of tonsillitis, but that study included only 38 patients. Other case series suggest that recurrence may be predicted based on a history of 2 to 3 episodes of acute tonsillitis in the year prior to the initial episode; such a history has been elicited in 15% to 30% of patients with PTA. Based on available evidence, it has been suggested that routine elective or quinsy tonsillectomy is not indicated for patients who present with their first PTA. However, if a patient is a candidate for elective tonsillectomy for other reasons (eg, 2 to 3 tonsillitis events in the previous 12 months), it seems rational to perform a quinsy tonsillectomy or to proceed with planned elective tonsillectomy after successful abscess drainage.

> **Pearl:** Tonsillectomy after peritonsillar abscess management is a consideration for patients who have had 2 to 3 episodes of tonsillitis in the previous year.

CHRONIC TONSILLITIS

Chronic tonsillitis is poorly defined in the literature but may be the appropriate terminology for sore throat of at least 3 months' duration accompanied by physical findings of tonsillar inflammation. Affected individuals may report symptoms of chronic sore throat, halitosis, or debris or concretions in the tonsil crypts known as *tonsilloliths*, in which the presence of biofilms has been implicated. Patients may also have persistent cervical adenopathy. Throat culture results in such cases are usually negative. Although no clinical trials have been conducted to help guide medical management of such patients, tonsillectomy is a reasonable consideration for those patients who do not respond to improved oropharyngeal hygiene and aggressive antibiotic therapy.

RECURRENT TONSILLITIS AND TONSILLECTOMY

When tonsils have been infected recurrently or chronically, the controlled process of antigen transport and presentation is altered because of shedding of the transporting M cells from the tonsil epithelium. As a result, tonsillar lymphocytes can theoretically become overwhelmed with persistent antigenic stimulation, rendering them unable to respond to antigens or function adequately in local protection or reinforcement of the upper respiratory secretory immune system. Furthermore, a direct influx of antigens disproportionately expands the population of mature B-cell clones, and, as a result, fewer early memory B cells go on to become J-chain–positive IgA immunocytes. There would therefore appear to be a therapeutic advantage to removing recurrently or chronically diseased tonsils. The surgeon should bear in mind, however, that tonsillectomy and adenoidectomy remove a source of immunocompetent cells, and some studies demonstrate minor alterations of immunoglobulin concentrations in adjacent tissues following tonsillectomy.

Cultures from deeper tissues of recurrently infected tonsils frequently reveal unusual pathogens, including *Staphylococcus aureus, H influenzae, Actinomycetes, Chlamydia, Mycoplasma,* and anaerobes; however, it remains unclear whether such cultures truly represent the offending organisms. Several studies suggest that bacteria in biofilms may be more important in recurrent tonsillitis than their planktonic counterparts.

Recurrent sore throat of a noninfectious nature is a hallmark of periodic fever, aphthous stomatitis, pharyngitis, and adenopathy (PFAPA), or Marshall syndrome. This disorder occurs primarily in children younger than 5 years, usually lasts more than 5 days, and recurs at regular intervals of 3 to 6 weeks. Systemic steroids and cimetidine have demonstrated efficacy in controlling the events. Two small, randomized, controlled trials demonstrated that tonsillectomy was effective for treating PFAPA, but children in the control groups also showed improvement. Tonsillectomy may be considered based on the frequency of illness, severity of infection, and child's response to medical management; however, a number of recent reports suggest that symptoms may recur after a period of initial improvement. The preponderance of recent data do not suggest a role for tonsillectomy in the management of pediatric acute-onset neuropsychiatric syndrome (PANS), previously known as PANDAS.

Appropriate medical and surgical management of children with recurrent infectious pharyngotonsillitis depends on accurate documentation of the cause and severity of individual episodes as well as the frequency of events. The PCC should record for each event a subjective assessment of the severity of illness; physical findings, including body temperature, pharyngeal or tonsillar erythema, tonsil size, tonsillar exudate, and cervical adenopathy (presence, size, and tenderness); and the results of microbiologic testing for GABHS. A summary of the documentation should be made available to the otolaryngologist to aid in medical decision-making about potential surgical intervention. In children with recurrent sore throat whose test results for GABHS are repeatedly positive, ruling out streptococcal carriage concurrent with viral infection may be desirable, as carriers are unlikely to transmit GABHS or develop suppurative complications or nonsuppurative sequelae of the disease such as acute rheumatic fever. Supportive documentation in children who meet criteria for tonsillectomy may include absence from school, spread of infection within the family, and family history of rheumatic heart disease or glomerulonephritis.

In all randomized controlled trials of tonsillectomy for infection, sore throat with each event was a necessary entrance criterion, and in most of these trials sore throat was the primary outcome studied. As a result, no claim can be made that tonsillectomy is indicated for children whose constellation of symptoms does not include sore throat, even when GABHS can be cultured from the throat. These studies also suggest that patients whose events are less severe or well documented do not gain sufficient benefit from tonsillectomy to justify the risk and morbidity of the procedure; in such patients, tonsillectomy should be considered only after a period of observation during which documentation of additional events may be made.

Children with frequent recurrences of throat infection over several months demonstrate high rates of spontaneous resolution. As a result, an observation period of at least 12 months is generally recommended before tonsillectomy is considered. In rare cases, early surgery may reasonably be considered for severely affected patients, such as those with histories of hospitalization for recurrent severe infections, those with rheumatic heart disease in the family or numerous repeated infections in a single household ("ping-pong spread"), or those with complications of infection such as PTA or Lemierre syndrome (thrombophlebitis of the internal jugular vein).

Observation of patients is also a reasonable management strategy in children who have had frequent recurrences of pharyngotonsillitis for more than 1 year. In several studies, children who had not had tonsillectomies demonstrated spontaneous improvement during the follow-up period, often with patients no longer meeting the original criteria for study entry. Additional information about the natural history of recurrent pharyngotonsillitis is found in case series describing outcomes for patients on wait-list tonsillectomy; many children who were reevaluated after months on such lists no longer met the criteria for surgery.

Tonsillectomy has been suggested for centuries as a means of controlling recurrent infection of the throat. However, clinical trials investigating the efficacy of tonsillectomy have had a high risk of bias because of poorly defined entrance criteria, nonrandom selection of participants who underwent surgery, exclusion of severely affected patients, or reliance on caregivers for postoperative data collection. In the most frequently cited and meticulous trial, Paradise and colleagues included only those patients whose episodes of throat infection met strict criteria, as outlined in **Table 10-2.** The key findings of their study were as follows:

● A mean rate reduction of 1.9 episodes of sore throat per year among children with tonsillectomies during the first year of follow-up compared with controls. However, sore throat associated with performance of the surgery (which would otherwise count as 1 episode) was excluded from the data. In the control group, patients' conditions also improved compared with their preenrollment infection frequency, experiencing a mean of only 3.1 annual events. Differences between groups were reduced in the second year and not significant by the third year of follow-up.

Table 10-2. Paradise Criteria for Tonsillectomy in Recurrent Tonsillitis	
Criterion	**Definition**
Frequency of sore throat events	7 or more episodes in the preceding year, *or* 5 or more episodes in each of the preceding 2 years, *or* 3 or more episodes in each of the preceding 3 years
Clinical features (1 required in addition to sore throat)	Temperature >38.3°C, *or* Cervical lymphadenopathy (tender lymph nodes or >2 cm), *or* Tonsillar exudate, *or* Positive culture for GABHS
Treatment	Antibiotics administered at an appropriate dose for proven or suspected episodes of GABHS
Documentation	Each episode and its qualifying characteristics are synchronously documented in the medical record, *or* In cases of insufficient documentation, 2 subsequent episodes of throat infection are observed by the clinician, with frequency and clinical features consistent with the initial history

Abbreviation: GABHS, group A β-hemolytic streptococcus.

From Baugh RF, Archer SM, Mitchell RB, et al. Clinical practice guideline: tonsillectomy in children. *Otolaryngol Head Neck Surg.* 2011;144(1 Suppl):S1–S30. Reprinted by permission of SAGE Publications.

- For episodes of *moderate* or *severe* throat infection, the control group experienced 1.2 episodes compared with 0.1 in the surgical group. Rate reductions diminished over the subsequent 2 years of follow-up and were not significant in the third year.
- Mean days with sore throat in the first 12 months were not statistically different between the 2 groups but included a predictable period of postoperative sore throat.

In a subsequent study by the same authors, entrance criteria were relaxed, with less rigorous criteria for the number of episodes, clinical features required, and documentation (ie, 4 to 6 episodes in the past year or 3 to 4 episodes per year in the past 2 years). In the 2 arms of the study (tonsillectomy or adenotonsillectomy vs control, and adenotonsillectomy vs control), patients undergoing surgery experienced rate reductions of 0.8 and 1.7 episodes, respectively, in the first year. Investigators concluded that the modest benefit conferred by tonsillectomy in children moderately affected with recurrent throat infection did not justify the inherent risks, morbidity, and cost of the surgery.

A randomized, controlled trial comparing tonsillectomy with watchful waiting in children aged 2 to 8 years examined temperature above 38.0°C for at least 1 day as the primary outcome measure. During a mean follow-up of 22 months, children in the tonsillectomy group had 0.2 fewer episodes of fever per person-year; from 6 to 24 months, there was no difference between the groups. The surgical group also demonstrated, per person-year, mild reductions in throat infections (0.2), sore throats (0.6), days with sore throat (5.9), and upper respiratory tract infections (0.5).

Pooled data from these studies were also analyzed in a Cochrane systematic review. Patients undergoing tonsillectomy experienced 1.4 fewer episodes of sore throat in the first year compared with the control group; however, the "cost" of this reduction was 1.0 episode of sore throat in the immediate postoperative period. Another systematic review suggested a 43% overall reduction in sore throat events. The number needed to treat with tonsillectomy to prevent 1 sore throat per month for the first year after surgery was 11. A third systematic review that included 13 randomized controlled trials and nonrandomized controlled studies on the efficacy of tonsillectomy in children reported pooled estimated risk differences favoring tonsillectomy over observation of 1.2 fewer episodes of sore throat, 2.8 fewer days of school absence, and 0.5 fewer episodes of upper respiratory infection per person-year.

Despite modest advantages conferred by tonsillectomy for sore throat, studies of quality of life universally suggest a significant improvement in patients undergoing the procedure. Only 2 of these studies enrolled children exclusively, and both reported improved scores in nearly all subscales. However, both studies also had numerous methodologic flaws, including enrollment of patients with "chronic tonsillitis" without definition based on signs and symptoms, absence of a control group, low response rates with potential selection bias, poor follow-up, and caregiver collection of data.

A recent guideline on tonsillectomy suggests that tonsillectomy for severely affected children with recurrent throat infection should be considered an option. Families of patients who meet appropriate criteria for tonsillectomy must weigh modest anticipated benefits of tonsillectomy for this indication against the natural history of resolution and risk of surgical morbidity and complications.

> **Pearl:** Tonsillectomy should be considered an option in the management of recurrent acute tonsillitis meeting the strict criteria of frequency, severity, and documentation. Tonsillectomy is *not* indicated for children who present without sore throat, even when group A β-hemolytic streptococcus can be cultured from the throat.

RECURRENT AND CHRONIC ADENOIDITIS

Disorders characterized in children as adenoiditis, rhinosinusitis, and nasopharyngitis are not easily distinguished from one another on the basis of symptoms. Most individuals in whom diagnosis is made present with nasal stuffiness, mucopurulent rhinorrhea, chronic cough, halitosis, and "snorting" or "gagging" on mucus throughout the day. Diagnosis of recurrent or chronic adenoiditis was based in 1 study on 3 or more months of chronic or recurrent nasal discharge associated with persistent or recurrent otitis media. In another study, the disorder was characterized by a constellation of findings including mucopurulent exudates on the adenoid surface with or without inflammation, recurrent fever or cold with persistent cough or serous otitis, and enlargement of posterior tonsillar lymph nodes. However, there are no established criteria for making this diagnosis or differentiating it from viral upper respiratory illness or acute sinusitis.

In chronic or recurrent nasopharyngitis, persistence of disease may be caused by colonization by pathogenic bacteria. *Haemophilus influenzae, Streptococcus pneumoniae, Streptococcus pyogenes,* and *S aureus* are commonly found in adenoid cultures and tissue samples among affected children. Rates of drug-resistant bacteria may be higher among patients with chronic or recurrent infection. Furthermore, molecular typing of paired bacterial isolates from the adenoid and lateral nasal wall in children undergoing adenoidectomy demonstrates a high degree of correlation, and sinonasal symptom scores appear to correlate with quantitative bacteriology of the adenoid core and not with adenoid size. Several studies have demonstrated bacterial biofilm formation in the adenoid; however, it is not clear if this is more common in persistent and recurrent nasopharyngitis than in obstructive adenoid hyperplasia. In some patients, sinonasal infection is more likely caused by stasis of secretions secondary to obstructive adenoid tissue than by bacterial factors, although the 2 may certainly be related. Gastroesophageal reflux has not been established as a cause of chronic adenoid inflammation.

Data suggest that adenoidectomy may be useful in management of children with persistent and recurrent sinonasal complaints, although a systematic review indicates that evidence is currently inadequate to firmly establish efficacy. Most PCCs favor adenoidectomy before consideration of endoscopic sinus surgery. The study by Weinberg et al suggests that children with recurrent acute symptoms may experience greater benefit from adenoidectomy than those with more chronic sinonasal disease.

> **Pearl:** Adenoidectomy is a reasonable alternative to repeated pharmacotherapy and endoscopic sinus surgery in patients with well-documented recurrent or chronic sinonasal illness.

OTITIS MEDIA AND ADENOIDITIS

Proximity of the adenoid pad to the eustachian tube has prompted a number of PCCs to study the potential benefits of adenoidectomy and adenotonsillectomy in the management of otitis media. The effect of the adenoid on the eustachian tube is likely one of regional inflammation or infection rather than of direct compression.

Since 1980, substantial evidence has shown that adenoidectomy and perhaps adenotonsillectomy have a role in the management of recurrent acute and chronic otitis media. However, some studies report results to the contrary, at least for recurrent acute otitis media. Benefit may be greatest for those children in whom the adenoid pad abuts the eustachian tube; however, such children can be identified only by preoperative nasopharyngoscopy.

Based on available data, it is reasonable to consider adenoidectomy along with the first set of tubes if the child has significant symptoms of nasal obstruction or recurrent rhinorrhea or, in children 4 years of age or older, when a second set of tubes is necessary, particularly for chronic middle-ear effusion. Children with tympanostomy tubes who develop otorrhea refractory to management with topical or systemic antibiotics may also reasonably be considered candidates for adenoidectomy. In children with a history of cleft palate, the procedure should be performed only when the otitis is relentless; in such cases, an inferior strip of adenoid should be preserved to avoid velopharyngeal insufficiency. Tonsillectomy with adenoidectomy carries additional morbidity and has less support in the literature. Tonsillectomy is a reasonable additional procedure when indications such as airway obstruction or recurrent pharyngitis are also present.

> **Pearl:** Adenoidectomy may be considered for the indication of chronic otitis media with the first set of tubes if the child has significant symptoms of nasal obstruction or recurrent rhinorrhea, when a second set of tubes is necessary for a child older than 4, and for children with refractory tympanostomy tube otorrhea.

▪ Hyperplasia of Tonsils and Adenoid

UPPER AIRWAY OBSTRUCTION AND SLEEP-RELATED BREATHING DISORDERS

When lymphoid tissue occupies a disproportionate amount of space in the pharynx, the upper airway becomes compromised. The condition can be exacerbated by other anatomical conditions, such as those seen in obesity, achondroplasia, mucopolysaccharidoses, or craniofacial syndromes. Children with diminished neuromuscular tone such as those with Down syndrome or cerebral palsy are also at increased risk of experiencing upper airway obstruction.

Hyperplasia of the tonsils and adenoid in children is commonly associated with pharyngeal obstruction. During the daytime, children with an enlarged adenoid demonstrate mouth breathing, rhinorrhea, and hyponasal speech, while those with tonsil hyperplasia may exhibit a muffled "hot potato" voice. However, the obstruction is even more apparent during sleep, when relaxation of pharyngeal musculature exacerbates resistance to airflow. Affected children often snore loudly and breathe primarily through the mouth, and they may have intermittent audible gasps, sternal retractions, and paradoxical motion of the chest. The physiologic sequelae of severely obstructed breathing may include hypoxemia, hypercapnia, and acidosis, which, in turn, signal central and peripheral chemoreceptors and baroreceptors to initiate pharyngeal dilation and arousals. Poor-quality sleep may result, and affected children often demonstrate daytime tiredness and/or hyperactivity as well as behavioral problems. Collectively, disturbances in sleep caused by obstruction are known as *sleep-related breathing disorders* (SRBD), which range in severity from primary snoring to obstructive sleep apnea (OSA), characterized by apneas and hypopneas during sleep. Patients with untreated OSA may, over time, develop cor pulmonale, right ventricular hypertrophy, congestive heart failure, alveolar hypoventilation, pulmonary hypertension, or failure to thrive and are at risk for permanent neurologic damage and even death. Although the prevalence of OSA in healthy school-aged children is 1% to 4%, as many as 10% of children have primary snoring.

Numerous sequelae have been linked to pediatric SRBD. Even mild OSA can have a significant impact on children's quality of life, with caregivers reporting poor school performance, behavioral problems, and poor focus. For example, numerous studies have shown that children with SRBD have significantly higher prevalence rates of both internalized behaviors (eg, withdrawal, shyness, anxiety) and externalized behaviors (eg, emotional lability, impulsivity, hyperactivity, aggressiveness, oppositional personality) compared with controls. Neurocognitive impairment is also noted in some children with SRBD, with research demonstrating deficits in language and visuospatial functions when compared with nonsnoring children. Finally, an association with enuresis has been demonstrated in up to 50% of children with SRBD. The mechanism by which this occurs has not been established, but theories include alterations in normal arousal and self-alerting mechanisms, hormonal changes (lower levels of antidiuretic hormone), and increased intra-abdominal pressure.

EVALUATION FOR SLEEP-RELATED BREATHING DISORDERS

The physical examination of children with SRBD should include assessment of the patient's weight and body mass index, as well as auscultation of the heart and lungs. A complete examination of the head and neck is critical, with special attention to potential nonlymphoid sites of obstruction, including hypoplasia of the midface and mandible and nasopharyngeal or choanal pathology. Patients with adenoid enlargement often present with adenoid facies (open mouth, flat midface, dark discoloration under the eyes).

The size of tonsils is best determined in a neutral state (ie, without the child gagging on a tongue depressor) to accurately estimate the volume of the pharynx they occupy. Tonsil hyperplasia is graded visually, most commonly using a scale of 1 to 4, as demonstrated in **Figure 10-1.** However, studies suggest that tonsil size as estimated by this scale does not always correlate with polysomnographic results and that even children with small tonsils can have significant OSA.

> **Pearl:** Tonsil size does not always correlate with severity of airway obstruction, as determined by polysomnography.

In the primary care setting, evaluation of adenoid size is best accomplished using lateral neck radiographs to assess the anteroposterior dimension of the adenoid; however, correlation between radiographically enlarged adenoid tissue and sleep apnea is lacking. In addition, results and interpretation are technique-sensitive, requiring an experienced radiology technician to achieve appropriate penetration and direct lateral projection without palate elevation. Another disadvantage is the exposure, though limited, to external-beam radiation. Direct visualization of the adenoid by means of fiber-optic endoscopy in the otolaryngologist's office is an alternative that is well tolerated and facilitates identification of other potential sites of upper airway obstruction, but the en face view of the

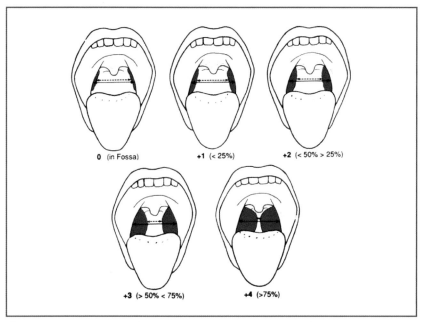

Figure 10-1. Assessment tool for tonsil size. Percentages represent the portion of transverse dimension of airway occupied by tonsil tissue.

From Brodsky L. Modern assessment of tonsils and adenoids. *Pediatr Clin North Am.* 1989;36(6):1551–1569, with permission from Elsevier.

tissue makes estimation of the degree of nasopharyngeal obstruction more difficult.

Hyperplasia of the tonsils and adenoid increases the likelihood of airway obstruction; consequently, most otolaryngologists will perform an adenotonsillectomy when the history correlates well with clinical findings of enlarged tonsils and adenoids. Otherwise healthy children with both typical nighttime symptoms of SRBD and daytime sequelae such as poor attention or daytime sleepiness are considered good candidates for adenotonsillectomy. Often, no further workup is performed before surgery in these children. Full-night polysomnography (PSG), which is considered the gold standard for diagnosis of OSA, is recommended prior to surgery for children with significant co-morbid medical conditions such as Down syndrome, obesity, and sickle cell disease. Polysomnography also can be useful if there is a discrepancy between the clinical history and physical examination findings. For example, a child with snoring and poor sleep in whom there is minimal tonsillar enlargement should be considered for PSG, as clinical evaluation yields a success rate of only 25% to 75% in predicting who has OSA syndrome. Current AAP guidelines recommend that children with habitual snoring (defined as more than 3 nights per week) and any additional signs or symptoms of sleep-disordered breathing including enlarged tonsils, obesity, or bedwetting be scheduled for a PSG or referred to an otolaryngologist or a sleep specialist for further evaluation.

Polysomnography objectively correlates ventilatory abnormalities with physiologic changes including electroencephalogram and electrocardiogram changes, limb movement, and body position. An obstructive apnea is defined as a greater than 90% drop in baseline airflow signal amplitude for a duration of at least 2 breaths. A hypopnea occurs when there is both a greater than 50% drop in airflow signal amplitude and either an arousal, an awakening, or a greater than 3% desaturation. The severity of OSA is generally quantified based on the obstructive apnea hypopnea index (OAHI). The OAHI is the total number of obstructive apneas and hypopneas divided by the total duration of sleep in hours. Although there is no consensus on the definition of OSA in children, an OAHI of less than 1 is considered within normal limits. An OAHI of 1 to 5 is defined as mild OSA, 5 to 10 is moderate OSA, and an OAHI greater than 10 is considered severe OSA. Unfortunately, pediatric PSG is expensive, time-consuming, and often unavailable. In addition, PSG parameters such as the OAHI fail to quantify the impact that SRBD has on a child's general health and quality of life. Other techniques of assessment, such as audiotaping, videotaping, pulse oximetry, and home PSG, may be helpful but are far less accurate.

> **Pearl:** In children with habitual snoring and tonsil enlargement, the PCC should schedule a polysomnogram or refer to an otolaryngologist or a sleep specialist for further evaluation. Polysomnography is most useful when the degree of lymphoid hyperplasia does not correlate with the severity of presenting symptoms, when children have significant comorbid medical conditions such as Down syndrome or obesity, and in the evaluation for continuous positive airway pressure in patients who have undergone adenotonsillectomy or who may not be good candidates for surgery.

TONSIL AND ADENOID SURGERY FOR SRBD

In children with mild SRBD (defined as an OAHI <5 with oxygen saturation >90 on PSG), nonsurgical treatment options such as watchful waiting, intranasal steroid sprays, and montelukast may be considered. However, the primary treatment of SRBD in symptomatic children with SRBD and at least mild adenotonsillar hyperplasia is adenotonsillectomy. In a recent randomized controlled trial comparing adenotonsillectomy with watchful waiting for pediatric OSA ("CHAT" [Childhood Adenotonsillectomy Trial] study), children in the surgical group had superior outcomes in terms of polysomnographic improvement and parent-reported behavior and quality of life. These results substantiate a large body of literature in which children with tonsillar disease (including those with throat infections or SRBD) have been shown to score significantly lower than their healthy counterparts in several quality-of-life subscales, including general health, physical functioning, behavior, bodily pain, and caregiver effect. A number of studies have reported dramatic improvements in quality-of-life scores following adenotonsillectomy, with follow-up as long as 3 years after surgery. Improvement reported by caregivers in most studies occurred irrespective of the severity of OSA syndrome. Similar improvements in behavior following adenotonsillectomy have also been demonstrated.

Additional studies have reported on decreased health care utilization and reduced costs as well as improvement in enuresis after removal of tonsils and adenoids. However, the impact of surgery on cognitive function is less clear. Short-term (7 months) neurocognitive outcomes were similar between children in the watchful waiting group and those in the adenotonsillectomy group in the CHAT study. However, the children in this study had relatively mild OSA and were older (5 to 9 years). Thus, further research is necessary to better understand the impact of adenotonsillectomy on cognitive function, as prior studies have described long-term residual neurocognitive impairments in children with more severe OSA. Children with behavioral problems, poor school performance, and hyperactivity should be considered for adenotonsillectomy even if they are found to have mild SRBD, as surgery has been shown to lead to significant improvements in these areas.

While adenotonsillectomy is considered first-line therapy for children with significant OSA, certain groups of children are at risk for persistent OSA following surgery. The CHAT study found that children with severe baseline OSA or obesity and those who are black were more likely to have residual sleep apnea after adenotonsillectomy. Children with craniofacial, neuromuscular, and genetic disorders are also known to be at high risk for persistent postoperative OSA. It is essential that PCCs be aware that surgery may not be curative in all children; patients with recurrent signs and symptoms of obstruction should be referred to an otolaryngologist or a sleep specialist for further evaluation.

> **Pearl:** Some patients, especially those who are obese, develop recurrent obstructive apnea after tonsillectomy; the PCC should inquire about recurrent symptoms at subsequent well-child visits.

▉ Malignancy of Tonsils or Adenoid

Pharyngeal malignancy, most notably lymphoma, may present as asymmetric tonsil hyperplasia. However, most children with apparent tonsil asymmetry more commonly have asymmetric effacement of the tonsils by tonsillar pillars or benign asymmetry of the tonsils. In a series of children with unilateral tonsil enlargement, Berkowitz and Mahadevan observed that all patients with lymphoma experienced enlargement of the tonsils within a 6-week period before diagnosis, and most had additional signs and symptoms, such as adenopathy greater than 3 cm, dysphagia, night sweats, and fevers, that distinguished their disease from benign tonsil hyperplasia. However, Dolev and Daniel reported that among 6 children identified with palatine tonsil lymphoma, all 6 exhibited no symptoms at their first visit. In studies including adults, the incidence of malignancy is low, and patients identified with tonsil malignancy have presented with symptoms. As a result, most children with tonsil asymmetry who do not have symptoms of obstruction are not likely candidates for tonsillectomy. However, children with asymptomatic tonsil asymmetry should be followed up for several months to monitor for symptoms suggestive of a malignant process.

> **Pearl:** Children with tonsil asymmetry are generally not candidates for tonsillectomy unless they have symptoms of obstruction or symptoms or findings suggestive of a malignant process.

◼ Other Tonsil and Adenoid Disorders

SPEECH IMPAIRMENT AND DYSPHAGIA

Hyperplasia of tonsil or adenoid tissue commonly results in decreased nasal airflow causing hyponasal or muffled speech. Language and articulation are not affected except in unusual cases in which patients have hypernasal speech due to impaired velopharyngeal closure secondary to tonsil enlargement. Rarely, severe enlargement of the tonsils or adenoid may cause dysphagia because of impairment of the pharyngeal phase of swallowing. Such patients usually have greater difficulty swallowing solids than liquids. When tonsil hyperplasia interferes with velopharyngeal closure, dysphagia is greater for liquids and is characterized by nasal regurgitation. In patients with adenoid hyperplasia, swallowing difficulties are more commonly related to poor coordination of breathing and swallowing. Dysphagia associated with failure to thrive and speech impairment due to unintelligible speech may be considered reasonable indications for adenotonsillectomy.

ABNORMAL DENTOFACIAL GROWTH

It has been postulated that chronic nasal obstruction from adenotonsillar hyperplasia may predispose some children to abnormalities of dentofacial growth. In such individuals, it is theorized that downward growth of the mandible and repositioning of the tongue compensate for the absence of nasal airflow by creating a larger oral airway. This results in an increased vertical facial dimension and increased gonial angle. Absence of contact between the tongue and palate causes a high and narrow palatal vault and a secondary posterior dental crossbite.

Medical and dental literature in this area has been extensively reviewed by Klein and by Smith and Gonzalez and continues to be an area of interest in orthodontic research. Though there is clearly a correlation between chronic nasal obstruction and long face syndrome, a cause-and-effect relationship has never been established in humans. Differences in study outcomes in animal models and humans are the result of inadequate means of determining the ratio of nasal breathing to mouth breathing; absence of normative data addressing nasal volume and resistance by age, sex, and body weight; and inadequate duration of follow-up. Although some data suggest that abnormalities of dentofacial growth in patients with adenotonsillar hyperplasia may be reversible, alterations may be minimal. Additional studies looking at more variables over a longer period of follow-up are necessary. In the interim, the otolaryngologist should evaluate children referred for adenotonsillectomy for orthodontic indications on a case-by-case basis and consider the procedure only for those with significant adenotonsillar hyperplasia.

HALITOSIS

Halitosis may result from food debris and bacteria retained within crypts of the tonsils and adenoid. However, although bad breath is often cited as an indication for adenotonsillectomy, a wide variety of other causes, including periodontal disease, debris of the tongue or lingual tonsils, sinonasal infection or foreign body, and gastroesophageal reflux, should also be considered. No clinical trials have been conducted to support adenotonsillectomy for this indication.

HEMORRHAGIC TONSILLITIS

Recurrent bleeding from prominent tonsil vessels may be controlled by cautery in most cooperative patients. However, patients who experience recurrence or cannot cooperate in the office setting may require tonsillectomy if bleeding becomes a nuisance or causes a significant reduction in the hemoglobin level or hematocrit.

■ Tonsillectomy and Adenoidectomy

Tonsillectomy and adenoidectomy remain among the most commonly performed operations in children. Between 1915 and the 1960s, these were the most frequently performed surgical procedures in the United States. Traditionally, their popularity resulted from a desire to control recurrent infection for which there was no appropriate medical therapy. Later, the focus of infection theory was the primary indication for surgery, which assumed that localized infections in these tissues could lead to systemic disease in other parts of the body.

Over the last 3 decades, clinical trials and systematic reviews have demonstrated that tonsillectomy and adenoidectomy have only modest efficacy in relieving recurrent or persistent upper respiratory infections and middle-ear disorders. However, during the same period there has been a greater awareness of the role of tonsil and adenoid hyperplasia in upper airway obstruction resulting in SRBD. As a result, incidence rates of tonsillectomy in the United States have increased significantly in the past 35 years, with SRBD being the primary indication for surgery. In 1970, the tonsillectomy rate was 126 procedures per 100,000 population, compared with 153 procedures per 100,000 in 2005. Coinciding with this increase has been a shift in indications for surgery from relief of recurrent infection to treatment of obstructive symptoms. In 1970, roughly 88% of tonsillectomies were performed because of infection, while approximately 23% were performed for this reason in 2005.

While adenotonsillectomy is considered to be a safe and effective surgery in the pediatric population, children typically experience several days of sore throat postoperatively. Ibuprofen and acetaminophen are recommended for pain control. Narcotics should be avoided as they may increase the risk of obstruction in the perioperative period. Additional complications such as dehydration, poor oral intake, and posttonsillectomy hemorrhage may also occur. Perioperative respiratory complications are more common in obese children, in those with severe baseline disease, and in patients younger than 3 years. Thus, current guidelines recommend an overnight hospital stay following adenotonsillectomy for these groups of children.

> **Pearl:** Current guidelines suggest overnight observation in the hospital following tonsillectomy in children younger than 3 years of age and in those with obesity, complex medical histories, or severe sleep apnea.

Primary care clinicians considering referral for tonsil or adenoid surgery must weigh the possibility that harm will result. Unfortunately, accurate statistics on mortality and morbidity in large patient populations are not readily available. Postadenotonsillectomy complications are divided into perioperative, immediate postoperative, and delayed postoperative periods. Perioperative complications include hemorrhage; intubation trauma causing laryngeal injury, laryngospasm, or laryngeal edema; respiratory compromise or cardiac arrest; aspiration; malignant hyperthermia; and trauma to the teeth, pharyngeal wall, soft palate, or lips. Burns of the oral commissure are the most common complication for which litigation occurs after tonsillectomy. Hemorrhage, infections, pain, edema and hematoma of the uvula, and pulmonary complications are common immediate postoperative complications, while postoperative scarring of the soft palate, nasopharyngeal stenosis, and tonsillar regrowth or remnant are delayed complications.

Primary (within 24 hours of surgery) or secondary (more than 24 hours after surgery) hemorrhage is the most common serious complication of adenotonsillar surgery and is more likely to result from tonsillectomy than adenoidectomy. In published reports, the rate of primary hemorrhage from tonsillectomy has ranged from 0.2% to 2.2%, and the rate of secondary hemorrhage has ranged from 0.1% to 3%. Fever is an accepted complication in the first 36 hours but will increase insensible water loss and predispose patients to dehydration. Parents need to be forewarned to maintain adequate hydration and should be given specific hydration goals as part of their discharge instructions. Dehydration may also result from nausea or vomiting secondary to anesthesia as well as from swallowed blood and decreased oral intake secondary to pain. Younger children are especially prone as they are less cooperative and have less volume reserve. Mortality from tonsillectomy is estimated at 1 per 16,000 to 35,000 tonsillectomies, with about one-third attributable to primary bleeding and the majority related to anesthetic mishaps.

The surgeon or a surrogate must have postoperative contact with patients or their caregivers to ensure there have been no postoperative complications. This may be accomplished at an office visit or by telephone assessment 2 to 8 weeks after surgery. Caregivers should be questioned about resolution of obstruction (if present preoperatively), return to normal diet, and evidence of velopharyngeal insufficiency (excessive air escape with speech). Patients also may develop recurrent obstruction or stenosis of the operated area months or years after the surgery; such patients have usually been discharged from the surgeon's care, and it is incumbent on the PCC to inquire about obstructive symptoms at follow-up visits.

Although some studies report minor alterations of immunoglobulin concentrations in the serum and adjacent tissues following tonsillectomy, no studies to date have demonstrated a significant clinical effect of tonsillectomy on the immune system. Heightened risk of poliomyelitis, which was an important deterrent to surgery before the advent of an effective vaccine and for which an immunologic basis was later elucidated, is no longer of practical concern in this era of virtually universal immunization. Finally, concern that tonsillectomy might predispose patients to the development of Hodgkin disease appears to have been dispelled by later epidemiologic investigations. Although it remains possible that the removal of immunologically active tonsils and adenoid will someday prove to undermine resistance to disease of some sort, the likelihood at present seems small.

> **Pearl:** No studies to date have demonstrated a significant clinical effect of tonsillectomy on the immune system.

■ Selected Readings

American Academy of Pediatrics. Group A streptococcal infections. In: Kimberlin DW, Brady MT, Jackson MA, Long SS, eds. *Red Book: 2018 Report of the Committee on Infectious Diseases*. 31st ed. Itasca, IL: American Academy of Pediatrics; 2018:748–762

Baldassari CM, Mitchell RB, Schubert C, Rudnick EF. Pediatric obstructive sleep apnea and quality of life: a meta-analysis. *Otolaryngol Head Neck Surg*. 2008;138(3):265–273

Berkowitz RG, Mahadevan M. Unilateral tonsillar enlargement and tonsillar lymphoma in children. *Ann Otol Rhinol Laryngol*. 1999;108(9):876–879

Böck A, Popp W, Herkner KR. Tonsillectomy and the immune system: a long-term follow up comparison between tonsillectomized and non-tonsillectomized children. *Eur Arch Otorhinolaryngol*. 1994;251(7):423–427

Burton MJ, Glasziou PP. Tonsillectomy or adeno-tonsillectomy versus non-surgical treatment for chronic/recurrent acute tonsillitis. *Cochrane Database Syst Rev*. 2009;1(1):CD001802

Dolev Y, Daniel SJ. The presence of unilateral tonsillar enlargement in patients diagnosed with palatine tonsil lymphoma: experience at a tertiary care pediatric hospital. *Int J Pediatr Otorhinolaryngol*. 2008;72(1):9–12

Garetz SL. Behavior, cognition, and quality of life after adenotonsillectomy for pediatric sleep-disordered breathing: summary of the literature. *Otolaryngol Head Neck Surg*. 2008;138(1 Suppl):S19–S26

Gerber MA, Baltimore RS, Eaton CB, et al. Prevention of rheumatic fever and diagnosis and treatment of acute Streptococcal pharyngitis: a scientific statement from the American Heart Association Rheumatic Fever, Endocarditis, and Kawasaki Disease Committee of the Council on Cardiovascular Disease in the Young, the Interdisciplinary Council on Functional Genomics and Translational Biology, and the Interdisciplinary Council on Quality of Care and Outcomes Research: endorsed by the American Academy of Pediatrics. *Circulation*. 2009;119(11):1541–1551

Hammarén-Malmi S, Saxen H, Tarkkanen J, Mattila PS. Adenoidectomy does not significantly reduce the incidence of otitis media in conjunction with the insertion of tympanostomy tubes in children who are younger than 4 years: a randomized trial. *Pediatrics*. 2005;116(1):185–189

Howard NS, Brietzke SE. Pediatric tonsil size: objective vs subjective measurements correlated to overnight polysomnogram. *Otolaryngol Head Neck Surg*. 2009;140(5):675–681

Kaplan EL, Johnson DR. Unexplained reduced microbiological efficacy of intramuscular benzathine penicillin G and of oral penicillin V in eradication of group a streptococci from children with acute pharyngitis. *Pediatrics*. 2001;108(5):1180–1186

Kaygusuz I, Gödekmerdan A, Karlidag T, et al. Early stage impacts of tonsillectomy on immune functions of children. *Int J Pediatr Otorhinolaryngol*. 2003;67(12): 1311–1315

Klein JC. Nasal respiratory function and craniofacial growth. *Arch Otolaryngol Head Neck Surg*. 1986;112(8):843–849

Kronenberg J, Wolf M, Leventon G. Peritonsillar abscess: recurrence rate and the indication for tonsillectomy. *Am J Otolaryngol*. 1987;8(2):82–84

Lehmann KJ, Nelson R, MacLellan D, Anderson P, Romao RLP. The role of adenotonsillectomy in the treatment of primary nocturnal enuresis in children: a systematic review. *J Pediatr Urol*. 2018;14(1):53.e1–53.e8

Marcus CL, Brooks LJ, Draper KA, et al; American Academy of Pediatrics Section on Pediatric Pulmonology, Subcommittee on Obstructive Sleep Apnea Syndrome. Diagnosis and management of childhood obstructive sleep apnea syndrome. *Pediatrics*. 2012;130(3): 576–584

Marcus CL, Moore RH, Rosen CL, et al; Childhood Adenotonsillectomy Trial (CHAT). A randomized trial of adenotonsillectomy for childhood sleep apnea. *N Engl J Med*. 2013;368(25):2366–2376

Mitchell RB, Archer SM, Ishman SL, Rosenfeld RM, et al. Clinical practice guideline: tonsillectomy in children (Update). *Otolaryngol Head Neck Surg*. 2019;160(1_Suppl): S1–S42

Mitchell RB, Boss EF. Pediatric obstructive sleep apnea in obese and normal-weight children: impact of adenotonsillectomy on quality-of-life and behavior. *Dev Neuropsychol*. 2009;34(5):650–661

Nguyen LH, Manoukian JJ, Yoskovitch A, Al-Sebeih KH. Adenoidectomy: selection criteria for surgical cases of otitis media. *Laryngoscope*. 2004;114(5):863–866

Oomen KP, Rovers MM, van den Akker EH, et al. Effect of adenotonsillectomy on middle ear status in children. *Laryngoscope*. 2005;115(4):731–734

Owens JA. Neurocognitive and behavioral impact of sleep disordered breathing in children. *Pediatr Pulmonol*. 2009;44(5):417–422

Paradise JL, Bluestone CD, Bachman RZ, et al. History of recurrent sore throat as an indication for tonsillectomy—predictive limitations of histories that are undocumented. *N Engl J Med*. 1978;298(8):409–413

Paradise JL, Bluestone CD, Colborn DK, et al. Adenoidectomy and adenotonsillectomy for recurrent acute otitis media: parallel randomized clinical trials in children not previously treated with tympanostomy tubes. *JAMA*. 1999;282(10):945–953

Paradise JL, Bluestone CD, Colborn DK, et al. Tonsillectomy and adenotonsillectomy for recurrent throat infection in moderately affected children. *Pediatrics*. 2002;110 (1 Pt 1):7–15

Paradise JL, Bluestone CD, Rogers KD, et al. Efficacy of adenoidectomy for recurrent otitis media in children previously treated with tympanostomy-tube placement. Results of parallel randomized and nonrandomized trials. *JAMA*. 1990;263(15): 2066–2073

Parker KG, Gandra S, Matushek S, et al. Comparison of 3 nucleic acid amplification tests and a rapid antigen test with culture for the detection of group A streptococci from throat swabs. *J Appl Lab Med.* 2019;4(2):164–169

Paulussen C, Claes J, Claes G, Jorissen M. Adenoids and tonsils, indications for surgery and immunological consequences of surgery. *Acta Otorhinolaryngol Belg.* 2000;54(3):403–408

Pichichero ME, Casey JR, Mayes T, et al. Penicillin failure in streptococcal tonsillopharyngitis: causes and remedies. *Pediatr Infect Dis J.* 2000;19(9):917–923

Randolph MF, Gerber MA, DeMeo KK, Wright L. Effect of antibiotic therapy on the clinical course of streptococcal pharyngitis. *J Pediatr.* 1985;106(6):870–875

Shapiro NL, Strocker AM, Bhattacharyya N. Risk factors for adenotonsillar hypertrophy in children following solid organ transplantation. *Int J Pediatr Otorhinolaryngol.* 2003;67(2):151–155

Shulman ST, Bisno AL, Clegg HW, et al. Clinical practice guideline for the diagnosis and management of group A streptococcal pharyngitis: 2012 update by the Infectious Diseases Society of America [published correction appears in *Clin Infect Dis.* 2014;58(10): 1496]. *Clin Infect Dis.* 2012;55(10):1279–1282

Smith RM, Gonzalez C. The relationship between nasal obstruction and craniofacial growth. *Pediatr Clin North Am.* 1989;36(6):1423–1434

van den Aardweg MT, Schilder AG, Herkert E, Boonacker CW, Rovers MM. Adenoidectomy for recurrent or chronic nasal symptoms in children. *Cochrane Database Syst Rev.* 2010; 1(1):CD008282

van der Horst C, Joncas J, Ahronheim G, et al. Lack of effect of peroral acyclovir for the treatment of acute infectious mononucleosis. *J Infect Dis.* 1991;164(4):788–792

van Staaij BK, van den Akker EH, Rovers MM, et al. Effectiveness of adenotonsillectomy in children with mild symptoms of throat infections or adenotonsillar hypertrophy: open, randomised controlled trial. *BMJ.* 2004;329(7467):651

CHAPTER 11

Pediatric Oropharyngeal Trauma

David L. Mandell, MD

Introduction
Epidemiology
Presenting Symptoms
Physical Examination
Diagnostic Imaging
Treatment Options
    Surgical Closure

Prophylactic Antibiotics
Hospital Admission and
    Observation
Natural History and
    Prognosis

▪ Introduction

Injuries to the oropharynx of children are thought to be quite commonplace. Many such injuries may not be witnessed or brought to medical attention because of the absence of any major symptoms. However, when oropharyngeal trauma is associated with bleeding, pain, or dysphagia, a caregiver is usually prompted to seek medical attention. Prophylactic antibiotics have often been recommended in cases in which the oropharyngeal mucosa has been lacerated. Most cases of oropharyngeal trauma in children heal with no lasting damage to the patient, usually without the need for surgical closure.

Although recovery from oropharyngeal trauma is usually uneventful, rare cases have been reported in which children have developed neurologic complications (eg, stroke, death) following such injuries, presumably because of occult internal carotid artery injury. Unfortunately, there is currently no definitive mechanism by which primary care clinicians (PCCs) can predict which children with oropharyngeal trauma might go on to develop these catastrophic neurologic complications. An imaging study is one way to attempt to assess the carotid artery, although there is no agreement as to which study should be performed (computed tomography [CT], CT angiography, magnetic resonance angiography [MRA], or no study at all). Even within institutions in which imaging is performed there is considerable variability regarding which patients undergo such studies.

> **Pearl:** Although most cases of pediatric oropharyngeal trauma result in rapid healing without complications, rare instances of internal carotid injury and delayed onset of severe neurologic sequelae have been reported.

▪ Epidemiology

Oropharyngeal injury in children occurs at an average age of 3.5 years. One theory why toddlers make up the highest-risk group for oropharyngeal injury is that they tend to run and fall with objects in their mouths. As with most types of trauma, boys are affected more often than girls, and they are 1.5 to 5.5 times more likely to experience oropharyngeal trauma. The most common objects that cause such injury are pens, pencils, musical instruments, pipes, tubes, toys, and sticks. Other offending objects include toothbrushes, straws, and lollipops. In approximately 5% of cases of pediatric oropharyngeal trauma, the object that caused the trauma is not witnessed and is unknown. A typical large tertiary care pediatric hospital may see approximately 18 such injuries per year.

> **Pearl:** Pediatric oropharyngeal injury is most common in male toddlers, who often run and fall with toys and other objects in their mouths.

▪ Presenting Symptoms

The median length of time that elapses from oropharyngeal injury to presentation to a PCC is 3 hours. Most children will have expectorated 5 to 20 mL of blood prior to arrival in the emergency department (ED). Some patients complain of pain or odynophagia, although most are asymptomatic by the time they are seen by a PCC. Typically, there are no neurologic symptoms at the time of presentation. If the patient complains of headache, blurred vision, or nausea, or if the parent or guardian describes the child as being unusually irritable, the PCC should suspect a potential neurovascular injury and initiate the appropriate imaging study.

> **Pearl:** Although bleeding after oropharyngeal trauma is the most common factor that prompts parents to bring their children for medical attention, by the time most of these children are seen, they are entirely asymptomatic.

■ Physical Examination

Hemodynamic stability is the norm on initial physical examination of children with oropharyngeal trauma. Although younger children and those who are mentally disabled may resist oropharyngeal examination, visualization of the site of potential injury is essential and may require parental-assisted restraint of the child and use of a tongue depressor and a headlight, with suction available to clear away oropharyngeal secretions. On oropharyngeal examination, the site of injury involves the lateral oropharynx in 70% to 81% of injuries, with the remainder occurring in the midline. Some authors have reported that the left side of the oropharynx is involved more often than the right side, theoretically because of the predominance of right-handedness among the general population (ie, children are running while their right hand is placing the offending object in the oral cavity). Lateral injuries are far more likely to be associated with vascular injuries.

The appearance of oropharyngeal injury can range from mild bruising with no mucosal disruption, to a large avulsed tissue flap with a fistula into the nasopharynx, to a great vessel exposure. A grading scale has been developed to help standardize the description of injuries. Grade I injuries consist of ecchymosis without mucosal penetration (7% of cases). Grade II injuries are puncture wounds or lacerations measuring 1 cm or less (64% of cases). Grade III injuries are lacerations larger than 1 cm or those with an oronasal fistula or avulsed tissue flap (29% of cases). In approximately 2% of patients who present to a PCC, the foreign body itself is noted to be protruding from the oropharyngeal wound.

Signs of neurologic dysfunction are usually absent. However, the PCC should closely assess for drowsiness and listlessness, irritability, confused speech, vision changes, vomiting, and arm or leg weakness. Also, auscultation for a carotid bruit should be performed, and the PCC should assess for any external neck swelling.

> **Pearl:** Clear visualization of the site of injury is recommended, and the severity of the injury appearance can be graded for descriptive purposes.

Diagnostic Imaging

Because of the rarity of neurologic sequelae, there is some debate about whether imaging studies should be routinely performed to look for potential carotid artery injury in children with otherwise benign-appearing oropharyngeal traumatic injury. The potential benefit of imaging is that if early intimal damage to the internal carotid artery can somehow be identified, anticoagulation therapy can be instituted, thus potentially decreasing the likelihood of thrombus formation and propagation and development of neurologic sequelae. Imaging is less likely to be required for midline traumatic palatal injuries because injuries in this location (ie, a wound at the hard palate–soft palate junction) are less likely to damage the great vessels. Lateral oropharyngeal lesions are thought to be associated with a higher risk of complications.

One mechanism for assessing potential internal carotid injury resulting from pediatric oropharyngeal trauma is CT with intravenous (IV) contrast. Although PCCs may be more inclined to order a radiographic study in cases in which the size and appearance of the wound are more severe, the mechanism of carotid injury in this scenario is from arterial compression, not penetration, so even grade I injuries (no mucosal penetration) can lead to a carotid intimal tear and subsequent thrombosis. Computed tomographic images can be reconstructed to create a CT angiogram; MRAs also may be used, although MRA studies cost more, take longer to perform (and thus are more likely to require sedation in young children), and may not be as readily available in the typical ED setting.

According to pooled data from the largest, most recently published series of children with oropharyngeal trauma, 89 of 358 patients underwent CT. Of these 89 patients, 2 (2.2%) were found to have intimal disruption of the internal carotid artery, which was confirmed with conventional angiography. The patients were treated expectantly with aspirin. In addition, 1 patient (1.1%) was found to have a carotid artery "spasm," and another was found to have a soft-tissue hematoma adjacent to the internal carotid artery, with no direct association with the artery on follow-up conventional angiography. Thus, among all recent large series in the literature (including all patients, even those who did not undergo scanning), the likelihood of discovering a true intimal carotid artery injury in the setting of pediatric oropharyngeal trauma is 2 of 358 (0.6%), and the likelihood of developing neurologic sequelae among all patients in these series combined was 0.0%. Because of these data, midline pharyngeal injuries do not generally require imaging. Imaging of lateral pharyngeal wall injuries should be considered case by case.

> **Pearl:** If an imaging study is performed to assess the status of the carotid artery in the setting of pediatric oropharyngeal trauma, the likelihood of finding a true intimal arterial tear is approximately 2.2%. Most pediatric patients with routine oropharyngeal trauma, however, have not undergone scanning.

▓ Treatment Options

SURGICAL CLOSURE

Most traumatic oropharyngeal injuries heal well spontaneously. Surgical closure is performed in only 4% to 8% of all cases. Patients who are more likely to require surgical closure are those with large avulsion flaps, those with an impaled foreign body still in the wound, and those rare patients in whom open neck exploration might be needed for great vessel access in the event of significant bleeding on foreign body extraction (**figures 11-1** and **11-2**).

PROPHYLACTIC ANTIBIOTICS

Prophylactic antibiotics are reportedly used in up to 88% of cases. Typically, a dose of IV antibiotics is administered while the patient is in the ED, followed by postdischarge oral antibiotics. The antibiotics should cover gram-positive organisms and anaerobes; a reasonable choice is IV ampicillin-sulbactam followed by oral amoxicillin-clavulanate.

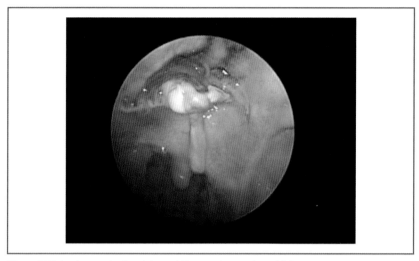

Figure 11-1. Acute penetrating injury of the oropharynx in a child.

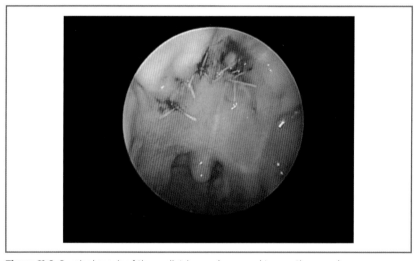

Figure 11-2. Surgical repair of the pediatric oropharyngeal traumatic wound.

HOSPITAL ADMISSION AND OBSERVATION

Most patients stay in the hospital less than 24 hours, and many are discharged home from the ED. Hospitalization with longer admissions may be required for patients who are younger than 1 year; who are mentally disabled (in whom assessment of changes in mental status may be more difficult); who have poor oral intake, infection, or pneumomediastinum; who are undergoing a child abuse workup or who have unsafe home situations; or who are recovering from surgical palatal repair. Neurologic complications are rare. When they do occur, there is often a delay of up to several days until symptom onset, such that overnight admission for observation may provide a false sense of security and generally is not recommended. When discharged home, patients should be given instructions similar to those given to patients who have experienced minor head trauma (**Box 11-1**). Parents are asked to closely monitor their child for any neurologic signs or symptoms for a few more days, with a follow-up outpatient office visit within a week.

> **Pearl:** Most oropharyngeal wounds heal well without surgery. Prophylactic antibiotics are often given if the mucosa of the oropharynx has been penetrated, and most children can be discharged home without hospital admission. Admitting the child overnight may provide a false sense of security because development of any neurologic symptoms can occur up to several days later.

■ Natural History and Prognosis

All but the most dramatic avulsed tissue flaps tend to heal spontaneously within 1 to 2 weeks without surgical closure, and symptoms such as pain and dysphagia are usually short lived. As innocuous as this type of trauma may appear, however, there is still the potential

Box 11-1. Warning Signs for Parents/Caregivers After Pediatric Oropharyngeal Trauma
Arm or leg weakness
Confused speech
Drowsiness
Irritability
Listlessness
Seizures
Vision changes
Vomiting

for devastating neurologic sequelae if any injury to the internal carotid artery has occurred. Fortunately, such complications are quite rare. In fact, of 358 cases of pediatric oropharyngeal trauma identified in the literature from the past 2 decades, not a single case with neurologic complications was noted. In addition, no specific clinical factors have been identified to help predict which patients may be at higher risk of developing neurologic complications.

Scattered throughout the medical literature are rare case reports of children developing neurologic signs and symptoms such as hemiparesis, hemiplegia, seizure, coma, and even death following lateral oropharyngeal trauma that initially seemed unassuming and benign. In these cases, it is believed that the foreign body didn't puncture the internal carotid artery but rather briefly compressed it against internal bony structures such as the skull base and the first 2 to 3 cervical vertebrae. As a result, the internal carotid artery can develop an intimal tear with subsequent gradual development of a mural thrombus. The thrombus eventually can lead to luminal occlusion, although in children this event alone is usually not enough to cause overt neurologic symptoms because of adequate circle of Willis collateral circulation. In some cases, the thrombus can propagate distally, growing to occlude the middle or anterior cerebral arteries, at which point cerebral infarction can occur. It can take up to 60 hours for such a thrombus to form and propagate distally, thus likely accounting for the so-called lucid period during which patients appear asymptomatic prior to onset of neurologic signs and symptoms.

Thus, when it comes to pediatric oropharyngeal trauma, a high level of suspicion has to be maintained regarding the potential for delayed onset of neurologic complications. A contrast CT scan of the neck seems to be the most efficient type of evaluation to use in attempting to detect early intimal damage to the internal carotid artery. However, imaging does not seem to have been used in most cases in the literature, and routine imaging cannot be emphatically recommended in light of the rarity of arterial injury.

Pearl: The natural history of pediatric oropharyngeal trauma is almost always favorable, with no lasting adverse effects, but primary care clinicians should keep in mind the rare possibility of intimal disruption of the internal carotid artery with delayed onset of neurologic signs and symptoms.

■ Selected References

Brietzke SE, Jones DT. Pediatric oropharyngeal trauma: what is the role of CT scan? *Int J Pediatr Otorhinolaryngol.* 2005;69(5):669–679

Hellmann JR, Shott SR, Gootee MJ. Impalement injuries of the palate in children: review of 131 cases. *Int J Pediatr Otorhinolaryngol.* 1993;26(2):157–163

Hengerer AS, DeGroot TR, Rivers RJ Jr, Pettee DS. Internal carotid artery thrombosis following soft palate injuries: a case report and review of 16 cases. *Laryngoscope.* 1984;94(12 Pt 1):1571–1575

Hennus MP, Speleman L. Internal maxillary artery pseudoaneurysm: a near fatal complication of seemingly innocuous pharyngeal trauma. *Case Rep Crit Care.* 2011;2011:241375

Marom T, Russo E, Ben-Yehuda Y, Roth Y. Oropharyngeal injuries in children. *Pediatr Emerg Care.* 2007;23(12):914–918

Pierrot S, Bernardeschi D, Morrisseau-Durand MP, Manach Y, Couloigner V. Dissection of the internal carotid artery following trauma of the soft palate in children. *Ann Otol Rhinol Laryngol.* 2006;115(5):323–329

Radkowski D, McGill TJ, Healy GB, Jones DT. Penetrating trauma of the oropharynx in children. *Laryngoscope.* 1993;103(9):991–994

Ratcliff DJ, Okada PJ, Murray AD. Evaluation of pediatric lateral oropharyngeal trauma. *Otolaryngol Head Neck Surg.* 2003;128(6):783–787

Schoem SR, Choi SS, Zalzal GH, Grundfast KM. Management of oropharyngeal trauma in children. *Arch Otolaryngol Head Neck Surg.* 1997;123(12):1267–1270

Soose RJ, Simons JP, Mandell DL. Evaluation and management of pediatric oropharyngeal trauma. *Arch Otolaryngol Head Neck Surg.* 2006;132(4):446–451

Suskind DL, Tavill MA, Keller JL, Austin MB. Management of the carotid artery following penetrating injuries of the soft palate. *Int J Pediatr Otorhinolaryngol.* 1997;39(1):41–49

Uchino H, Kuriyama A, Kimura K, Ikegami T, Fukuoka T. Accidental oropharyngeal impalement injury in children: a report of two cases. *J Emerg Trauma Shock.* 2015; 8(2):115–118

Umibe A, Omura K, Hachisu T, Anazawa U, Tanaka Y. Life-threatening injury caused by complete impalement of a toothbrush: case report. *Dent Traumatol.* 2017;33(4):317–320

Zonfrillo MR, Roy AD, Walsh SA. Management of pediatric penetrating oropharyngeal trauma. *Pediatr Emerg Care.* 2008;24(3):172–175

CHAPTER 12

Cleft Lip and Palate

Adam B. Johnson, MD, PhD, and Charles M. Bower, MD

Introduction
Epidemiology
Presenting Symptoms
Physical Examination
   Findings

Diagnosis
Treatment Options
Natural History and
   Prognosis

■ Introduction

Orofacial clefting is the most common congenital craniofacial malformation. Although most clefts are isolated anomalies, cleft lip and palate (CL/P) may be associated with other malformations or defined syndromes. The primary care clinician (PCC) is essential in the initial diagnosis and continued coordinated care of a child with CL/P. Because most CL/Ps are diagnosed prenatally or soon postnatally, the PCC's role can be invaluable when dealing with issues such as feeding, developmental delays, behavior problems, and recurrent infections. Following identification of a child with a cleft, referral to a CL/P multidisciplinary team is essential. Caring for clefts requires experienced professionals from multiple specialties and often several surgeries over a span of years to optimize patient outcomes. The American Cleft Palate-Craniofacial Association (ACPA) recommends referral to credentialed teams in which care is delivered by professionals with a sufficient number of patients per year to ensure optimal care.

One in 800 children are born with a cleft lip or palate, which means that PCCs will likely encounter these children throughout their career. A recent survey of PCCs indicated that they currently treated a mean of 1.1 children with clefts. Additionally, 87% of survey respondents gave appropriate referrals to a tertiary center within 2 weeks of birth. Despite this experience, 67% desired a medical update concerning clefts. The goal of this review is to provide a firm foundation for understanding the diagnosis and presenting symptoms of clefts and the appropriate time line for medical and surgical management.

Epidemiology

Cleft lip and palate is the most common congenital facial malformation. It is more common in boys, while cleft palate alone is more common in girls. The incidence of CL/P varies by ethnicity—American Indians, 3.7 per 1,000 live births; Chinese, 2.0 per 1,000; whites, 1.7 per 1,000; and blacks, 0.4 per 1,000. Reports indicate the breakdown of cleft type as CL/P, 35%; isolated cleft lip, 26%; and isolated cleft palate, 39%.

Clefts are typically isolated defects, related to several genetic and environmental factors. Most CL/P occurs in children with no family history of CL/P. Only a small percentage of defects have been attributed to a known environmental teratogenic agent (eg, sodium valproate). Approximately 20% to 25% of children with clefts will have an associated malformation. Craniofacial, skeletal/extremity, and cardiovascular anomalies can occur. Clefting is associated with more than 400 syndromes, including velocardiofacial syndrome (22q11 deletion), Stickler syndrome, Van der Woude syndrome, Kabuki syndrome, trisomy 13 (Patau syndrome), trisomy 18 (Edwards syndrome), and Pierre Robin sequence. Children with clefts should be thoroughly examined to detect other anomalies. Consultation with a geneticist is appropriate.

> **Pearl:** While a cleft lip or palate is usually an isolated anomaly, the PCC should be alert for findings consistent with associated syndromes.

Presenting Symptoms

An embryologic understanding of cleft development provides the anatomical basis for symptom presentation. The location and severity of the cleft will predict associated clinical manifestations of which the PCC should be aware. Starting at 5 weeks' gestation, the embryonic midfacial structures are organized from the 5 facial prominences. The maxillary processes from each side of the face grow toward each other until they meet and fuse in front of the medial nasal passages, forming the upper lip (**Figure 12-1**). The frontonasal process develops into the primary palate and primary nasal septum. The inner aspect of the maxillary process on each side develops into palatine shelves, which fuse in the midline, forming the secondary palate. A CL/P deformity results from an interruption of fusion of the prominences and subsequent failure of mesoderm ingrowth. Thus, an isolated cleft lip, an isolated cleft palate, or a combined CL/P may form, depending on the disruption in embryonic development.

The initial presentation in children with clefts is an anatomical malformation found on physical examination. While often discovered at an initial postnatal examination, an increasing number of clefts (unilateral, bilateral, and midline CL/P) are detected on prenatal ultrasonography. Ultrasound has been used for 30 years, with enhanced detection based on classification schemes and technological improvement. A 2010 systematic review revealed that 2-dimensional ultrasound screening for CL/P has a relatively low detection rate and is associated with a few false-positive results; 3-dimensional (3-D) ultrasound, however, achieved a 90% detection rate for cleft lip and a variably

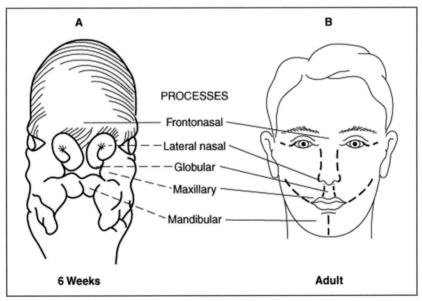

Figure 12-1. Embryologic fusion of the facial prominences leads to normal facial development.

From Lalwani AK. *Current Diagnosis & Treatment in Otolaryngology—Head and Neck Surgery.* 2nd Ed. New York, NY: McGraw-Hill; 2008. Reprinted by permission of the McGraw-Hill Companies.

lower rate for cleft palate. With continued experience, caregivers will likely see a rise in clefts, especially cleft lip, diagnosed prenatally.

Despite improvements in prenatal ultrasound detection, CL/P typically is discovered on postnatal examination. A cleft lip usually is obvious, and an appropriate palatal examination will demonstrate most clefts of the palate. Occasionally, submucous cleft palates (ie, secondary palate intact but muscles not joined properly) will present late, with failure to thrive, or even later, with speech problems. During the initial examination, concomitant feeding issues become the central presenting symptom. Although most children with an isolated cleft lip have little difficulty with feeding, children with a cleft palate often require assistance because of significant problems generating negative intraoral pressure, which creates difficulty with breastfeeding and bottle-feeding. Reduced efficiency of nutritive sucking can lead to lengthy feeding times, the ingestion of excessive amounts of air, and fatigue for infants and parents. Moreover, it may be difficult for the infant to stabilize the nipple in the mouth because the opposing palatal tissue surface for tongue compression is absent. Most cleft palate teams include a feeding specialist who can assist the PCC in managing feeding issues in infancy. Ways to overcome these feeding deficiencies are covered in the treatment section of this chapter.

> **Pearl:** Increasing numbers of clefts are detected with prenatal ultrasound, with the remainder detected by proper physical examination at birth.

▧ Physical Examination Findings

A complete physical examination in a child with a cleft serves as a bridge to further diagnostic and therapeutic interventions. As with any newborn seen for the first time, Apgar scores, vital signs, and weight should be obtained. Respiratory distress may be present in children with Pierre Robin sequence and requires evaluation and management for airway obstruction. Pierre Robin sequence is a condition involving a combination of micrognathia (small mandible), glossoptosis (posterior displacement of the tongue), and airway obstruction. While cleft palate is not a part of the original description, it is often present in these patients. In these children, a prone position, a nasal airway, or intubation may be necessary to support the airway. Such patients should be referred to an otolaryngologist or a cleft palate team for evaluation and intervention as indicated. Providing that the child is in stable condition, the PCC can conduct a more thorough examination.

The upper lip should be examined, and the cleft should be classified as unilateral or bilateral and as complete or incomplete. In a complete unilateral cleft lip, the orbicularis oris sphincter is interrupted and muscle fibers turn upward at the cleft to insert partly onto its margin, while other fibers extend to the anterior nasal spine and alar base of the nose. In an incomplete cleft lip, the orbicularis is also interrupted, but often a bridge of skin and mucosa spans the cleft (**Figure 12-2A**). In a complete bilateral cleft lip, there is no functional orbicularis muscle in the central soft tissue (prolabium) (**Figure 12-2B**). In a complete unilateral cleft lip, the nose is also disrupted by the cleft, with septal deviation and displaced lower lateral nasal cartilage leading to a slumped nasal contour on the side of the cleft (**Figure 12-2C**). The gumline (alveolar ridge) and palate should then be inspected for a cleft. Complete cleft palates (unilateral or bilateral) affect the primary and secondary palate (**Figure 12-3**). Incomplete cleft palates may involve a variable amount of the soft and hard palate. Submucous cleft palates may present with only a bifid uvula, a muscular diastasis of the soft palate in the midline (zona pellucida, often noted by a bluish hue), or a V-shaped notch that can be palpated at the junction of the hard and soft palate. The posterior palatal muscles form the velum, a muscular sling that acts to lengthen the soft palate and narrow the pharynx. In a cleft palate, this musculature is not joined in the midline and abnormally inserts at the posterior edge of the hard palate. This disruption helps to explain the feeding, speech, and eustachian tube dysfunction in children with cleft palate.

In children with Pierre Robin sequence, the examination must begin with an evaluation of the airway. Severe airway obstruction can be present, prompting immediate intervention. After determination of a safe airway, other anomalies can be addressed. An ophthalmologist should examine the child's eyes, as some patients have Sticklers syndrome, which is associated with retinal problems. The mandible should be palpated and the temporomandibular joints examined. Attention to the degree of discrepancy between the upper jaw and the lower jaw is important to estimate the anticipated severity of airway and feeding problems. Normal temporomandibular joints are necessary if a mandibular distraction is to be performed. Flexible

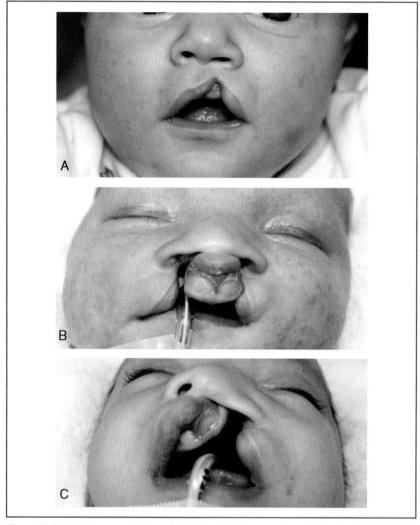

Figure 12-2. Variable presentations of cleft lip. A, Left incomplete cleft lip. B, Bilateral cleft lip. C, Left complete cleft lip.

nasopharyngoscopy can be helpful to evaluate the airway and predict the need for intervention.

The PCC should examine the ears and assess for otitis media with effusion (OME) via pneumatic otoscopy. In children with cleft palate, the insertion of the tensor veli palatini into the eustachian tube is abnormal, an abnormality commonly resulting in both poor ventilation of the ear and OME, which manifests with hearing loss at an early age and has a prolonged course and high rate of recurrence.

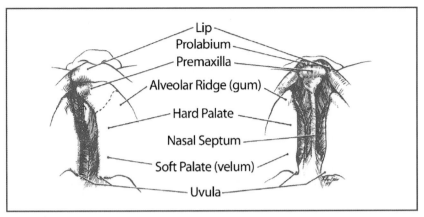

Figure 12-3. Unilateral and bilateral cleft palate.

Reprinted by permission from American Cleft Palate-Craniofacial Association, Chapel Hill, NC.

Because the prognosis for children with isolated clefts is good, whereas the prognosis for those with associated anomalies varies, a complete craniofacial, cardiopulmonary, and extremity examination also should be performed. Pits of the lower lip are seen in Van der Woude syndrome. Pierre Robin sequence in a child with a flat nasal bridge and myopia typifies Stickler syndrome. Velocardiofacial syndrome presents variably with cleft palate, velopharyngeal insufficiency (VPI), cardiac anomalies, unusual facial appearance, and learning difficulties. Children with Treacher Collins syndrome often exhibit auricular anomalies, midfacial hypoplasia, down-slanting palpebral fissures, and cleft palate. Many more syndromes are associated with CL/P, and genetic consultation is appropriate for further diagnostic workup and parental counseling.

> **Pearl:** The disruption of the normal palatal muscular anatomy seen in cleft palates explains the feeding, speech, and otologic difficulties that arise.

Diagnosis

The diagnosis of CL/P is usually made via prenatal ultrasound or in the early postnatal period. If detected on prenatal ultrasound, a prenatal consultation with a cleft team is appropriate. Parents of infants with clefts are often shocked and confused. To cope with these feelings, they find it useful to have a prenatal meeting with the cleft team who will be caring for their child after birth. After birth, a previously undiagnosed cleft is typically recognized at the initial physical examination. The PCC should examine the inside of the mouth with a tongue depressor and palpate the palate. Small posterior or submucous cleft palates initially may go unrecognized. These infants may present with failure to thrive, feeding difficulties, inability to nurse, or hypernasal speech (VPI) later in life. A diagnosis of CL/P following birth is equally traumatic to parents, with similar feelings of bereavement and loss while the family copes with all the typical issues of having a new infant.

Proper physical diagnosis will lead to appropriate classification of the cleft. In 1962, the ACPA introduced a complex classification, and many more have been introduced since that time. While these are important for the cleft team and for monitoring specific patient outcomes, they are not critical for effective communication between the caregiver and provider. A more straightforward scheme stratifies patients into 3 categories: isolated cleft lip (including the alveolus), isolated cleft palate (occurring posterior to the incisive foramen), and CL/P (**Box 12-1**). The description of the lip and/or the palate should also indicate whether the cleft is unilateral or bilateral and whether it is complete or incomplete. Simplifying the classification allows for improved communication between the PCC and cleft team, as well as enhanced communication with parents regarding their child's diagnosis.

In addition to the diagnostic aspects of the physical examination in classifying CL/P, assessment of hearing is important. Universal

---

Box 12-1. Classification of Cleft Lip and Palate

Cleft Lip
- Unilateral or bilateral
- Complete or incomplete

Cleft Palate
- Unilateral or bilateral
- Complete or incomplete
- Primary palate: alveolus to the incisive foramen
- Secondary palate: incisive foramen posteriorly
- Submucous cleft palate: muscle dehiscence only (may present as a bifid uvula)

Cleft Lip and Cleft Palate

newborn hearing screening should identify those children with moderate to severe hearing loss. The increased incidence of OME, glue ear, and conductive hearing loss in patients with cleft palate has long been recognized. Because OME occurs essentially in all patients with cleft palate, early recognition, treatment, and audio-logic follow-up are crucial. Although speech is not assessed at the initial evaluation, because of the potential impairments in velo-pharyngeal function and hearing, speech development should be assessed early. Children with cleft palate who are at risk can be identified by a cleft-trained speech pathologist at 18 months of age in 98% of cases.

> **Pearl:** A simple classification for clefts includes isolated cleft lip, isolated cleft palate, and cleft lip and palate. The cleft should be described further as unilateral or bilateral.

■ Treatment Options

Children with CL/P often require an ongoing treatment plan spanning from birth to late adolescence. This treatment follows a sequence of staged surgical procedures associated with rehabilitative speech, orthodontic measures, and attention to psychosocial needs. The PCC is often pivotal in coordinating the care of a child with CL/P. Parents should have the opportunity to meet with a cleft team member soon after diagnosis for appropriate counseling (**Box 12-2**). When a new-born is found to have a CL/P, most parents experience shock, denial, sadness, anger, and anxiety before they are able to bond with their

---

Box 12-2. Topic Areas to Discuss With Parents of Newborns With Cleft Lip or Palate

♦ Explain that the cleft is not their fault.
♦ Use proper medical terminology (ie, cleft lip or palate).
♦ Demonstrate normal aspects of the physical examination.
♦ Discuss feeding difficulties and demonstrate feeding techniques.
♦ Reassure parents that the child is not in pain.
♦ Discuss and arrange cleft team consultation.
♦ Reassure parents that cleft lip or palate is correctable with surgery.

---

child. Early interaction with a cleft team can reassure parents and address their fears. Team members typically include a cleft surgeon, an audiologist, a speech pathologist, a dentist, an orthodontist, a social worker, an otolaryngologist, an oral and maxillofacial surgeon, a geneticist, a psychologist, a pediatrician, a nutritionist, and a patient care coordinator.

When a neonate is born with a cleft (especially cleft palate), initial treatment should focus on feeding. Although infants with clefts may require modifications in feeding practices prior to surgical closure of the defect, few changes in dietary recommendations are necessary. A feeding assessment ideally should be performed by a feeding specialist (eg, speech pathologist) within 24 hours of birth. Only in very rare cases are children with cleft palates able to breastfeed. A variety of nipples and bottles are specially designed to assist a child with a cleft palate to effectively feed. No single device is superior to others, and the feeding specialist can aid parents or other caregivers in determining what works best for their child. Common feeders used in the United States include the cleft-specific Dr Brown's bottle, Haberman feeder, Mead Johnson Cleft Lip/Palate Nurser, and Pigeon Nipple. Most children can consume an adequate number of calories strictly on oral feeding. Close follow-up is required after hospital discharge to ensure adequate weight gain. An increased number of calories in the formula or substitution of assisted devices may be required if weight gain is poor. A nutritionist can be a valuable resource in treating feeding difficulties.

Depending on the anomaly, children with CL/P will follow a general time line of surgical interventions throughout the first 20 years after birth (**Figure 12-4**). The cleft surgeon, under the recommendations of the cleft team, performs the initial surgeries. If a cleft lip is present, it is typically repaired at 2 to 3 months of age. A generally quoted parameter for surgery is the rule of 10s: the child is older than 10 weeks, weighs more than 10 lbs, and has a hemoglobin level greater than 10 g/dL. Occasionally, if the cleft lip is wide, techniques will first be used to narrow the cleft gap. These include lip taping, nasal alveolar molding, or lip adhesion. After the cleft lip repair, children are often placed in soft arm restraints to limit digital trauma to the surgical site.

Cleft palate repair is usually performed at about 9 to 12 months of age to allow sufficient palatal and maxillary growth and to minimize subsequent growth problems, but before the child develops speech. Surgery may be delayed until age 15 months or later in patients with Pierre Robin sequence. The palate muscles are detached and moved

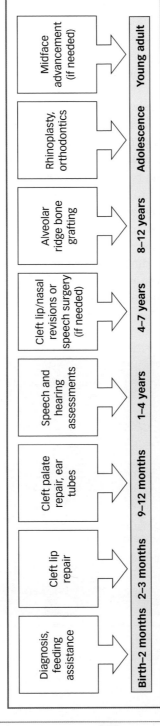

Figure 12-4. General time line for cleft lip and palate care.

from their abnormal lateral insertion to form a more normally functioning sling across the midline. Realigning the soft palate musculature and lengthening the palate decrease the risk of future speech problems (**Figure 12-5**). Nasal and oral mucosal flaps are joined in the midline to prevent oronasal communication. Patients are admitted postoperatively, often with a stitch placed in the tongue in case of airway obstruction (so as not to use an oral airway). The infant's oxygen saturation is monitored overnight, and he or she can usually be discharged the following day if taking adequate nutrition by mouth. Avoiding bottles, pacifiers, and straws minimizes sucking, which potentially could disrupt the palate repair. Arm restraints are again used to avoid digital trauma to the palate.

Airway support is necessary in about one-third of infants with Pierre Robin sequence. Prone positioning, oxygen, a nasal airway, or intubation may be necessary early interventions. Many patients require nasogastric tube feeding early on. Problems that may require more aggressive intervention include frequent desaturations, elevated pCO_2, overt respiratory distress, or inability to extubate. Patients with failure to thrive and poor feeding may also benefit from surgical

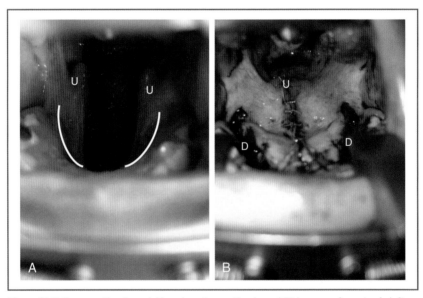

Figure 12-5. Preoperative (panel A) and postoperative (panel B) images of repair of cleft of hard and soft palates. Palatal incisions (white lines) are made laterally along the alveolar ridge, and mucosal flaps are raised. The elevated flaps are advanced medially and posteriorly toward the uvula (U), with suture closure in the midline. The donor sites in the lateral palate (D) heal by secondary intention.

intervention. Polysomnography can be helpful in defining the degree of airway compromise in patients with moderate levels of obstruction. A maxillofacial computed tomographic scan with 3-D reconstruction is helpful to define bony anatomy.

Airway management depends not only on the severity of obstruction, but also on resources, training, and skill of the care team. Prone positioning can be used in mild cases to get through the neonatal period, with the caveat that airway obstruction may worsen within the first few weeks after birth. Nasal trumpets also may be used to relieve obstruction. They are a good noninvasive way to overcome the obstruction, but require the family to keep the trumpet in place after going home. In tongue-lip adhesion, the anterior tongue tip is surgically secured to the lower lip. Although the procedure is straightforward, the possibility of avoiding a tracheotomy and progressing to oral feeding is less likely than that with the more invasive mandibular distraction osteogenesis (MDO). This technique relies on "catch-up growth" of the mandible and requires the adhesion to be retained for approximately 1 year. Second airway procedures are necessary in up to 45% of lip-tongue adhesions because mandibular growth is uncertain. The most common complication is dehiscence of the adhesion.

Mandibular distraction osteogenesis has gained in popularity in recent years. This procedure consists of osteotomies in the mandible with placement of distractors to advance the mandible anteriorly and inferiorly. While the immediate complications are minimal, the procedure can result in temporomandibular joint ankylosis, trauma to developing teeth, and marginal mandibular nerve paralysis secondary to removal of the devices through scar tissue. With MDO, the skeletal deficiency is corrected, resulting in a higher probability of achieving oral feedings and avoiding tracheotomy. Sleep apnea and failure to thrive are commonly resolved with MDO. Patients with concomitant syndromes are less likely to be treated successfully with MDO and may be better candidates for tracheotomy as the initial airway surgery. Central nervous system abnormalities, laryngomalacia, and preoperative intubation may increase the failure rate of MDO. Tracheotomy should be considered as an alternative surgery in these children, in children whose parents wish to prevent the stated risks, and in patients with significant comorbidities who cannot undergo multiple or lengthy surgeries. For some patients with significant feeding difficulty but a good airway, gastrostomy tube placement may be appropriate.

Eustachian tube dysfunction is common in children with cleft palate because of the altered muscle position of the palate and anomalies of the eustachian tube. Close medical and audiologic follow-up during the first 5 years after birth ensures detection of significant hearing loss. The American Academy of Pediatrics clinical practice guideline on OME places children with cleft palate in an at-risk group for development delays. Thus, consideration for early placement of ventilation ear tubes is recommended. A recent study provides evidence that most children with cleft palate have reduced hearing levels unless ventilation tubes have been inserted. Most ventilation tubes are placed at the time of cleft palate repair, although some are placed earlier at the time of cleft lip repair. The role of the audiologist and otolaryngologist is to continue monitoring hearing and eustachian tube function when patients return to the cleft team.

After the initial surgical repairs of the clefts and placement of ear tubes, patients are typically followed up by the cleft team every 9 to 12 months. A hearing and speech assessment at those visits will determine any deficits. From 18 months on, the patient will be regularly monitored for speech development and proper function of the palate. The specific structural deficiencies of a cleft palate can impose articulatory constraints on speech development. These include VPI, residual clefts or fistula after initial repair, nasal obstruction, and dental/occlusal anomalies. An estimated two-thirds of children with cleft palate repairs are advised to receive speech therapy, which often is all that is required to overcome articulation problems. Velopharyngeal insufficiency is characterized by hypernasal resonance, weak pressure consonants, or nasal emission accompanying pressure-consonant production. A dysfunctional palate with incomplete closure of the velopharyngeal sphincter can lead to VPI. Approximately 5% to 30% of children require secondary speech surgery following cleft palate repair because of VPI. Most surgeons perform the repair with a pharyngeal flap or sphincter pharyngoplasty, essentially narrowing the nasopharyngeal inlet. The goal is eliminating velopharyngeal dysfunction without creating obstructive sleep apnea, which is a known adverse effect of the surgeries. The role of the speech pathologist on a cleft team is to identify problems and recommend appropriate treatment.

General dentists, orthodontists, and oral and maxillofacial surgeons play an important role in the care of a child with a cleft of the palate or alveolus. Children with CL/P may have missing or extra teeth. They also have an increased incidence of tooth decay, so earlier cleanings and preventive dental care are important. While the child is in the mixed dentition stage (7–10 years of age) and prior to eruption of the cleft canine, the cleft alveolus is typically closed with a bone graft obtained from autologous cancellous bone from the iliac crest. Formal orthodontics can then proceed to improve dental occlusion. Occasionally, patients develop midface retrusion because of impaired maxillary growth after CL/P repair. The need for maxillary advancement surgery to bring the midface forward occurs in about 5% to 25% of patients with CL/P. The oral and maxillofacial surgeon or cleft surgeon performs this surgery.

Children with cleft lip deformities often have underlying nasal deformities caused by the altered anatomy. To improve the appearance and function of the nose, most cleft surgeons will perform septorhinoplasty. A primary rhinoplasty is often performed at the time of cleft lip repair. Further nasal tip work may be performed to achieve symmetry with other future surgeries. A definitive secondary septorhinoplasty that includes improvement of septal and bony abnormalities is reserved until adolescence to ensure that nasal development is not interrupted and an appropriate-sized nose has formed. Revisions of cleft lip (to improve the lip scar) and palate (close fistulas) can also be combined with these secondary procedures if necessary.

> **Pearl:** Early referral to a cleft team can ensure the proper stepwise treatment plan necessary for children with clefts.

■ Natural History and Prognosis

The natural history of an unrepaired CL/P is that of continued facial deformity, speech and feeding difficulties, and ear problems into adulthood. Studies of young adults with unrepaired CL/P demonstrate less facial growth restriction than that in those with early repair. Treating the facial disfigurement and speech and feeding impairments far outweighs any potential midface growth restriction challenges. Based on refinements of technique and successful outcomes, the question has not been whether to repair but the appropriate timing of surgery.

Regarding cleft lip repair, studies have shown that neonatal surgery does not provide better results or any psychological benefit for parents. In addition, permitting the child to grow and tolerate surgery at 3 months of age gives the parents time to get to know their child and adjust to the appearance of the cleft. Children who cope well later in life are those whose parents are psychologically well-adjusted to the CL/P.

Following cleft lip surgery at age 2 to 3 months, the timing of cleft palate repair must be decided. Early studies have shown that a child has a better chance of developing normal speech if the cleft palate is repaired early. Unfortunately, surgery to the bony cleft alveolus and palate has been shown to interfere with maxillary growth. Despite this paradox, evidence exists that good facial growth and good speech can be achieved after closure of the palate in a single stage before 1 year of age—thus, the selection of a 9- to 12-month window for closure of the cleft palate. Cleft palate repair may need to be delayed until 15 months of age or later in patients with Pierre Robin sequence and airway difficulties. If cleft palate repair is delayed, speech development may be worse. Even when these parameters are followed, 20% to 30% of children will require prolonged intensive speech therapy or secondary speech surgery because of articulation errors and VPI.

The natural otologic history of children with cleft palate includes OME and eustachian tube dysfunction. Prospective trials in which myringotomy has been undertaken routinely at the same time as cleft repair demonstrate an incidence of OME of 92%, compared with a prevalence of 20% in children without cleft palate. Eustachian tube function improves in older children with cleft palates, and after age 6 years, there is likely to be resolution of OME. Otologic examination in older children with cleft palate should evaluate for tympanic membrane perforations, persistent OME, severe eardrum retractions, and retraction pocket cholesteatomas. Referral to an otolaryngologist is appropriate if the ear examination raises concern about possible otologic pathology.

By following an appropriate surgical and intervention time line in children with CL/P, excellent results are achieved. Early referral to a cleft team will place the child under the umbrella of many trained professionals. Their common goal is to attain as much normalcy for the child with CL/P as possible, and the reported outcome studies demonstrate that this is achievable.

■ Selected References

Abel F, Bajaj Y, Wyatt M, Wallis C. The successful use of the nasopharyngeal airway in Pierre Robin sequence: an 11-year experience. *Arch Dis Child*. 2012;97(4):331–334

American Academy of Family Physicians, American Academy of Otolaryngology-Head and Neck Surgery, American Academy of Pediatrics Subcommittee on Otitis Media With Effusion. Otitis media with effusion. *Pediatrics.* 2004;113(5):1412–1429

Atkinson M. Surgical management of otitis media with effusion in children—NICE guideline: what paediatricians need to know. *Arch Dis Child Educ Pract Ed.* 2009; 94(4):115–117

Bender PL. Genetics of cleft lip and palate. *J Pediatr Nurs.* 2000;15(4):242–249

Bluestone CD. Eustachian tube obstruction in the infant with cleft palate. *Ann Otol Rhinol Laryngol.* 1971;80(Suppl 2):1–30

Boyne PJ, Sands NR. Secondary bone grafting of residual alveolar and palatal clefts. *J Oral Surg.* 1972;30(2):87–92

Broen PA, Moller KT, Carlstrom J, Doyle SS, Devers M, Keenan KM. Comparison of the hearing histories of children with and without cleft palate. *Cleft Palate Craniofac J.* 1996;33(2):127–133

Coy K, Speltz ML, Jones K. Facial appearance and attachment in infants with orofacial clefts: a replication. *Cleft Palate Craniofac J.* 2002;39(1):66–72

Dalston RM. Communication skills of children with cleft lip and palate: a status report. In: Bardach J, Morris HL, eds. *Multidisciplinary Management of Cleft Lip and Palate.* Philadelphia, PA: Saunders; 746–749

Flores RL, Tholpady SS, Sati S, et al. The surgical correction of Pierre Robin sequence: mandibular distraction osteogenesis versus tongue-lip adhesion. *Plast Reconstr Surg.* 2014;133(6):1433–1439

Fraser GR, Calnan JS. Cleft lip and palate: seasonal incidence, birth weight, birth rank, sex, site, associated malformations and parental age. A statistical survey. *Arch Dis Child.* 1961;36(188):420–423

Gómez OJ, Barón OI, Peñarredonda ML. Pierre Robin Sequence: an evidence-based treatment proposal. *J Craniofac Surg.* 2018;29(2):332–338

Grow JL, Lehman JA Jr. A local perspective on the initial management of children with cleft lip and palate by primary care physicians. *Cleft Palate Craniofac J.* 2002; 39(5):535–540

Horton CE, Crawford HH, Adamson JE, Ashbell TS. Tongue-tie. *Cleft Palate J.* 1969; 6:8–23

Jorgenson RJ, Shapiro SD, Salinas CF, Levin LS. Intraoral findings and anomalies in neonates. *Pediatrics.* 1982;69(5):577–582

Kaufman FL. Managing the cleft lip and palate patient. *Pediatr Clin North Am.* 1991; 38(5):1127–1147

Lees M. Genetics of cleft lip and palate. In: Watson ACH, Sell DA, Grunwell P, eds. *Management of Cleft Lip and Palate.* London, England: Whurr Publishers; 2001

Maarse W, Bergé SJ, Pistorius L, et al. Diagnostic accuracy of transabdominal ultrasound in detecting prenatal cleft lip and palate: a systematic review. *Ultrasound Obstet Gynecol.* 2010;35(4):495–502

Milerad J, Larson O, Hagberg C, Ideberg M. Associated malformations in infants with cleft lip and palate: a prospective, population-based study. *Pediatrics.* 1997;100(2 Pt 1): 180–186

Noar JH. Questionnaire survey of attitudes and concerns of patients with cleft lip and palate and their parents. *Cleft Palate Craniofac J.* 1991;28(3):279–284

Nyberg DA, Sickler GK, Hegge FN, Kramer DJ, Kropp RJ. Fetal cleft lip with and without cleft palate: US classification and correlation with outcome. *Radiology.* 1995;195(3): 677–684

Paradise JL, Bluestone CD, Felder H. The universality of otitis media in 50 infants with cleft palate. *Pediatrics.* 1969;44(1):35–42

Randall P, LaRossa DD, Fakhraee SM, Cohen MA. Cleft palate closure at 3 to 7 months of age: a preliminary report. *Plast Reconstr Surg.* 1983;71(5):624–628

Redford-Badwal DA, Mabry K, Frassinelli JD. Impact of cleft lip and/or palate on nutritional health and oral-motor development. *Dent Clin North Am.* 2003;47(2):305–317

Robinson PJ, Lodge S, Jones BM, Walker CC, Grant HR. The effect of palate repair on otitis media with effusion. *Plast Reconstr Surg.* 1992;89(4):640–645

Senders CW, Peterson EC, Hendrickx AG, Cukierski MA. Development of the upper lip. *Arch Facial Plast Surg.* 2003;5(1):16–25

Slade P, Emerson DJ, Freedlander E. A longitudinal comparison of the psychological impact on mothers of neonatal and 3 month repair of cleft lip. *Br J Plast Surg.* 1999; 52(1):1–5

Strauss RP, Sharp MC, Lorch SC, Kachalia B. Physicians and the communication of "bad news": parent experiences of being informed of their child's cleft lip and/or palate. *Pediatrics.* 1995;96(1 Pt 1):82–89

Suslak L, Desposito F. Infants with cleft lip/cleft palate. *Pediatr Rev.* 1988;9(10):331–334

Vanderas AP. Incidence of cleft lip, cleft palate, and cleft lip and palate among races: a review. *Cleft Palate J.* 1987;24(3):216–225

Young JL, O'Riordan M, Goldstein JA, Robin NH. What information do parents of newborns with cleft lip, palate, or both want to know? *Cleft Palate Craniofac J.* 2001; 38(1):55–58

Neck

CHAPTER 13

Neck Masses and Adenopathy

Randall A. Bly, MD and Sanjay R. Parikh, MD

▓ Introduction

Neck masses in children represent a variety of pathologies, encompassing many possible etiologies, ranging from congenital to infectious to neoplastic. Masses can be present anywhere in the head and neck, with varying rates of growth and age at onset. Initial assessment must include evaluation of the airway because compression can occur with some masses. Infectious masses may present with septicemia and the patient may be acutely ill. Certainly, in these cases urgent treatment should be initiated, typically with referral to an emergency department and otolaryngology consultation.

In general, the differential diagnosis favors infectious and congenital etiologies because of the rarity of neoplasms in the pediatric population. Palpable cervical lymphadenitis is common and prevalent in nearly half of all healthy children. Fortunately, in most cases these represent benign processes. However, a level of suspicion must be maintained for cases in which the history, physical examination findings, or imaging results are concerning. In many of these cases, additional workup or biopsy may be necessary.

To formulate a differential diagnosis and begin treatment, the primary care clinician (PCC) can classify the mass according to its clinical presentation and history. A useful way to organize the neck mass is by location, whether it is midline or lateral in the neck (**Figure 13-1**). In general, midline neck masses represent a congenital etiology. Any mass that is not located near the anterior midline is referred to as lateral, including masses that arise in the posterior neck. Lateral neck masses are more variable in their etiology, but infectious cause is the most likely. When combined with the clinical history and examination findings, the differential diagnosis can be made to guide the workup of neck masses in children.

> **Pearl:** Midline neck masses are more likely to be caused by congenital malformations, whereas lateral neck masses are often seen with infectious etiologies.

Epidemiology

Cervical adenopathy is the most common presentation of masses in the neck. A study in Sweden demonstrated that up to 45% of healthy schoolchildren had palpable cervical lymphadenopathy on examination. When symptomatic patients who seek treatment for cervical lymphadenopathy are studied, up to 75% of cases are due to reactive lymph nodes caused by bacterial or viral infections. In most of these cases, neck masses were located in the lateral neck.

Multiple studies have reported that congenital etiologies such as thyroglossal duct cysts, branchial cleft cysts, and lymphatic malformations represent 12% to 22% of all neck masses.

Neoplastic processes such as lymphoma, sarcoma, or metastatic lesions account for less than 8% of neck masses in the pediatric population.

Presenting Symptoms

Masses can present in a variety of ways, including painless lumps noted incidentally or acute, painful, erythematous masses in the neck. Cervical adenopathy can be discrete or diffuse, with or without local

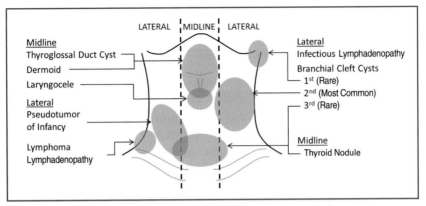

Figure 13-1. Typical location regions for common midline and lateral pediatric neck masses. There is significant variability in the location for many etiologies. Infectious lymphadenopathy can occur anywhere but is more likely to be located in the lateral neck. Lymphoma lymphadenopathy may present anywhere in the neck but typically occurs laterally in the posterior triangle. Note: Region locations drawn for clarity in labeling and can occur on the left or right side (slight left- or right-sided propensities for certain congenital etiologies not necessarily depicted).

inflammation. The PCC should obtain a detailed clinical history about the mass or masses. Additional information such as tuberculosis exposure, prior bacille Calmette-Guérin vaccination, or cat exposure can be helpful. Abscesses can occur anywhere in the head and neck and can be superficial or deep.

Congenital etiologies may manifest with infectious symptoms. A tender midline neck mass in a patient with fevers and localized erythema may represent a previously subclinical thyroglossal duct cyst or dermoid cyst that has become acutely infected.

Because of the wide variety of pathologies that can manifest as neck masses, presenting symptoms discussed as follows relate to the specific diagnosis.

■ Physical Examination Findings

Careful attention should be paid to vital signs, including the growth curve to assess trends in weight loss. This is particularly important in more chronic processes. Neck masses are characterized by location, quality, size, and appearance.

In young children, many neck masses can be seen with simple visual inspection if the patient looks up toward the ceiling. Doing so will stretch the skin, bring the larynx forward, and help to reveal midline masses (**Figure 13-2**). Palpation with the pads of the index and middle fingers is best to appreciate subtle masses underlying the skin and to assess the mobility of the mass. The latter is most important in distinguishing a dermoid cyst, which usually can be rolled around like a marble under the skin, from a thyroglossal duct cyst, which is deeper and not easily displaced so that only the dome of the cyst is palpable. Palpation of all regions of the neck can discover a diffuse process that the patient initially thought was a single mass. In these cases especially, the PCC should examine lymph node regions outside the neck, including supraclavicular, axillary, and inguinal lymph node groups.

A thorough head and neck examination is essential, including testing of cranial nerves. For example, a rare first branchial cleft cyst presents as a mass near the angle of the mandible, but a sinus tract may also be seen in the external auditory canal on otoscopy. This finding provides important clues about etiology. A mass in a similar location over the parotid gland may be associated with peritonsillar swelling and may represent a mass in the deep lobe of the parotid. In addition, there are systemic inflammatory etiologies that cause cervical adenopathy. Thus, a complete history and physical examination can help elucidate these challenging diagnoses.

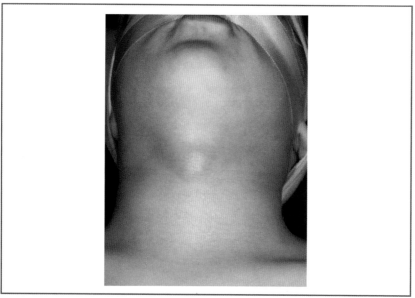

Figure 13-2. Midline neck mass in a 14-year-old boy confirmed to be a thyroglossal duct cyst on pathological analysis after a sistrunk procedure.

■ Differential Diagnosis of Midline Neck Masses

THYROGLOSSAL DUCT CYSTS

Thyroglossal duct cysts represent nearly 75% of all midline neck masses in children. These cysts are remnants of the embryologic descent of the thyroid gland, which begins at the foramen caecum at the base of the tongue. In nearly 70% of cases, the initial presentation is a midline, nontender neck mass at the level of the thyroid cartilage. About 20% of the time it presents with an infection.

Ultrasound is the diagnostic imaging modality of choice. It can often confirm that the mass is cystic and predict its contents as well as confirm that the thyroid gland is present in its normal position lower in the neck. This is important because in 1% to 2% of cases the cyst may contain ectopic thyroid tissue that is the patient's only thyroid tissue. When no thyroid gland can be identified, radionuclide scanning and thyroid function tests should be considered preoperatively. Computed tomography (CT) is useful when the diagnosis remains in doubt.

Treatment options are observation versus surgical removal via the Sistrunk procedure, which also removes a portion of the hyoid bone and the tract that extends into the origin of the lesion at the base of the tongue. The recurrence rate is extremely high if only the cyst is removed. If a patient has an infected cyst, antibiotic therapy is the best initial management, and a Sistrunk procedure should be considered when inflammation has reduced. Performing a simple incision and drainage on an acutely infected cyst may cause scarring, make the Sistrunk procedure more challenging, and increase the risk of recurrence. Regardless, incision and drainage may be necessary for infections that are refractory to medical therapy. Typically, if the mass is bothersome or has become infected, it should be surgically removed to prevent future problems.

> **Pearl:** An acutely inflamed thyroglossal duct cyst is best managed with medical therapy to avoid scarring. This will improve the outcome of a complete resection later when there is less inflammation.

DERMOID CYSTS

Dermoid cysts are part of a spectrum of benign germ cell neoplasms. They are the most common type, and are composed of ectoderm and mesoderm tissue. Only 7% of all dermoid cysts occur in the head and neck, and the periorbital region is the most common location. Other locations include the nasal tip and neck, and they are often found near the midline.

Dermoid cysts in the neck present similarly to thyroglossal duct cysts with palpable mass, frequently with noted recent change and firm consistency. Unlike thyroglossal duct cysts, however, dermoid cysts generally present with progressive indolent growth and no history of fluctuating size. Ultrasound may not be able to discern between the 2, but, as noted earlier, physical examination often does. Treatment is complete surgical resection, but observation is an option if the patient is asymptomatic and the mass is small. Acute infectious episodes should be managed medically with antibiotics; surgical excision should be considered when an acute infection has resolved.

Other lesions in the spectrum are rare and include teratoid tumors (contain poorly differentiated ectoderm, mesoderm, and endoderm), true teratomas (contains well-differentiated tissue from all 3 layers), and epignathus, in which identifiable fetal organs, such as limbs, may be seen within the mass. These tumors may be very large and present at birth. Some may cause airway obstruction. When possible, complete surgical resection is the best treatment option.

THYROID AND PARATHYROID MASSES

Thyroid and parathyroid masses are rare in the pediatric population. Thyroid nodules occur in 0.05% to 1.8% of children, and it is estimated that malignant thyroid disease occurs in fewer than 2 per 100,000 children per year. Such masses are usually discovered as a visible and/or palpable mass that moves in conjunction with the larynx during swallowing. Initial serologic evaluation to establish the nature of the nodule includes thyroid function tests and determination of calcium levels.

Ultrasound is the study of choice to confirm the presence of a thyroid nodule and to establish its size. For lesions larger than 1 cm, the American Thyroid Association recommends biopsy by fine needle aspiration for euthyroid or hypothyroid patients to rule out malignancy (**Figure 13-3**). In cases considered likely to require

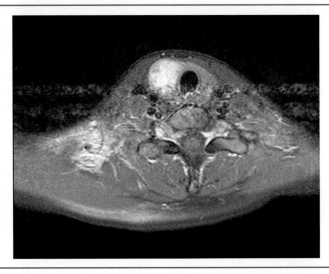

Figure 13-3. Axial T1-weighted magnetic resonance imaging with contrast in a 15-year-old girl with a right thyroid lobe mass who underwent total thyroidectomy after suspicious fine-needle biopsy finding suggested papillary carcinoma, which was confirmed on final pathological analysis.

biopsy, it may be prudent for the PCC to request that an interventional radiologist biopsy the lesion at the same time as the initial ultrasound. The study may require sedation or general anesthesia. Some otolaryngologists, especially those with ultrasound equipment in their offices, will perform FNA in the office in select patients using only topical anesthetic. If the patient and family have already decided on surgical excision, or if general anesthesia is needed for FNA, there may be limited utility in obtaining the test. Conversely, when FNA reveals a cystic lesion with no atypical cells, this finding may obviate the need for surgical intervention. In a recent study of 30 pediatric patients undergoing FNA biopsy, there was 1 false-negative result and 5 that were inconclusive. When FNA is not performed with the initial ultrasound, the decision to perform it is best discussed with the patient and family.

Malignant lesions generally require surgical removal. Nodules with associated hyperthyroidism also should be considered for removal, as hyperfunctioning nodules have been associated with a risk of malignancy. Thyroid lobectomy is performed when open surgery is required for a tissue diagnosis. When a malignant diagnosis is confirmed, total thyroidectomy with or without nodal dissection of the neck is indicated depending on clinical staging and pathological findings. In patients with multiple endocrine neoplasia type 2A, total thyroidectomy is recommended before age 5 years to prevent medullary thyroid carcinoma.

Parathyroid masses are exceedingly rare. Only 7 cases have been recorded in the literature, and they may not even present with a palpable neck mass.

INFANTILE HEMANGIOMAS

Infantile hemangiomas are the most common benign neoplasm of childhood, affecting up to 10% of children in the first 12 months after birth. They can occur anywhere in the body, but the most common location is the central portion of the face. Hemangiomas characteristically present with a proliferative stage, followed by an involution phase that begins in late infancy and may continue for several years. In recent years, propranolol therapy has become the mainstay of medical treatment for lesions associated with severe symptoms, functional compromise, or a high risk of permanent cosmetic deformity. Surgery is indicated when a hemangioma does not improve with observation or medical therapy, when a hemangioma is focal and in a favorable location, or when elective surgery would leave a scar that would be the same if the lesion were removed after involution. Children should be referred to an institution where multidisciplinary evaluation can occur with a dermatologist, a surgeon, and other specialists familiar with the pathology. Vascular malformations are discussed in Chapter 25.

LARYNGOCELES

Laryngoceles are rare and caused by outpouchings of the saccule of the larynx. They typically develop in patients who regularly breathe out forcefully with the mouth and nostrils closed, such as musicians who play wind instruments and may have nasal obstruction. They can present as a midline neck mass if herniation extends beyond the thyroid cartilage. They may protrude through the thyrohyoid membrane, palpable just above the thyroid cartilage. If outpouching is internal, infants or children may present with stridor and airway obstruction. Ultrasound and CT may help delineate the extent of the mass. Flexible or direct laryngoscopy should be performed to assess for internal components. Surgical resection is the recommended treatment.

■ Differential Diagnosis of Lateral Neck Masses

Studies have demonstrated that nearly half of healthy children have a palpable neck mass on examination. Most are hyperplastic lymph nodes with no associated signs or symptoms of illness and require no evaluation or intervention. When an etiology can be identified, it is usually an infectious illness, but most cases are benign and self-limited. Congenital etiologies are the next most frequently encountered cause of lateral neck masses. Malignancies and inflammatory syndromes are less common but represent a broad spectrum of causes.

INFECTIOUS CAUSES OF LATERAL NECK MASSES

Acute Lymphadenitis

Acutely enlarged lymph nodes are usually submandibular or high deep cervical nodes to which most of the lymphatics of the head and neck drain. Pharyngeal, dental, and scalp infections are sources that commonly lead to reactive cervical lymphadenopathy. Bilateral or diffuse acute lymphadenitis is usually caused by viral infection, but bacterial sources such as *Streptococcus pyogenes* or *Mycoplasma pneumoniae* can also be the pathogens. Clinical clues such as coexisting inflammation of the gingiva and oral cavity or rash suggest viral sources such as herpes simplex and cytomegalovirus. Occipital or posterior lymphadenitis is frequently associated with concurrent infection or inflammation of the scalp, but it also may be associated with rubella infection. Most viral causes are benign and resolve spontaneously.

Mononucleosis infection is a possibility and should be considered in the differential diagnosis. Imaging tests often will reveal multiple lymph nodes, which can be significant in size (6–12 cm). Diagnosis is suggested by elevated atypical lymphocytes on a complete blood cell count and confirmed by a heterophile antibody test (monospot, 87% sensitive, 91% specific). Antibody testing to viral-specific antibodies (97% sensitive, 94% specific) is preferred to the monospot in children younger than 5 years. If test results are negative but clinical suspicion remains, additional testing, such as polymerase chain reaction (PCR) for Epstein-Barr virus DNA, can be useful. Confirming the diagnosis is important so that other concerning processes, such as neoplasm, can be determined to be less likely on the differential diagnosis. In addition, confirmation of the diagnosis may obviate the need for surgical biopsy to rule out malignancy.

Unilateral or focal acute lymphadenitis is typically caused by bacterial infection. The 2 most common organisms are *Staphylococcus aureus* and *S pyogenes*. There appears to be a trend toward an increasing incidence of community-acquired methicillin-resistant *S aureus* in many populations. These bacterial infections can progress to form phlegmon or abscess, which causes increased tenderness, decreased neck range of motion, and a palpable, tender neck mass. Sometimes, there is overlying skin erythema and hyperemia. Ultrasound or CT scan with contrast is often indicated to assess the extent of infection. Depending on the patient's clinical stability, surgical drainage may be indicated. Intravenous antibiotic therapy with appropriate coverage based on local antibiograms should be initiated. If a patient's condition is clinically stable, a trial of antibiotic therapy prior to surgical drainage has the potential to avoid a surgical procedure. In these cases, the family and patient must be well informed, and the patient should be monitored in the inpatient setting so that reimaging or surgical drainage can be performed quickly if needed. Additional information about deep neck space infections is provided in Chapter 14.

In neonates, acute unilateral lymphadenitis can be caused by group B streptococcal infection. This typically occurs in males who are febrile with erythematous skin changes and ipsilateral otitis media.

Pearl: Palpable cervical lymphadenopathy is a common finding in children and is usually caused by reactions to viral infections in the head and neck. Most episodes resolve spontaneously.

Chronic Lymphadenitis

Chronically enlarged lymph nodes are usually jugulodigastric or posterior triangle nodes. In many cases of cervical lymphadenopathy in healthy patients with no associated symptoms or clinical findings, it is not necessary to reach a definitive diagnosis if the patient can be closely followed clinically. In most such cases, the biopsy will return a diagnosis of reactive adenopathy with no other specific diagnosis. However, in cases of persistent adenopathy in a child with current or previous acute illness, or when a node is larger than 2 cm, diagnosis should be sought. Depending on the clinical presentation, blood and fungal cultures, PCR for *Bartonella henselae,* and a purified protein derivative (PPD) test should be considered. Ultrasound and CT scan also may be helpful. If the diagnosis is still uncertain and symptoms persist, FNA or open biopsy, with specimens sent for microbiological and histopathologic evaluation, is the best way to reach a definitive diagnosis.

Suspicion of a neoplastic process must be maintained for cases of chronic lymphadenopathy refractory to medical management. Regular follow-up is necessary to track progress and order additional tests or place referrals as necessary. Lymphoma (discussed in detail later) is 1 of the most common diagnoses that present similarly to chronic lymphadenitis. More than 50% of patients with head and neck lymphoma also have involvement of extranodal sites including oropharynx, paranasal sinuses, orbit, nasal cavity, and salivary glands. Further, there often are radiographic clues suggesting a neoplastic process. A combination of clinical history and suspicion, thorough physical examination, and radiographic results will guide the decision regarding a tissue biopsy.

The following is a list of pathogens, their presentation, and treatment strategies for infectious, benign, chronic lymphadenitis.

ATYPICAL MYCOBACTERIA (NONTUBERCULOUS MYCOBACTERIA)

These can be the cause of unilateral chronic lateral neck masses in children. Atypical mycobacteria include ubiquitous bacteria such as *Mycobacterium avium-intracellulare* and *Mycobacterium scrofulaceum* that are found particularly in midwestern and southwestern United States. These bacteria can breach mucosal and skin barriers through cuts or the teething process, which explains why cervical lymph nodes are most likely to be involved.

Patients usually present with a single neck mass located near the body or angle of the mandible and characteristic overlying violaceous skin changes. Often, there is some fluctuance within the mass. There also can be spontaneous drainage resulting in a chronic fistula tract. Atypical mycobacteria lymphadenitis must be distinguished from active tuberculosis lymphadenitis. Unlike active tuberculosis, atypical infections generally exhibit the following clinical characteristics:
1. No history of contact with active tuberculosis
2. PPD test result smaller than 15 mm
3. Normal findings on chest radiography
4. Younger than 4 years

There have been reports of PPD cross-reactivity in the presence of atypical mycobacterial infections. Thus, definitive diagnosis must be made with histopathologic and microbiological analysis, which can be achieved with FNA or open biopsy. Treatment traditionally has been surgical excision or curettage, with excellent results, but recent studies have demonstrated success with medical therapy or even observation alone in immunocompetent children. Once an accurate diagnosis has been reached through biopsy or culture, a discussion should be held with the family to decide the best option for management. Referrals should be made to an infectious disease specialist or otolaryngologist, or possibly both, to fully discuss options, including observation, antibiotic therapy, and surgical excision.

TOXOPLASMA GONDII

Toxoplasma gondii is widespread, with a prevalence as high as 90% depending on location. Humans can become infected by ingesting oocytes, often from cats or uncooked meats. Examination almost always reveals lymphadenopathy in the neck, with varying incidences of palpable lymphadenopathy in other lymph node regions. Most cases are asymptomatic and self-limiting. Serology testing is available but is rarely indicated, and it can be difficult to prove that acute infection is responsible for current lymphadenopathy.

BARTONELLA HENSELAE

A small gram-negative bacterium responsible for cat-scratch disease, *B henselae* typically causes infections in patients younger than 10 years, with regional lymphadenopathy being the predominant clinical feature. A history of exposure to cats, usually younger than 6 months, or flea bites and evidence of a pustule at the inoculation site make this diagnosis more likely. Diagnosis can be confirmed with PCR. Antibiotic therapy (macrolides or trimethoprim-sulfamethoxazole) is effective but often not necessary because many cases are self-limiting. Incision and drainage should be avoided because this can cause skin fistula tracts. If medical therapy is refractory, complete surgical excision should be performed.

HIV

HIV in children can present with chronic, generalized lymphadenopathy, which is often associated with splenomegaly. Serologic testing for HIV is part of the complete workup of chronic cervical lymphadenitis.

CONGENITAL CAUSES OF LATERAL NECK MASSES

Branchial Cleft Cysts

Relatively common, branchial cleft cysts account for nearly one-third of all congenital neck masses. The exact mechanism is not clear, but they are most likely caused by incomplete obliteration of branchial clefts in embryogenesis. They typically present in late childhood but can also first become clinically apparent in adulthood. Branchial cleft sinuses—epithelialized tracts connecting to the pharynx, dermis of neck, or external auditory canal—more commonly present in the first few years after birth (**Figure 13-4**). In contrast, branchial cleft cysts without a skin opening typically present at older ages. Cysts of the second branchial cleft account for 95% of these cysts. Second cleft cysts occur in the lateral neck anterior to the sternocleidomastoid (SCM) muscle (**Figure 13-5**). They may present as nontender cystic masses or as acute infections with localized erythema and tenderness. A history of fluctuating mass size supports congenital etiology. First branchial cleft anomalies present as masses or sinuses at or near the angle of the mandible and can communicate with the external auditory canal. Third branchial cleft cysts and sinuses are also rare and typically present as recurrent localized infections in the lower lateral neck adjacent to the ipsilateral lobe of the thyroid gland. They can communicate with the pyriform sinus in the pharynx (**Figure 13-6**) and are sometimes referred to as pyriform fossa sinus tract anomalies. Recurrent infections of the low anterior neck should prompt a laryngoscopy to look for a sinus tract at the time of incision and drainage. Transoral endoscopic cauterization of the sinus tract and simple incision and drainage without excision of the cyst wall have been reported to be successful in treating these specific pyriform fossa abnormalities. Avoiding complete excision reduces morbidity and the duration of surgery significantly. However, most types of branchial anomalies still require complete excision.

Ultrasound, CT, and magnetic resonance imaging (MRI) are useful to further evaluate the mass in relation to surrounding structures. Ultrasound is a good initial test to confirm that the mass is cystic, but additional cross-sectional imaging may be required.

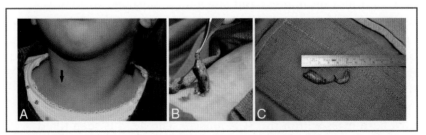

Figure 13-4. A, Small, nearly imperceptible, skin opening (punctum, arrow) in the lower neck of a child noted only when draining. B, Intraoperative photograph of 4-cm long sinus tract partially removed. C, Specimen showing the entirety of the sinus tract.

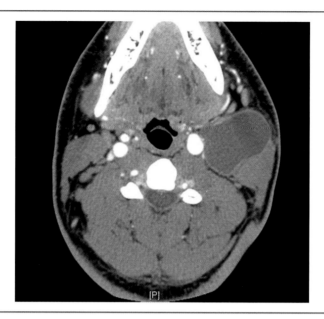

Figure 13-5. Axial computed tomography with contrast of a 16-year-old boy with persistent fluctuating left neck mass. The final pathological evaluation after complete excision confirmed a second branchial cleft anomaly.

Treatment is most commonly complete surgical resection. In the case of acute infection, antibiotic treatment is preferred because incision and drainage may cause scarring. In some cases, this cannot be avoided, and needle aspiration is often attempted to minimize scarring. Complete surgical resection can be performed with a high success rate if tissue is not actively inflamed.

Fibromatosis Colli and Congenital Muscular Torticollis

Fibromatosis colli (FC) (also referred to as pseudotumor of infancy or SCM tumor of infancy) and congenital muscular torticollis (CMT) are rare disorders involving dysfunction of the SCM muscle. Fibromatosis colli and CMT are similar entities, and distinction between the 2 has been vague. Recent literature has referred to the disorder as FC in patients younger than 6 weeks and as CMT if the patient is older at the time of diagnosis.

Fibromatosis colli typically presents in infants as a congenital rock-hard mass within the SCM muscle. The head is seen tilted toward the affected side, while the chin is turned away from the affected side, because the SCM muscle acts to rotate the head to the opposite side. The lesion can masquerade as a neoplasm

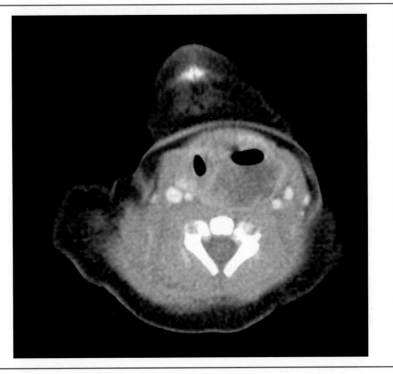

Figure 13-6. Axial computed tomography with contrast of a 3-year-old boy with acute onset of a left neck mass. Note involvement of the thyroid gland and air in mass consistent with an infected pharyngeal pyriform sinus tract anomaly (also referred to as a third branchial cleft anomaly).

(particularly rhabdomyosarcoma) or cervical lymphadenitis. Fibromatosis colli has a prevalence of 0.4% and is the third most common congenital musculoskeletal anomaly, after hip dislocation and clubfoot.

The pathogenesis of FC is unclear; theories point to mechanical factors of fetal positioning in utero or birth-related trauma. This is supported by associations with breech presentations and traumatic births. Ultrasonography typically demonstrates fusiform enlargement of the SCM muscle but will not differentiate the lesion from rhabdomyosarcoma.

Many FC cases resolve spontaneously, although physical therapy is likely to improve outcomes. Initial treatment involves range-of-motion exercises for the infant younger than 2 months. For symptoms that persist despite therapy, further imaging can be performed and surgical intervention is possible. Sternocleidomastoid tenotomy has been shown to be effective at releasing muscle heads. Surgical intervention should be performed when the patient is at least 12 to 18 months old. If symptoms persist past this period, facial and skull asymmetry may develop. The 12- to 18-month window allows ample time for spontaneous improvement to occur, but also permits early surgical intervention, if necessary, to prevent facial asymmetry.

Thymic Cysts

Thymic cysts result from thymic tissue implanting anywhere along the embryologic descent of the thymus from the third pharyngeal pouch. They are rarely reported in the literature, but may be more prevalent as they are often asymptomatic and noted incidentally. They are cystic and located to the left of midline. Occasionally, they are large and present with airway obstruction. Evaluation should begin with ultrasound in a patient in stable condition. Surgical excision is the recommended treatment for symptomatic masses. Observation is an option in some cases if there are no symptoms.

Vascular and Lymphatic Malformations

These are discussed in Chapter 15.

MALIGNANT CAUSES OF LATERAL NECK MASSES

Malignancies occur at an incidence of 1 in every 7,000 children younger than 14 years; they represent the second leading cause of death in the 1- to 14-year-old age group, following accidents. Within the head and neck, lymphomas are the most common malignancy encountered. There are many other types of rare malignant neoplasms that can present primarily or as metastatic lesions. Sarcomas and neuroblastomas make up a large portion of these uncommon malignancies.

Lymphoma

Lymphoma in the pediatric population accounts for 10% of all solid tumors in the United States. In regions where Epstein-Barr virus is endemic, Burkitt lymphoma is much more prevalent. According to a recent study in Korea, nearly half of pediatric lymphoma cases can present as a mass in the head and neck. Other characteristics of lymphoma were found to be male predominance (2.5:1) and age older than 10 years. Hodgkin lymphoma usually presents with painless cervical lymphadenopathy. Follicular and small lymphocytic lymphomas are more likely to present with bilateral, painless, soft, discrete, and small cervical nodes. Mucosa-associated lymphoid-tissue lymphomas can present as an isolated swelling of the thyroid or salivary glands, and are sometimes associated with autoimmune disorders.

Imaging studies can show multiple, solid, enlarged lymph nodes (**Figure 13-7**). High clinical suspicion is warranted in patients who first present with concerning signs. They should be followed up closely and be referred to a center where imaging studies to determine stage and best location for biopsy can be coordinated. Fine needle aspiration and core biopsy are only useful if the lymphoma evaluation results in a positive finding. Interpretation of cytologic test results and tissue samples must be done at an experienced laboratory, and the family must understand that the tissue sample may be inadequate for diagnosis. Open biopsy allows for the most accurate diagnosis.

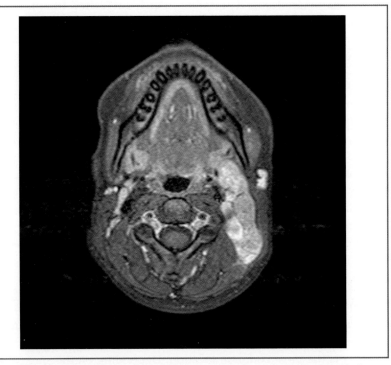

Figure 13-7. Axial image of T1-weighted magnetic resonance imaging with contrast of a 13-year-old girl with a lateral neck mass confirmed to be Hodgkin lymphoma on biopsy.

Lymphoma can present similarly to benign cervical adenopathy, but careful attention to details of clinical presentation, examination findings, and worrisome imaging results permit appropriate workup and consideration for referral. More than half of patients with head and neck lymphoma also have involvement at extranodal sites, including the posterior pharynx and Waldeyer ring, maxilla/mandible, paranasal sinuses, orbit, nasal cavity, and salivary glands. Radiologic findings suggestive of malignancy on ultrasound include displacement of vessels, aberrant vessels, an avascular focus, and subcapsular vessels. These physical examination and radiologic findings, coupled with a history of progressive cervical adenopathy or constitutional symptoms, warrant a biopsy to obtain a diagnosis. Retrospective studies of cervical adenopathy have based the decision to perform a biopsy on abnormal ultrasound findings and persistence of the mass after 4 to 6 weeks despite antibiotic therapy. Fewer than 15% of patients met the criteria for biopsy, and the majority of biopsy results show infectious or congenital etiologies. About 20% of patients who met the criteria and underwent biopsy received a diagnosis of lymphoma, which correlated to approximately 2% of all patients who presented with cervical lymphadenopathy. Treatment is usually chemotherapy. Cure rates for Hodgkin lymphoma approach 90%.

Sarcoma

Sarcoma soft tissue tumors make up fewer than 20% of pediatric head and neck malignancies; rhabdomyosarcoma is the most common type encountered. It usually presents in patients younger than 6 years. The orbit is involved in one-third of cases and may cause proptosis. Treatment is usually multimodal, with surgery, chemotherapy, and/or radiotherapy. Prognosis is a function of many factors, including the ability to obtain negative margins on surgical resection. Nonrhabdomyosarcomas are very rare, with an incidence of 2 to 3 cases per million. There are many types, including fibrosarcoma, chondrosarcoma, osteosarcoma, liposarcoma, leiomyosarcoma, and hemangiopericytoma.

Neuroblastomas

These neural tumors account for approximately 25% of malignant head and neck tumors in the pediatric population. The adrenal medulla is the most common location. Depending on the stage at presentation, a combined treatment plan of surgery, chemotherapy, and radiotherapy can be developed. However, despite advances in chemotherapy regimens, prognosis is poor overall because of the advanced stage at which many neuroblastomas become clinically apparent and are diagnosed.

Salivary Gland Tumors

These are discussed in Chapter 15.

INFLAMMATORY SYNDROMES

Chronic cervical lymphadenopathy may also be a manifestation of a number of inflammatory syndromes. A thorough history and physical examination can provide clues to systemic etiologies. Sarcoidosis, juvenile systemic lupus erythematous, Kawasaki disease, juvenile rheumatoid arthritis, Graves disease, and Rosai-Dorfman disease (histiocytosis) may present with cervical lymphadenopathy. Cervical adenitis has been reported after phenytoin injection or after vaccinations. Periodic fever, aphthous stomatitis, pharyngitis, and cervical adenitis (PFAPA) syndrome should be included in the differential diagnosis in the setting of this constellation of symptoms. Many other rare diseases, such as Kikuchi-Fujimoto disease and Kimura disease, are possible causes of cervical adenitis with systemic symptoms.

▓ Imaging

In cases in which diagnosis is uncertain and for possible surgical planning, imaging may be extremely helpful. For soft tissue masses, ultrasonography is the initial imaging modality of choice because of its ability to delineate borders and relationship to vessels, as well as provide accurate descriptions of size, shape, and vascularity. There is no radiation exposure, and it is relatively inexpensive and can be performed without sedation. If the mass is too large to be captured on ultrasound or if more detail is required, CT or MRI may be indicated.

> **Pearl:** Ultrasonography is the initial imaging modality of choice for evaluation of soft tissue neck masses in the pediatric population.

■ Treatment Options

Most persistent masses in the head and neck should undergo imaging and be evaluated by an otolaryngologist. Treatment options vary significantly. Observation may be the best initial management for many benign-appearing cervical adenopathies. Enteric and intravenous antimicrobial therapies play a large role in the treatment of infectious etiologies. Surgical resection is the best option for problematic congenital neck masses. Open biopsy plays an important role in accurate tissue diagnosis of malignancies.

■ Natural History and Prognosis

Benign cervical adenopathy that resolves is not associated with any significant long-term negative sequelae. Surgical interventions for acute infections or congenital masses are associated with short hospital stays and minimal morbidity. The prognosis for malignancies of the head and neck varies greatly; they are best examined individually with a patient and family once staging and histopathologic information is available.

■ Selected References

Albright JT, Pransky SM. Nontuberculous mycobacterial infections of the head and neck. *Pediatr Clin North Am.* 2003;50(2):503–514

Albright JT, Topham AK, Reilly JS. Pediatric head and neck malignancies: US incidence and trends over 2 decades. *Arch Otolaryngol Head Neck Surg.* 2002;128(6):655–659

Al-Dajani N, Wootton SH. Cervical lymphadenitis, suppurative parotitis, thyroiditis, and infected cysts. *Infect Dis Clin North Am.* 2007;21(2):523–541, viii

Al-Khateeb TH, Al Zoubi F. Congenital neck masses: a descriptive retrospective study of 252 cases. *J Oral Maxillofac Surg.* 2007;65(11):2242–2247

Altincik A, Demir K, Abacı A, Böber E, Büyükgebiz A. Fine-needle aspiration biopsy in the diagnosis and follow-up of thyroid nodules in childhood. *J Clin Res Pediatr Endocrinol.* 2010;2(2):78–80

Ayugi JW, Ogeng'o JA, Macharia IM. Pattern of congenital neck masses in a Kenyan paediatric population. *Int J Pediatr Otorhinolaryngol.* 2010;74(1):64–66

Bell AT, Fortune B, Sheeler R. Clinical inquiries. What test is the best for diagnosing infectious mononucleosis? *J Fam Pract.* 2006;55(9):799–802

Chen EY, Inglis AF, Ou H, et al. Endoscopic electrocauterization of pyriform fossa sinus tracts as definitive treatment. *Int J Pediatr Otorhinolaryngol.* 2009;73(8):1151–1156

Citak EC, Koku N, Demirci M, Tanyeri B, Deniz H. A retrospective chart review of evaluation of the cervical lymphadenopathies in children. *Auris Nasus Larynx.* 2011;38(5):618–621

Coppit GL III, Perkins JA, Manning SC. Nasopharyngeal teratomas and dermoids: a review of the literature and case series. *Int J Pediatr Otorhinolaryngol.* 2000;52(3): 219–227

Coventry MB, Harris LE. Congenital muscular torticollis in infancy: some observations regarding treatment. *J Bone Joint Surg Am.* 1959;41-A(5):815–822

Cushing SL, Boucek RJ, Manning SC, Sidbury R, Perkins JA. Initial experience with a multidisciplinary strategy for initiation of propranolol therapy for infantile hemangiomas. *Otolaryngol Head Neck Surg.* 2011;144(1):78–84

Emery C. The determinants of treatment duration for congenital muscular torticollis. *Phys Ther.* 1994;74(10):921–929

Fiedler AG, Rossi C, Gingalewski CA. Parathyroid carcinoma in a child: an unusual case of an ectopically located malignant parathyroid gland with tumor invading the thymus. *J Pediatr Surg.* 2009;44(8):1649–1652

Francis GL, Waguespack SG, Bauer AJ, et al; American Thyroid Association Guidelines Task Force. Management guidelines for children with thyroid nodules and differentiated thyroid cancer. *Thyroid.* 2015;25(7):716–759

Harris RL, Modayil P, Adam J, et al. Cervicofacial nontuberculous mycobacterium lymphadenitis in children: is surgery always necessary? *Int J Pediatr Otorhinolaryngol.* 2009;73(9):1297–1301

Herold BC, Immergluck LC, Maranan MC, et al. Community-acquired methicillin-resistant *Staphylococcus aureus* in children with no identified predisposing risk. *JAMA.* 1998;279(8):593–598

Hill DE, Chirukandoth S, Dubey JP. Biology and epidemiology of *Toxoplasma gondii* in man and animals. *Anim Health Res Rev.* 2005;6(1):41–61

Josefson J, Zimmerman D. Thyroid nodules and cancers in children. *Pediatr Endocrinol Rev.* 2008;6(1):14–23

Larsson LO, Bentzon MW, Berg-Kelly K, et al. Palpable lymph nodes of the neck in Swedish schoolchildren. *Acta Paediatr.* 1994;83(10):1091–1094

Niedzielska G, Kotowski M, Niedzielski A, Dybiec E, Wieczorek P. Cervical lymph-adenopathy in children: incidence and diagnostic management. *Int J Pediatr Otorhinolaryngol.* 2007;71(1):51–56

Nogová L, Reineke T, Eich HT, et al. Extended field radiotherapy, combined modality treatment or involved field radiotherapy for patients with stage IA lymphocyte-predominant Hodgkin's lymphoma: a retrospective analysis from the German Hodgkin Study Group (GHSG). *Ann Oncol.* 2005;16(10):1683–1687

Papadopouli E, Michailidi E, Papadopoulou E, Paspalaki P, Vlahakis I, Kalmanti M. Cervical lymphadenopathy in childhood epidemiology and management. *Pediatr Hematol Oncol.* 2009;26(6):454–460

Pryor SG, Lewis JE, Weaver AL, Orvidas LJ. Pediatric dermoid cysts of the head and neck. *Otolaryngol Head Neck Surg.* 2005;132(6):938–942

Ren W, Zhi K, Zhao L, Gao L. Presentations and management of thyroglossal duct cyst in children versus adults: a review of 106 cases. *Oral Surg Oral Med Oral Pathol Oral Radiol Endod.* 2011;111(2):e1–e6

Robson CD. Imaging of head and neck neoplasms in children. *Pediatr Radiol.* 2010; 40(4):499–509

Roh JL, Huh J, Moon HN. Lymphomas of the head and neck in the pediatric population. *Int J Pediatr Otorhinolaryngol.* 2007;71(9):1471–1477

Rosenberg HK. Sonography of pediatric neck masses. *Ultrasound Q.* 2009;25(3):111–127

Scott KJ, Schroeder AA, Greinwald JH Jr. Ectopic cervical thymus: an uncommon diagnosis in the evaluation of pediatric neck masses. *Arch Otolaryngol Head Neck Surg.* 2002;128(6):714–717

Sridhara SK, Shah RK. Rosai-Dorfman in the submandibular salivary glands of a pediatric patient. *Laryngoscope.* 2010;120(Suppl 4):S228

Szinnai G, Meier C, Komminoth P, Zumsteg UW. Review of multiple endocrine neoplasia type 2A in children: therapeutic results of early thyroidectomy and prognostic value of codon analysis. *Pediatrics.* 2003;111(2):e132–e139

Tunkel DE, Domenech EE. Radioisotope scanning of the thyroid gland prior to thyroglossal duct cyst excision. *Arch Otolaryngol Head Neck Surg.* 1998;124(5):597–599

Wei JL, Schwartz KM, Weaver AL, Orvidas LJ. Pseudotumor of infancy and congenital muscular torticollis: 170 cases. *Laryngoscope.* 2001;111(4 Pt 1):688–695

Wexler LH, Helman LJ. Pediatric soft tissue sarcomas. *CA Cancer J Clin.* 1994;44(4):211–247

Wiersinga WM. Thyroid cancer in children and adolescents: consequences in later life. *J Pediatr Endocrinol Metab.* 2001;14(Suppl 5):1289–1296

Wolinsky E. Mycobacterial lymphadenitis in children: a prospective study of 105 nontuberculous cases with long-term follow-up. *Clin Infect Dis.* 1995;20(4):954–963

Zeharia A, Eidlitz-Markus T, Haimi-Cohen Y, Samra Z, Kaufman L, Amir J. Management of nontuberculous mycobacteria-induced cervical lymphadenitis with observation alone. *Pediatr Infect Dis J.* 2008;27(10):920–922

CHAPTER 14

Deep Neck Space Infection

Amy Hughes, MD, and Sukgi S. Choi, MD, MBA

▧ Introduction

Deep neck infections (DNIs) are common among pediatric patients and occur most frequently after dental or upper respiratory tract infections, often in the presence of a congenital neck mass. While the frequency of these infections has decreased with the advent and expansion of antimicrobial therapy, the problem still exists and requires a team approach using medical and surgical management. The proximity of DNIs to major vascular structures, the mediastinum, and the central nervous system makes early diagnosis and treatment imperative owing to the potential for catastrophic complications, including devastating neurologic sequalae and even death.

There is a lack of consensus and a dearth of literature regarding the diagnosis and management of DNI. Frequent questions arise about the selection of the imaging modality, timing and duration of antibiotic therapy, and role of surgical intervention in treatment. The aim of this chapter is to summarize the literature and provide recommendations for the management of patients with a DNI.

▓ Epidemiology

The incidence of DNI in the United States is estimated to be 4.6 per 100,000 children. Most cases occur in children younger than 6 years. Coticchia et al reported an average age of 4.1 years in their series of 169 pediatric patients. There was a male predominance (56% vs 44%), and white (54%) and black (43%) children were most commonly affected.

▓ Anatomy

The neck is divided into compartments by the cervical fascia and anatomical structures (**Figure 14-1**). Knowledge of these compartments and their contents is critical to understanding routes of spread between compartments and potential complications. The cervical fascia is separated into superficial and deep layers. The superficial layer of the cervical fascia underlies the skin, surrounds the platysma muscle, and is continuous with the superficial muscular aponeurotic system, which invests the musculature of the face. This continues cranially as the temporoparietal fascia. While the superficial layer of the cervical fascia is straightforward, the deep cervical fascia is more complex. The deep layer of the cervical fascia is divided into 3 distinct layers: superficial, middle, and deep.

SPACES

The neck is divided into several spaces, which act as natural barriers to help contain deep neck space abscesses. Most commonly, DNIs are described as being in the parapharyngeal and retropharyngeal spaces; however, a basic knowledge of neck compartments allows primary care clinicians (PCCs) to have increased awareness of potential complications based on the location of the infection (**Figure 14-2**).

Submandibular

The submandibular space comprises 2 spaces separated by the mylohyoid muscle: the sublingual space and the submylohyoid (or submaxillary) space. Importantly, the tooth roots of the second and third

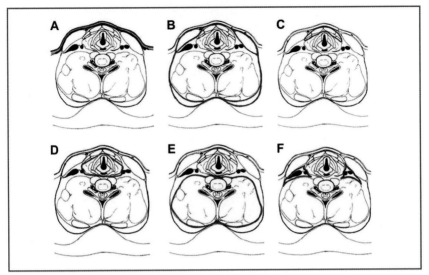

Figure 14-1. Cervical fascial planes highlighted in red. A, Superficial cervical fascia. B, Superficial layer of deep cervical fascia. C, Muscular division of the middle layer of deep cervical fascia. D, Visceral division of the middle layer of deep cervical fascia. E, Deep layer of deep cervical fascia. F, Carotid sheath.

Modified from Vieira, Allen SM, Stocks RM, Thompson JW. Deep neck infection. *Otolaryngol Clin North Am.* 2008;41(3):459–483, with permission from Elsevier.

molars lie below the mylohyoid line of the mandible, allowing infections of these teeth to spread directly into the submylohyoid compartment. The submylohyoid space contains the submental space, which is the space confined by the anterior belly of the digastric muscle bilaterally, mandible anteriorly, and hyoid bone posteriorly and inferiorly.

Parapharyngeal

The parapharyngeal space, or lateral pharyngeal space, is immediately subjacent to the lateral pharyngeal wall. It is the shape of an inverted pyramid that extends from the skull base down to its apex at the level of the hyoid bone (**Figure 14-2**). The medial border is the pharyngeal musculature, consisting of the superior pharyngeal constrictor muscle and its surrounding pharyngobasilar fascia. The lateral border is the mandible and pterygoid musculature. The parapharyngeal space is divided into the prestyloid space, which contains the deep lobe of the parotid, fat, and lymph nodes, and the poststyloid space, which contains the internal jugular vein, internal carotid artery, cranial nerves IX to XII, the sympathetic trunk, the superior sympathetic ganglion, the ascending pharyngeal artery, and lymph nodes.

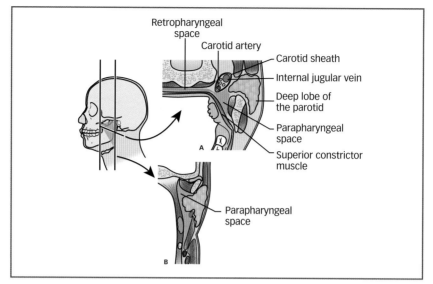

Figure 14-2. A, Axial section at the level of the oral cavity demonstrating the contents of the parapharyngeal space. B, Coronal section through the oropharynx showing the vertical boundaries of the parapharyngeal space.

Based on Blumberg JM, Judson BL. Surgical management of parapharyngeal space infections. *Oper Tech Otolaryngol-Head Neck Surg.* 2014;25(3):304–309.

Peritonsillar

The peritonsillar space is the space immediately lateral to the tonsil capsule. It separates the tonsil from the pharyngeal musculature. As such, the pharyngeal musculature lies between the peritonsillar and parapharyngeal spaces.

Retropharyngeal

The retropharyngeal space is bordered posteriorly by the alar fascia, a component of the deep layer of the deep cervical fascia, and anteriorly by the visceral layer of the middle layer of the deep cervical fascia (**Figure 14-3**). The retropharyngeal space extends from the skull base to the mediastinum. Undiagnosed or inadequately treated infections within this space can lead to catastrophic intrathoracic complications. The retropharyngeal space is divided into a right and left side by a midline raphe. As such, processes involving the retropharyngeal space generally resect the midline.

The retropharyngeal space contains lymph nodes that can be the origins of pathology within the space. Upper respiratory infections (URIs) can manifest with lymphadenopathy in the retropharyngeal nodes and ultimately suppurate. Similarly, other pathology, including upper aerodigestive

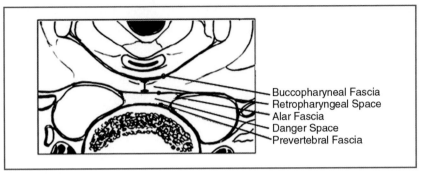

Buccopharyneal Fascia
Retropharyngeal Space
Alar Fascia
Danger Space
Prevertebral Fascia

Figure 14-3. Divisions of the deep cervical fascia delineating the retropharyngeal and danger spaces. Note the midline raphe dividing the right and left retropharyngeal space, which is absent in the danger space.

Modified from Vieira, Allen SM, Stocks RM, Thompson JW Deep neck infection. *Otolaryngol Clin North Am.* 2008;41(3):459–483, with permission from Elsevier.

tract malignancies, can hide within these lymph nodes, so lymph node enlargement in this area is not necessarily caused by an infection.

Prevertebral

The prevertebral space is defined anteriorly by the prevertebral fascia. Its posterior border is the vertebral bodies of the spine and the anterior longitudinal ligament.

Danger

The danger space is defined anteriorly by the alar fascia and posteriorly by the prevertebral fascia. This space extends from the skull base to the coccyx. In contrast to the retropharyngeal space, infections in the danger or prevertebral spaces can occur in the midline.

Vascular (Carotid)

The carotid space, also known as the visceral vascular space, is that which is contained by the carotid sheath. Beyond the major vascular structures, this space also contains the vagus nerve and the sympathetic trunk. The glossopharyngeal, spinal accessory, and hypoglossal nerves also exit the skull base into the carotid space and travel within the space until their exit at various points along its length.

Spaces of the Face

The spaces of the face are included here to establish their relationship to the spaces of the neck:

- The masticator space lies between the masseter muscle laterally and the lateral pterygoid muscle medially. It is an extension of the temporal space and includes branches of the third division of the trigeminal nerve as well as the internal maxillary artery.

- The buccal space is contained between the buccopharyngeal fascia on the medial aspect of the buccinator muscle and the skin of the cheek laterally. It contains the parotid duct, facial artery, and buccal fat pad.
- The parotid space is connected with the parapharyngeal or lateral pharyngeal space. The lateral border is the parotidomasseteric fascia, which is a component of the superficial layer of the deep cervical fascia. It contains the facial nerve and external carotid artery branches as well as the parotid gland.

▒ Diagnosis

HISTORY AND PHYSICAL EXAMINATION FINDINGS

Deep neck infections are frequently preceded by infections of the ears, nose, or throat, given their continuity with the deep neck spaces and their lymphatic drainage pathways. Odontogenic sources are also common, with the submandibular space most frequently involved when the infection is dental in origin. The presenting signs and symptoms of DNI in children may be subtle and can vary widely. These are detailed in **Table 14-1,** with fever and neck mass the most common presenting symptoms, followed by a lymphadenopathy, sore throat, poor oral intake, and neck stiffness. Coticchia et al reported respiratory distress in about 4% of their patient population. The mean (standard deviation) duration of symptoms before presentation has been reported to be 3.5 (3.05) days (**Table 14-1**).

The most common physical examination findings include cervical lymphadenopathy, decreased neck range of motion, torticollis, tonsillitis, and tonsillar displacement. Drooling, stridor, and dyspnea are less commonly present at admission. In their review, Adil et al found that patients with dyspnea/stridor were 2.7 times more likely to undergo surgical intervention. In contrast, patients with lymphadenopathy and fever were twice as likely to be managed medically.

Primary care clinicians should consider the diagnosis of a congenital neck mass in patients who present with a neck abscess during infancy or a neck abscess that is recurrent in nature. These patients also may be asymptomatic, with the exception of the palpable neck mass on examination. Abscesses or fluid collections that are present in the midline are most commonly infected thyroglossal duct cysts, while infected branchial cleft cysts occur laterally and are typically unilocular collections with a well-circumscribed circular shape (**Figure 14-4**).

Table 14-1. Most Common Presenting Signs, Symptoms, and Investigations of Deep Neck Infection by Age Group

Age Group (y)	Duration of Symptoms Prior to Admission (d)	Common Presenting Signs or Symptoms				
		Most Common				Less Common
<1	3.1	Fever	LAD	Rhinorrhea	Poor oral intake	Agitation	Neck stiffness
≥1 to <4	5.1	LAD	Neck mass	Fever	Poor oral intake	Sore throat	Neck stiffness
≥4 to <10	4.8	Neck mass	Fever	LAD	Neck stiffness	Oropharyngeal abnormalities	Poor oral intake
≥10 to <19	6.3	Neck mass	Fever	Sore throat	Dysphagia	Neck stiffness	Poor oral intake
All patients	4.7	Neck mass	Fever	LAD	Poor oral intake	Sore throat	Neck stiffness

Abbreviation: LAD, lymphadenopathy.
Data from Coticchia JM, Getnick GS, Yun RD, Arnold JE. Age-, site-, and time-specific differences in pediatric deep neck abscesses. *Arch Otolaryngol Head Neck Surg.* 2004;130(2):201–207.

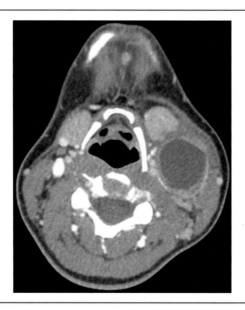

Figure 14-4. Axial contrast-enhanced computed tomographic image showing an infected second branchial cleft cyst.

LABORATORY STUDIES

Laboratory evaluation may include a complete blood cell count, C-reactive protein (CRP) level, and erythrocyte sedimentation rate. These tests may be useful in the diagnosis of a DNI as well as in clinical monitoring of a patient's response to treatment. Several authors have reported a significantly higher white blood cell count in infected patients with abscess formation compared with those without an abscess (22.0 vs 18.4). With regard to CRP levels, no statistically significant differences were found between groups.

DIAGNOSTIC IMAGING

Diagnostic imaging is integral to the management of DNI. Reviewed here are the various imaging modalities, including their advantages and disadvantages. **Table 14-2** details radiographic findings in patients with deep neck abscesses.

Lateral Neck Radiography

Lateral neck radiography was once the cornerstone of diagnostic imaging for DNI; however, with the advent of computed tomography (CT), its utility in diagnosing deep neck space infections has been

Table 14-2. Investigative Findings of Patients with Deep Neck Infections by Age Group

Age Group (y)	Investigative Findings			
	Mean WBC Count (× 10³ cells/ μL)	Mean Temperature (Celsius)	Positive Lateral Neck Radiograph (% patients)	Positive Neck CT (% patients)
<1	23.2	38.6	100	91
≥1 to <4	20.6	38.6	89	95
≥4 to <10	18.5	38.4	90	85
≥10 to <19	14.9	38.3	100	79
All patients	20.1	38.5	91	90

Abbreviations: CT, computed tomography; WBC, white blood cell.
Data from Coticchia JM, Getnick GS, Yun RD, Arnold JE. Age-, site-, and time-specific differences in pediatric deep neck abscesses. *Arch Otolaryngol Head Neck Surg.* 2004; 130(2):201–207.

debated. Nagy and Backstrom reported that lateral neck radiographs had a sensitivity of 83% for determining the presence of a DNI, compared with a 100% sensitivity for contrast-enhanced CT imaging. While lateral neck radiography is simple, quick, and easily accessible, its limited role in making an accurate diagnosis and allowing for surgical planning has made it less relevant today.

Ultrasound

As otolaryngologists become increasingly familiar with ultrasound, an increasing emphasis is being placed on its use. Evidence suggests that ultrasound may be more accurate than CT in differentiating an abscess from a phlegmon; however, it is operator dependent, does not provide surgeons with extensive anatomical detail for operative planning, and is not as reliable for evaluation of deeper neck space infections.

Computed Tomography

Contrast-enhanced CT scan is the gold-standard imaging modality for the evaluation of DNI. It provides a fast and accurate diagnosis, allowing for timely treatment planning. Computed tomography also provides important information about the adjacent anatomy for use in evaluating surgical approaches and the presence of complications, such as internal jugular vein thrombosis and mediastinitis.

Multiple studies have been published correlating CT with intraoperative findings. The outcomes have suggested that the sensitivity of CT for diagnosing an abscess ranges from 87.9% to 95%, but, overall, CT is not as specific. While rim enhancement is a commonly used CT characteristic for differentiating between an abscess and a phlegmon, some studies have shown no significant difference between the degree of rim enhancement and incidence of surgical drainage; however, irregularity or scalloping of the abscess wall (**Figure 14-5**) did have a positive predictive value of 94% for finding pus at the time of incision and drainage. Hypodensity volume measurements of 2,000 mm³ or greater also have been suggested as a predictor of the need for surgical drainage; however, this too is controversial.

Magnetic Resonance Imaging

Although the use of magnetic resonance imaging (MRI) in evaluating DNI is documented and it is potentially useful, the practicality of performing MRI in all patients in whom a DNI is suspected is limited. The expense and time required for imaging, particularly in the pediatric age group in which general anesthesia is frequently required for scanning, outweigh the enhanced soft-tissue definition.

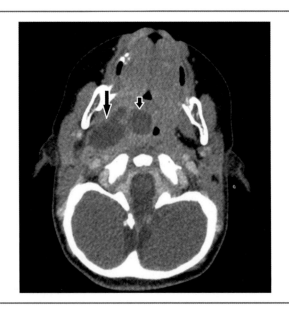

Figure 14-5. Axial contrast-enhanced computed tomographic image showing a right retropharyngeal (small arrow) fluid collection with rim enhancement and a right parapharyngeal (large arrow) fluid collection with scalloped edges.

> **Pearl:** Contrast-enhanced computed tomography is the preferred study for evaluation of deep neck infections. Irregularity or scalloping of the abscess wall may predict the presence of pus at the time of incision and drainage.

▣ Microbiology

The microbiology of DNI can be divided into groups based on the source of infection. Infections of odontogenic origin are distinctly different from nonodontogenic infections in terms of the inciting pathogen.

ODONTOGENIC INFECTIONS

Mixed anaerobic and aerobic bacteria are often isolated from odontogenic infections, with *Streptococcus viridans* a commonly isolated aerobic organism. *Prevotella, Staphylococcus,* and *Peptostreptococcus* have also been described. In a 2006 study, sensitivity data for these organisms demonstrated a high susceptibility of *S viridans* to penicillin and ampicillin, while the staphylococci were significantly less susceptible. Staphylococci were highly susceptible to ciprofloxacin (95%), clindamycin (90%), and vancomycin (100%). Sensitivity data for anaerobic isolates were not available.

NONODONTOGENIC INFECTIONS

Several studies have looked at the microbiological makeup of deep neck space abscesses. Brook collected data from 14 patients; he isolated anaerobic bacteria in all patients and mixed flora in 12 of the 14 patients. *Peptostreptococcus* and *Bacteroides* species were the most commonly isolated anaerobic bacteria, whereas commonly isolated aerobic bacteria included alpha- and gamma-hemolytic streptococci, *Staphylococcus aureus, Haemophilus influenzae*, and group A hemolytic streptococci. Similar results were published by Asmar, who also reported isolating mixed organisms and anaerobes in 53% of cases. Of note, other studies have isolated largely aerobic bacteria, specifically group A streptococcus and *S aureus*, with rare anaerobic bacteria noted. Patients treated with antibiotics before drainage may have negative cultures.

Resistant organisms, namely methicillin-resistant *S aureus* (MRSA), appear to be increasing in prevalence in DNI. In a study of 245 patients undergoing incision and drainage of neck abscesses, Thomason et al reported an increase in the proportion of MRSA isolates from 9% in 2001 to 40% in 2005. This finding is concerning given that this organism is not covered by first-line antibiotic therapy for refractory lymphadenitis or other URIs. Evidence also suggests that MRSA may be more aggressive than its nonresistant counterparts.

Importantly, the microbiology of neck abscesses in patients with diabetes differs from that in nondiabetic patients. These patients often have infections related to *Klebsiella pneumoniae.* Care must be taken when treating patients with diabetes to cover *Klebsiella,* as clindamycin alone is not an effective therapy in these cases.

In summary, the microbiology of DNI varies in the location and suspected etiology of the infection. Anaerobic and aerobic organisms, including the possibility of MRSA, must be considered when selecting antimicrobial therapy. Most PCCs start treatment with intravenous (IV) clindamycin or ampicillin/sulbactam until cultures become available or treatment failure occurs.

■ Treatment

MEDICAL THERAPY

Antibiotic therapy is the cornerstone of treatment for all DNIs. The decision to treat with antibiotics alone should be based on clinical and radiographic data and may be considered in patients who are antibiotic naïve, have small abscesses, or have no evidence of airway compromise. While it would be ideal to tailor antimicrobial therapy to cases in which the origin of infection is known, frequently it is difficult to determine the exact source of the infection and, as a result, comprehensive coverage of the most common organisms responsible for DNIs is an appropriate first step.

McClay et al reported a series of 11 patients with parapharyngeal, retropharyngeal, or combined abscesses defined by CT scan with a diameter greater than 1 cm in all dimensions. The maximum-diameter abscess in this series was 3.9 cm. The patients were treated with clindamycin and, in most cases, cefuroxime. Ten of 11 patients (91%) experienced resolution of their symptoms with medical therapy alone by 8 days. The 1 patient whose infection did not resolve underwent successful surgical drainage of purulence. Importantly, none of the patients in this series had evidence of airway compromise. The authors reassessed patients' conditions at 48 hours after the initiation of IV antibiotic therapy for signs of improvement. If none were noted, surgical intervention was considered.

In a larger series, Al-Sabah et al retrospectively reviewed 68 patients with a retropharyngeal infection based on CT scan. All patients received empirical clindamycin therapy. Only 25% of patients required surgical intervention. They concluded that all patients should receive a trial of conservative medical management for 72 hours, with surgery reserved for those who do not respond. On average, patients in the medical group received 5 days of IV antibiotic therapy and 10 days of oral therapy after discharge. The surgical patients received 6.5 days of IV therapy followed by 10 days of oral therapy after discharge. There were no recurrences.

The increasing incidence of MRSA has resulted in the evolution of routine antibiotic therapy. Many PCCs now recommend the empirical use of clindamycin, with possible addition of a cephalosporin (cefuroxime or ceftriaxone) to account for this trend. Care must be taken to distinguish between community-acquired and hospital-acquired strains, which are frequently resistant to clindamycin and trimethoprim-sulfamethoxazole.

> **Pearl:** Antimicrobial therapy may be considered as first-line management for DNI in patients who are antibiotic naïve, have small abscesses, or have no evidence of airway compromise.

SURGICAL THERAPY

Surgical management of DNIs should be considered in patients with airway symptoms, evidence of an associated complication (ie, mediastinitis), and possibly a larger abscess (>2.2 cm). Additionally, patients who have not shown improvement after 48 hours of IV antibiotic treatment should be re-evaluated for surgical management.

The role of needle aspiration in the treatment of DNI has shown variable success, with 56% to 80% of patients responding to needle aspiration and antibiotic treatment alone. This treatment modality has shown greater success in unilocular abscesses and should be considered in patients with presumed congenital neck masses. The benefit of performing needle aspiration in this population is preservation of the surgical plane for future surgical interventions. In children, needle aspiration is often performed using imaging guidance, most commonly ultrasound.

When proceeding to incision and drainage of a DNI, surgeons must consider whether to approach the abscess transorally or transcervically or whether to use a combined approach. The general consensus has been that patients with abscesses extending lateral to the great vessels or abscesses that involve multiple deep neck spaces are best approached transcervically. For patients with abscesses limited to the parapharyngeal space and medial to the great vessels, an intraoral approach is both safe and effective. It has also been suggested that patients undergoing an intraoral incision and drainage have decreased postoperative hospital stays when compared with their transcervical counterparts.

■ Complications and Special Considerations

MEDIASTINITIS

Mediastinitis is a potentially life-threatening complication of DNI (**Figure 14-6**). While mediastinitis is more of a problem for adults, it can be seen in children; if treated appropriately, children are more apt to recover fully without significant morbidity. *Staphylococcus aureus* appears to be the major pathogen in this process, and MRSA is a significant contributor. Although most cases of mediastinitis are secondary to retropharyngeal space infections, direct extension of infection from an odontogenic source (Ludwig angina) may also occur.

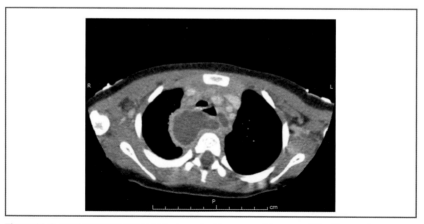

Figure 14-6. Axial contrast-enhanced computed tomographic scan of the thorax demonstrating the extension of a retropharyngeal abscess into the mediastinum.

> **Pearl:** The important factor in mediastinitis is the rapidity with which it can occur. If computed tomography is concerning for mediastinal inflammation or suggests extension of the infectious process from the neck toward the chest, prompt surgical consultation with an otolaryngologist is paramount. When there is evidence of extension into the mediastinum, a thoracic surgeon should be consulted as well.

CAROTID ARTERY RUPTURE AND PSEUDOANEURYSM

Carotid artery complications are rare but life-threatening sequelae of DNI. There are few reported cases of carotid artery rupture in the literature, particularly within the past decade. Pathogenesis is believed to be secondary to an arteritis, which ultimately results in pseudoaneurysm formation (**Figure 14-7**) and subsequent rupture. The mortality from these complications may be as high as 83%. While some signs of carotid artery pseudoaneurysm, such as an expanding pulsatile mass in the neck, worsening anemia, or a loud neck bruit, are obvious, other subtle findings include oropharyngeal ecchymoses, palsy of cranial nerves IX to XII, and an ipsilateral Horner syndrome. Assessment of the carotid artery on initial imaging and prompt surgical treatment of DNIs in the absence of improvement with conservative medical management are important.

LUDWIG ANGINA

First described by Wilhelm Frederick von Ludwig in 1836, Ludwig angina is a rapidly progressive cellulitis of the floor of the mouth that, in Ludwig's time, was nearly universally fatal. Most cases are odontogenic in origin; however, the disorder may also occur without a discernible etiology. Airway management in Ludwig angina is controversial. In 2000, Britt et al published a review suggesting that not all patients required tracheostomy (only 2 in their series of 28 patients underwent tracheotomy) and that select patients may be monitored closely without intubation or tracheotomy. Treatment includes antimicrobial therapy targeting odontogenic organisms such as *Streptococcus* species, followed by gram-negative rods and anaerobes. Antimicrobial therapy, when initiated early, is the cornerstone of treatment, with surgery now an adjunctive treatment modality.

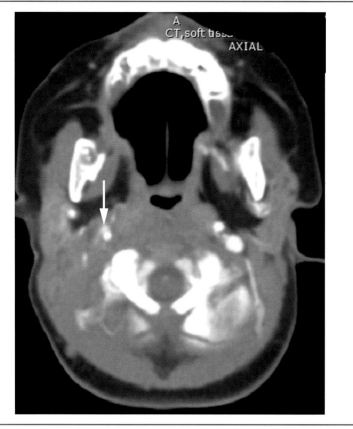

Figure 14-7. Axial contrast-enhanced computed tomographic scan demonstrating an area of enhancement around the right carotid artery consistent with carotid pseudoaneurysm, which was confirmed by angiography.

LEMIERRE SYNDROME

Lemierre syndrome is characterized by anaerobic bacteremia, internal jugular vein thrombosis, and septic embolization secondary to infections in the head and neck. The disorder, characterized by Dr André-Alfred Lemierre in 1936, occurs secondary to an infection with the bacteria *Fusobacterium necrophorum*. While uncommon, with an estimated incidence of between 0.6 and 2.3 per million population, it can have potentially devastating consequences. Treatment is surgical and medical. Surgery should be aimed at draining any pus that may be present in the surrounding deep neck spaces. Medical therapy is directed at treating the infection. While most cases are secondary to infection with *Fusobacterium,* there are an increasing number of reports of *S aureus* being isolated, and, thus, coverage must address both organisms. Clindamycin is a good first-line choice for *Fusobacterium* and also covers sensitive and resistant strains of *S aureus*. Treatment with anticoagulation therapy is controversial.

▓ Conclusion

A team approach to medical and surgical management of DNIs is required for early diagnosis and intervention. Common presenting signs and symptoms include fever, neck pain, and torticollis. If the clinical history and examination findings are concerning for a DNI, contrast-enhanced CT is highly sensitive and provides ideal anatomical definition, making it the preferred imaging modality. In general, patients with DNI should undergo a trial of antibiotic therapy in the form of a combination penicillin/beta-lactamase inhibitor or clindamycin, with or without a cephalosporin. If a patient presents with dyspnea or stridor or fails to respond to medical therapy within 24 to 72 hours, surgical intervention should be considered. Primary care clinicians should monitor for rare, but potentially fatal, complications.

▓ Selected References

Adil E, Tarshish Y, Roberson D, Jang J, Licameli G, Kenna M. The public health impact of pediatric deep neck space infections. *Otolaryngol Head Neck Surg.* 2015;153(6): 1036–1041

Al-Sabah B, Bin Salleen H, Hagr A, Choi-Rosen J, Manoukian JJ, Tewfik TL. Retropharyngeal abscess in children: 10-year study. *J Otolaryngol.* 2004;33(6):352–355

Amar YG, Manoukian JJ. Intraoral drainage: recommended as the initial approach for the treatment of parapharyngeal abscesses. *Otolaryngol Head Neck Surg.* 2004;130(6):676–680

Asmar BI. Bacteriology of retropharyngeal abscess in children. *Pediatr Infect Dis J.* 1990;9(8):595–597

Beningfield A, Nehus E, Chen AY, Yellin S. Pseudoaneurysm of the internal carotid artery after retropharyngeal abscess. *Otolaryngol Head Neck Surg.* 2006;134(2):338–339

Britt JC, Josephson GD, Gross CW. Ludwig's angina in the pediatric population: report of a case and review of the literature. *Int J Pediatr Otorhinolaryngol.* 2000;52(1):79–87

Brodsky L, Belles W, Brody A, Squire R, Stanievich J, Volk M. Needle aspiration of neck abscesses in children. *Clin Pediatr (Phila).* 1992;31(2):71–76

Brook I. Microbiology of retropharyngeal abscesses in children. *Am J Dis Child.* 1987; 141(2):202–204

Coticchia JM, Getnick GS, Yun RD, Arnold JE. Age-, site-, and time-specific differences in pediatric deep neck abscesses. *Arch Otolaryngol Head Neck Surg.* 2004;130(2):201–207

Davis GG. III. Acute septic infection of the throat and neck: Ludwig's angina. *Ann Surg.* 1906;44(2):175–192

Grisaru-Soen G, Komisar O, Aizenstein O, Soudack M, Schwartz D, Paret G. Retropharyngeal and parapharyngeal abscess in children: epidemiology, clinical features and treatment. *Int J Pediatr Otorhinolaryngol.* 2010;74(9):1016–1020

Har-El G, Aroesty JH, Shaha A, Lucente FE. Changing trends in deep neck abscess: a retrospective study of 110 patients. *Oral Surg Oral Med Oral Pathol.* 1994;77(5):446–450

Herzon FS. Needle aspiration of nonperitonsillar head and neck abscesses: a six-year experience. *Arch Otolaryngol Head Neck Surg.* 1988;114(11):1312–1314

Lemierre A. On certain septicemias due to anaerobic organisms. *Lancet.* 1936;227(5874): 701–703

Malloy KM, Christenson T, Meyer JS, et al. Lack of association of CT findings and surgical drainage in pediatric neck abscesses. *Int J Pediatr Otorhinolaryngol.* 2008; 72(2):235–239

McClay JE, Murray AD, Booth T. Intravenous antibiotic therapy for deep neck abscesses defined by computed tomography. *Arch Otolaryngol Head Neck Surg.* 2003;129(11):1207–1212

Meyer AC, Kimbrough TG, Finkelstein M, Sidman JD. Symptom duration and CT findings in pediatric deep neck infection. *Otolaryngol Head Neck Surg.* 2009;140(2):183–186

Miller WD, Furst IM, Sàndor GK, Keller MA. A prospective, blinded comparison of clinical examination and computed tomography in deep neck infections. *Laryngoscope.* 1999; 109(11):1873–1879

Nagy M, Backstrom J. Comparison of the sensitivity of lateral neck radiographs and computed tomography scanning in pediatric deep-neck infections. *Laryngoscope.* 1999;109(5):775–779

Naidu SI, Donepudi SK, Stocks RM, Buckingham SC, Thompson JW. Methicillin-resistant *Staphylococcus aureus* as a pathogen in deep neck abscesses: a pediatric case series. *Int J Pediatr Otorhinolaryngol.* 2005;69(10):1367–1371

Rega AJ, Aziz SR, Ziccardi VB. Microbiology and antibiotic sensitivities of head and neck space infections of odontogenic origin. *J Oral Maxillofac Surg.* 2006;64(9):1377–1380

Shah RK, Chun R, Choi SS. Mediastinitis in infants from deep neck space infections. *Otolaryngol Head Neck Surg.* 2009;140(6):936–938

Thomason TS, Brenski A, McClay J, Ehmer D. The rising incidence of methicillin-resistant *Staphylococcus aureus* in pediatric neck abscesses. *Otolaryngol Head Neck Surg.* 2007;137(3):459–464

Thompson JW, Cohen SR, Reddix P. Retropharyngeal abscess in children: a retrospective and historical analysis. *Laryngoscope.* 1988;98(6 Pt 1):589–592

Vieira F, Allen SM, Stocks RM, Thompson JW. Deep neck infection. *Otolaryngol Clin North Am.* 2008;41(3):459–483

Wright CT, Stocks RM, Armstrong DL, Arnold SR, Gould HJ. Pediatric mediastinitis as a complication of methicillin-resistant *Staphylococcus aureus* retropharyngeal abscess. *Arch Otolaryngol Head Neck Surg.* 2008;134(4):408–413

CHAPTER 15

Salivary Gland Disorders in Children

Daniel L. Wohl, MD, and Eileen Raynor, MD

■ Introduction

Salivary glands are exocrine glands that produce and secrete saliva through their ducts into the oral cavity and oropharynx. Saliva provides lubrication and enzymes in support of food digestion, along with having protective basic pH and anti-infectious properties. Salivary gland disorders in children are a relatively less common constellation of signs and symptoms encountered in a general pediatric practice. As one gains a clearer understanding of their basic cellular components and function and recognizes their role in head and neck physiology, identifying and managing benign and pathologic salivary gland disorders will become a more straightforward process. This chapter is intended to discuss specific disorders of the salivary glands and their management. The etiology and management of sialorrhea is covered in Chapter 17, Feeding Disorders and Ankyloglossia in Infants and Children and is beyond the scope of this chapter.

▦ Salivary Gland Developmental Anatomy

There are 3 major paired salivary glands—parotid, submandibular, and sublingual glands—plus hundreds of small, minor salivary glands, predominantly within hard and soft palate mucosa. Embryologically, all of these glandular structures are derived from ectoderm (stomodeum) or endoderm (foregut), which differentiate into the internal mucosal lining of the oral cavity and oropharynx. Major salivary glands secrete in response to autonomic nervous system stimulation during eating, with intrinsic parasympathetic and sympathetic postganglionic innervation.

Parotid glands are the largest salivary glands. They occupy space lateral to the mandibular ramus and have deep lobes that extend (external) to the upper lateral pharynx—the parapharyngeal space. The relatively short parotid duct (Stensen duct) runs roughly horizontally and empties into the oral cavity opposite the permanent maxillary second molar (or where it will be when it erupts). The facial nerve (cranial nerve VII) courses through the parotid gland and begins to separate into multiple branches within the body of the gland, creating a potential risk that must be accounted for in the diagnosis of parotid gland pathology, and when surgery is considered.

Submandibular glands are the second largest of the 3 major salivary glands. They develop lateral to the tongue and are located within the submandibular triangle. The relatively long submandibular duct (Wharton duct) courses horizontally through the floor of the mouth to exit near the midline, with paired left and right puncta anterior to the lingual hilum. The submandibular gland resides immediately anterior to the hypoglossal nerve (cranial nerve XII—tongue movement) and envelops a portion of the facial artery, which ascends through the deeper aspect.

Sublingual glands are the smallest of the major salivary glands. They are relatively superficial, lying just deep to the mucosa of the anterior floor of the mouth. The sublingual glands empty their secretions via several short ducts (ducts of Rivinus) into the floor of the mouth posterior to, but sometimes directly into, the submandibular gland ducts. Several hundred minor salivary glands also are present throughout the oral cavity and oropharynx. These glands are relatively small and have very short excretory ducts that empty saliva directly through the mucosa into their anatomical space.

▓ Salivary Gland Physiology

Salivary gland physiology is a function of its cellular components. Each salivary gland is a variably sized aggregate of multiple salivary gland units that empty into collecting ducts that progressively coalesce into a common ductal structure. Each salivary gland unit is an organized multicellular complex with a proximal secretory acinus connected to a distal ductal element. Saliva is produced and stored by highly specialized serous and mucous glands in the acinus, with surrounding myoepithelial cells able to help propel the fluid, when stimulated, through a less complex but still metabolically active ductal apparatus.

Saliva is a complex solution of electrolytes, proteins, and enzymes, plus histocompatible antimicrobials and clotting factors. It has a high bicarbonate ion content, which creates alkaline pH. Saliva is mostly water; in general, the smaller the gland, the thicker the secretions. The parotid gland is composed almost entirely of serous glands, and its secretion has the highest water content with relatively lower mucin content, although it is still rich in enzymes. In contrast, the submandibular glands are a mixture of serous and mucous glands, and the sublingual glands are composed primarily of mucous glands, with much greater viscosity to their secretions. Saliva has a baseline slow, steady production rate with production and flow stimulated first with the sight and smell of food, augmented by chewing and taste sensations, and continuing with esophageal- and gastric reflex–mediated responses. Depending on the size of the child, as much as between 250 and 1,500 mL of saliva may be secreted daily.

▓ Salivary Gland Function

Components of saliva underscore their purpose. Saliva maintains moisture within the oral cavity and oropharynx, lubricating food, which helps with swallowing and solubilizing dry food to create taste. Its relative alkaline pH of 7.4 protects against acidic compounds, including regurgitated gastric secretions. Enzymes in saliva, such as starch amylases and lysozymes, help begin the food digestion process and inhibit bacterial growth. Additional antimicrobial activity, including IgA secretion, makes saliva a locally efficient component of the body's immune system. Overall, the multiple properties of saliva help protect against dental caries formation and provide insight into why minor mucosal injuries to the oral cavity and oropharyngeal mucosa generally heal on their own without infection.

Salivary gland dysfunction and disease, therefore, can manifest with altered salivary production, flow, or content with the potential for dry mouth (xerostomia), mucosal ulceration, and increased susceptibility to oral cavity or oropharyngeal infection. Dysfunction can result from primary or secondary ductal obstruction, such as from local inflammation, lithiasis (stones), or an intrinsic mass, with pain from ductal distension the primary presenting symptom, generally worse with eating. Although relatively uncommon in children, benign and malignant tumors may arise from any of the cellular components of salivary glands themselves or from any of the nonglandular components contained within the capsule (eg, within parotid glands that embryologically envelope lymph nodes and related vascular structures). In cases of salivary gland tumors, it is often the presence of asymmetric swelling that brings the lesion to clinical attention. **Box 15-1** is a list of salivary gland disorders.

■ Physical Examination of Salivary Glands

The examination includes an external and intraoral assessment of major salivary glands and visible oral cavity mucosa. Externally, the primary care clinician (PCC) should first look for any asymmetric swelling and the general appearance. Overlying skin should be observed for erythema, tenderness, dermal involvement, and edema. Bimanual palpation, with 1 hand placed externally and a gloved finger placed intraorally, can determine the consistency, how much of the gland is involved, whether there is a fixed or mobile mass versus diffuse enlargement, and the general texture of the gland.

Intraorally, inspection of the ducts should include assessment of the buccal mucosa and floor of the mouth. Trauma related to cheek biting or dental appliances may cause ductal obstruction, leading to fullness and erythema of the puncta as well as erythema and inflammation of surrounding mucosa. Salivary gland stones may be visible or palpable at the distal end of the duct and will look yellow or white. These stones are relatively firm to palpation and often tender to touch. Similarly, congenital atresia of the submandibular duct also presents with a whitish dilation of the distal portion of the duct (**Figure 15-1**). Evaluation of the ducts should also include visualization of salivary flow. By "milking" the suspicious gland from posterior to anterior in the parotid gland or pushing cranially for the submandibular gland, salivary flow can be noted from the puncta. An

Box 15-1. Salivary Gland Disorders

Inflammatory

Acute
Bacterial
  Suppurative sialadenitis
  Lymphadenitis/abscess
Viral
  Mumps
  HIV
  Other
Chronic
Obstructive
  Sialectasis
  Sialolithiasis
  Mucocele
Granulomatous
  Mycobacterial
  Actinomycosis
  Cat-scratch disease
  Sarcoidosis
  Toxoplasmosis
  Histoplasmosis
Necrotizing sialometaplasia

Congenital

Dermoid
Branchial cleft cyst
Congenital ductal cyst
Agenesis of salivary gland

Autoimmune/Systemic

Benign lymphoepithelial disease
Sjögren syndrome
Chronic sialorrhea
Cystic fibrosis
Allergy (shellfish, strawberry)

Neoplastic

Benign
  Pleomorphic adenoma
  Warthin tumor
  Lipoma
Malignant
  Mucoepidermoid carcinoma
  Acinic cell carcinoma
  Adenocarcinoma
  Adenoid cystic carcinoma
  Rhabdomyosarcoma
  Lymphoma
  Other
Vascular malformations
  Hemangioma
  Lymphatic malformations
  Arteriovenous malformations
  Other

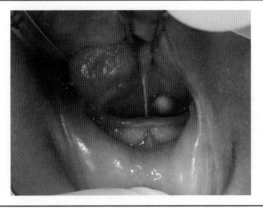

Figure 15-1. Congenital atresia of the left submandibular duct.

obstructed duct will not demonstrate adequate flow, and the PCC may note an increase in edema around the ducts or puncta. Ductal fluid with sialadenitis appears milky or purulent, and systemic disorders that affect saliva, such as Sjögren syndrome or cystic fibrosis, may demonstrate thick mucoid saliva. Punctal erythema with clear saliva generally suggests viral etiology.

The PCC also needs to assess and document cranial nerve function. Facial nerve function in all divisions should be noted (cranial nerve VII). Tongue mobility and general somatic sensation should also be identified (cranial nerves XIII and V). Facial or tongue weakness is a concerning sign and suggests a neoplastic process.

> **Pearl:** Facial nerve weakness and rapid enlargement of a salivary gland are highly suspicious of a malignant process. Solid lesions are more likely to be malignant in children than in adults.

Diagnosis of Salivary Gland Disorders

DIAGNOSTIC IMAGING

Radiologic studies can provide useful information about the diagnosis of a salivary gland disorder. Potential studies include plain radiography, sialography, ultrasonography, computed tomography (CT), and magnetic resonance imaging (MRI).

Plain radiographs have limited utility in salivary gland disorders but may be useful in identifying calcifications and sialoliths. Plain radiographs may also be obtained with contrast sialography to identify strictures within the salivary ductal system. However, sialography is also performed in conjunction with CT scanning, which provides more information about the relationship of a stricture to the surrounding soft tissues. Furthermore, sialography requires cannulation of the parotid or submandibular duct, which is difficult to accomplish in a child on an outpatient basis.

Computed tomography is used in imaging salivary glands to identify strictures and stones, to differentiate salivary gland enlargement from disorders of the surrounding tissues, and to assess fluid collections and abscesses within the glands. For most PCCs, noncontrast CT is the study of choice for identifying and localizing sialoliths (**Figure 15-2**),

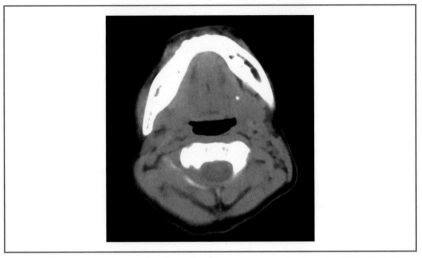

Figure 15-2. Noncontrast computed tomographic scan demonstrating sialolith in the left submandibular duct of a 12-year-old.

and CT is commonly used in sialography to identify ductal strictures and their soft tissue relationships. Imaging is also often necessary in assessing the soft tissues around the salivary glands. While MRI provides excellent detail and does not expose the child to external beam radiation, it usually requires sedation or anesthesia, and contrast-enhanced CT will often suffice to evaluate fluid collections such as abscesses and branchial cleft cysts. Early abscesses can be readily identified by CT imaging demonstrating a central hypodense area with ring enhancement. Salivary gland masses also may be initially evaluated with CT imaging.

Magnetic resonance imaging provides excellent soft tissue detail and can directly identify the facial nerve within the confines of the parotid gland. Magnetic resonance imaging is also generally preferred to evaluate vascular lesions. Flow voids can be identified, which helps in characterizing vascular malformations. High-flow lesions, such as arteriovenous malformations, are more readily delineated than are low-flow lesions, such as hemangiomas and lymphatic or venous malformations. Sedation and general anesthesia in infants and young children are usually necessary to achieve good-quality images free of motion artifact.

Ultrasonography is noninvasive and does not require radiation exposure or sedation but has limited utility in evaluating salivary gland conditions.

LABORATORY STUDIES

A variety of diagnostic laboratory studies assist in the diagnosis of salivary gland pathology. An elevated white blood cell count and C-reactive protein are useful in tracking infectious processes. Culture of saliva from an infected gland may identify pathogenic bacteria; however, the PCC should be aware of the high frequency of cross-contamination with normal oral flora. A number of viral infections are associated with salivary gland swelling, and serologic testing for cyto-megalovirus, Epstein-Barr virus, Coxsackie virus, and mumps should be considered based on clinical assessment. In cases of bilateral parotid cystic lesions, HIV testing may be considered. Serology and other clinical testing should be considered to evaluate for other causes of salivary gland swelling, such as sarcoidosis, Sjögren syndrome, and other autoimmune disorders, as well as diabetes and hypothyroidism.

Biopsy

In cases of suspected neoplastic involvement of the salivary gland, fine-needle aspiration (FNA) biopsy may be useful in making a diagnosis. The procedure is usually performed on an outpatient basis, although most children require sedation. Fine-needle aspiration has an overall diagnostic accuracy of 84%, and concomitant use of ultrasonography to guide the biopsy improves specificity, which ranges from 95% to 100% for malignancies. When FNA is not feasible, surgical incisional biopsy to obtain a small sample is generally not recommended; rather, excisional biopsy is preferred in cases in which there is a risk of tumor spillage or the lesion is too small to access by needle biopsy. Fine-needle aspiration also may be useful in cases of mycobacterial infection to obtain a DNA sample in which the offending organism can be identified by polymerase chain reaction (PCR). Sjögren syndrome can be confirmed via excision of a minor salivary gland from the lip; the gland can demonstrate the same histopathologic features as larger salivary glands, thereby obviating the need for open biopsy with a greater potential risk in major glands.

■ Treatment Options for Salivary Gland Disorders

INFLAMMATORY CONDITIONS

Viral Infections

MUMPS

Before widespread vaccination, mumps was the most common salivary gland inflammatory disease in children around 5 years of age. It is an acute, contagious illness causing painful bilateral parotid enlargement, fever, headache, and malaise. It is transmitted by contact with salivary droplets and has an 18- to 21-day incubation period. Saliva can shed the virus up to 6 days before noticeable parotid swelling and 9 days afterward. Mumps can affect the central nervous system (CNS) and cause meningoencephalitis in 2% to 3% of patients. Pancreatitis, sensorineural hearing loss, and orchitis are potentially severe sequelae. Treatment is usually supportive, consisting of adequate hydration, rest, respiratory isolation, and antipyretics. Vaccination is advocated for prevention, and immunity is lifelong.

HIV

Up to 30% of HIV-positive children have parotid involvement, consisting of lymphocytic infiltrates. Intraglandular lymphadenopathy and non-Hodgkin B-cell lymphoma are more common in these patients. Lymphoepithelial cysts can result in bilateral parotid enlargement. Aspiration of these cysts is indicated in patients with enlargement, causing significant discomfort.

OTHER VIRUSES

Epstein-Barr virus may cause enlargement of intraparotid lymph nodes. Coxsackie A virus, echovirus, and cytomegalovirus can all cause viral parotitis. In cases of cytomegalovirus parotitis, the CNS, liver, and kidneys are also often affected.

Bacterial Infections

ACUTE BACTERIAL SIALADENITIS

Acute sialadenitis usually affects the parotid gland but can also be seen in the submandibular gland. It occurs in children of all ages and may be a solitary episode or recurrent. Patients have an acutely swollen, firm, and tender gland, associated with fever, difficulty eating owing to pain, and dysgeusia. Dehydration and immunosuppression are common etiologies. Purulent saliva is expressed from the duct, and culture is diagnostic. *Streptococcus viridans* and *Staphylococcus aureus* are the most common pathogens. Anaerobes are found in up to 50% of patients. Treatment consists of systemic antimicrobial coverage, hydration, heat, massage, and sialogogues such as lemon drops or pickles, which stimulate salivary flow. In cases that do not resolve with these measures, progression to abscess formation needs to be considered. The gland will remain swollen and painful with overlying erythema. Imaging usually is not necessary, but CT scanning can be diagnostic. Surgical drainage of the abscess is necessary to clear infection. Recurrent sialadenitis can lead to fibrosis of the gland and discomfort, in some cases necessitating salivary gland resection. In these cases, surgical excision is usually curative.

ACUTE PAROTITIS OF INFANCY

This disease usually affects premature newborns and the parotid glands preferentially because of the serous nature of saliva. The bacteriology is similar to that found in bacterial sialadenitis, and treatment consists of antimicrobials and hydration. Resolution usually occurs within a week.

Chronic Inflammatory Conditions

JUVENILE RECURRENT PAROTITIS

Juvenile recurrent parotitis is reported to be the second most common salivary gland inflammatory disease in children following mumps. It is characterized by periods of painful parotid gland swelling, fever, and malaise and usually occurs unilaterally. Children with juvenile recurrent parotitis often have intervening normal periods. There is a higher likelihood of congenital ductal abnormality, dental trauma, dehydration, or sialoliths. Children aged 3 to 6 years are most affected, and there is a male preponderance. Most cases resolve spontaneously around adolescence. *Streptococcus pneumoniae* and *Haemophilus influenzae* are the usual organisms isolated.

Treatment of juvenile recurrent parotitis is the same as that of suppurative parotitis. In recalcitrant cases, sialendoscopy, lavage, dilation, or cortisone injection may be indicated. There are no data to suggest that systemic corticosteroids provide any additional benefit; however, duct lavage with corticosteroids has shown some promise. In recent studies, sialendoscopy demonstrated a low rate of symptom recurrence (25%); however, these studies were not random-ized controlled trials and, therefore, one cannot determine whether those patients would have experienced spontaneous improvement. Endoscopy will demonstrate a white appearance of the ductal lay-ers without a normal vascular cover. Ultrasonography can identify punctuate sialectasis found in recurrent parotitis as well as enlarged intraparotid lymph nodes. Computed tomography demonstrates fibrosis of the gland and microcalcifications in the ductal system. In severe cases, total gland resection may be indicated. Recurrent par-otitis can be the initial manifestation of Sjögren syndrome.

SIALECTASIS

Dilation of the small intercalated ducts can lead to salivary stasis and secondary bacterial infection. Symptoms are usually unilateral, although abnormal ducts are often found in both parotids. Clinical presentation is similar to that of acute parotitis. Sialectasis can be an isolated finding or can occur in association with juvenile recurrent parotitis.

STRICTURE

Generally related to trauma and occasionally the result of infection, intraductal calculi can also lead to stricture formation. Proximal dilation of the duct may be seen on radiographic imaging. Gland swelling is related to oral intake and slowly resolves over 1 to 2 hours after feeding. Endoscopic dilation often can resolve strictures of major ducts; gland excision is reserved for refractory cases.

SIALOLITHIASIS

More common in adolescents than younger children, 80% of sialoliths occur in the submandibular gland. Boys are affected more often than girls (3:1). Saliva from the submandibular gland is more viscous and contains more calcium and phosphorus. The duct has a longer, uphill course and takes a right-angle turn from the hilum of the gland. Stones usually contain a high concentration of calcium and are radiopaque. Children with cystic fibrosis do not have an increased preponderance to developing sialoliths. Symptoms include painful gland enlargement after eating, which subsides over several hours. The stone may be visualized at the duct puncta or palpated along the duct, but also may be lodged within the gland at the hilum. Peripheral sialoliths may extrude spontaneously or may need to be removed surgically, which usually consists of dilation of the duct and stone extraction. Hilar stones are generally larger and not palpable, causing diffuse gland enlargement. Treatment of these stones is usually gland excision. Plain radiography can identify 80% of submandibular calculi. Noncontrast CT is useful in equivocal cases (see **Figure 15-2**).

Sialendoscopy is a relatively new technique that is useful for stone removal and stricture dilation, as well as in the management of juvenile recurrent parotitis. This procedure is performed under general anesthesia and involves salivary duct dilation followed by placement of a small endoscope, which allows for irrigation, infusion of steroids, laser and mechanical fragmentation of stones, or basket retrieval of ductal stones. In general, the parotid ducts are easier to cannulate as they are larger and more horizontally oriented than the submandibular gland ducts. Ductal perforation is the most frequently reported complication of this procedure.

Granulomatous Diseases

Granulomatous diseases of the salivary gland usually occur within intraparotid lymph nodes and can be localized or diffuse. Usually, these diseases are slowly progressive, and saliva appears normal.

Mycobacterial infections can cause overlying skin to become erythematous, often with a characteristic purple hue, with eventual skin breakdown and suppurative drainage with progressive growth. Nontuberculous mycobacteria cause 90% of such cases. Acid-fast bacillus staining may be positive, but it is not diagnostic of the strain of mycobacteria. Cultures are not always positive and can take up to 6 weeks to demonstrate growth. Fine-needle aspiration and PCR amplification of DNA may be useful for early identification of species. Treatment consists of complete curettage or surgical excision of the granulomatous lesion to minimize facial nerve disruption. In cases of diffuse infection or infection with *Mycobacterium tuberculosis,* long-term multidrug therapy also is usually indicated.

Actinomycosis involves salivary glands and results from intraoral trauma. Presentation is a painless mass, and cutaneous fistulae are common (61%). Yellow-white inclusions known as *sulfur granules* are diagnostic. Treatment consists of 6 courses of intravenous penicillin or erythromycin followed by multiple courses of oral antibiotics.

Cat-scratch disease, brucellosis, and histoplasmosis are other causes of granulomatous sialadenitis. Fine-needle aspirate biopsy can often confirm tissue diagnosis. In cases of sarcoidosis, parotid swelling may be the initial presentation in up to 40% of patients. Swelling is persistent, and there is minimal discomfort. Facial paresis may be present in rare cases. Differentiation from a malignant process is necessary.

Prognosis usually depends on management of the underlying systemic condition. For atypical mycobacterial infections, gland removal or intralesional curettage and addition of antimycobacterial therapy in extensive disease is usually curative, with no long-term sequelae. Management of salivary gland involvement due to sarcoidosis, Sjögren syndrome, or cystic fibrosis is aimed at supportive measures and systemic treatment of the specific disorder. Allergic reactions are usually managed by means of symptomatic medication intervention and avoidance of the offending food item.

CYSTIC LESIONS

Most cystic lesions of the salivary glands occur within the parotids, but they can occur in any glandular structure. They may be congenital or related to trauma or inflammatory conditions.

Surgical excision or marsupialization usually results in cure. The exception may be a lymphoepithelial cystic lesion related to an HIV infection. These cysts may recur with variable frequency and are usually bilateral. Treatment in these cases is supportive and may involve needle aspiration for symptomatic lesions; prognosis is related to the overall condition of the patient.

Congenital, Nonacquired

RANULA

These mucous-retention cysts of the sublingual glands can present as a swelling in the floor of the mouth or in the submandibular triangle as they extend around the mylohyoid muscle (plunging ranula [**Figure 15-3**]). Treatment consists of marsupialization or complete surgical excision of the cyst as well as excision of the offending sublingual gland.

FIRST BRANCHIAL ARCH CYSTS

These uncommon lesions can present as parotid masses. Type 1 lesions are duplications of the external auditory canal and usually occur in the conchal bowl of the ear or in the postauricular sulcus, although they may present in the preauricular region near the parotid gland as a draining sinus. Type 2 first branchial arch anomalies are

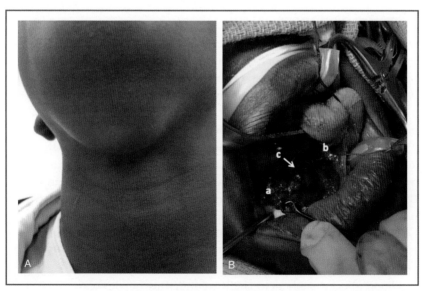

Figure 15-3. A, Plunging ranula presenting as a submental mass. B, Transoral treatment of a plunging ranula. Sublingual salivary gland (a), submandibular salivary duct (b), ranula (c). The lesion was marsupialized, decompressing the submental mass.

even less common. They course from the infra-auricular region to the upper neck behind the mandible. The tract passes in close approximation to the facial nerve (cranial nerve VII), and abscess formation or chronically draining sinuses are common. Treatment consists of superficial parotidectomy with facial nerve preservation. Computed tomography or MRI can demonstrate duplication of the external auditory canal or cystic lesions adjacent to the external auditory canal or parotid gland. Type 1 first branchial cleft cysts may demonstrate a cystic mass superior to the main trunk of the facial nerve, whereas type 2 cysts may demonstrate cartilage and cysts within the parotid gland itself. These lesions generally enhance in T2-weighted MRI images.

Acquired

TRAUMA

Blunt trauma may result in an intraglandular hematoma that can mimic a cyst. Penetrating trauma can result in disruption of the ductal structures, leading to salivary leakage or ductal cyst and stricture formation. Treatment is supportive for blunt trauma but may require evacuation of a sialocele or hematoma. In penetrating trauma, repair of the duct over a stent will often allow for good function of the salivary system. Direct repair of the facial nerve may be necessary in cases of parotid or cheek-penetrating traumatic injuries.

SYSTEMIC DISORDERS

Diffuse parotid swelling may be seen in a variety of conditions. Fatty infiltration of the gland may be found in diabetes. In up to 30% of patients with bulimia, bilateral symmetric parotid hypertrophy is demonstrated. Ninety percent of patients with cystic fibrosis have enlargement of the submandibular gland. Multiple agents such as iodine and heavy metals can cause asymptomatic salivary gland enlargement.

Sjögren syndrome, an autoimmune disorder manifested by xerostomia, keratoconjunctivitis, and connective tissue disease, also produces diffuse nonpainful enlargement of the salivary glands. Biopsy specimens exhibit lymphocytic infiltration and gland atrophy. Patients have an increased incidence of non-Hodgkin B-cell lymphoma and other lymphoproliferative disorders. Diagnosis is made based on positive serologic test results for SS-A or SS-B antibodies.

Food allergy, such as to shellfish and strawberries, can cause significant, sudden parotid gland edema, along with urticaria, angioedema, or rash and an acute change in salivary viscosity. Patients usually have an immediate type 1 hypersensitivity to the offending allergen, and parents and older children are often able to relate acute onset of swelling to the specific food.

> **Pearl:** Recurrent sialadenitis may indicate ductal stricture or a systemic disorder that requires further workup and evaluation. Subspecialty referral is indicated in these situations.

SOLID LESIONS

Infantile hemangiomas account for 50% to 60% of pediatric salivary gland tumors. With the exception of these lesions, less than 5% of salivary gland tumors occur in children younger than 16 years. However, solid salivary gland tumors in children are more likely to be malignant, and most of these occur in parotid glands. These lesions can be subdivided into benign, low-grade malignancies, and high-grade malignancies.

Hemangiomas

Hemangiomas generally present within the first year after birth and have a rapid proliferative growth phase, followed an involution period that is mostly completed between 4 years of age and 6 years of age. Hemangiomas are composed of capillary spaces and solid cellular masses within glandular secretory segments. Up to 80% occur in the parotid gland (**Figure 15-4**) and 18% to 20% in the submandibular gland. Up to 20% of patients have multiple lesions. They present as erythematous, warm, compressible masses and do not cause facial nerve weakness. Saliva is normal on expression.

Ultrasound can suggest a diagnosis of hemangioma; MRI provides better detail but is rarely necessary. Hemangiomas usually regress spontaneously and may resolve completely without any treatment. However, treatment of larger lesions is usually advisable to reduce the likelihood of surgical intervention in the future. The preferred treatment modalities are systemic propranolol and/or intralesional injection of steroids. Long-term sequelae may include scarring of affected areas or persistent cosmetic deformity.

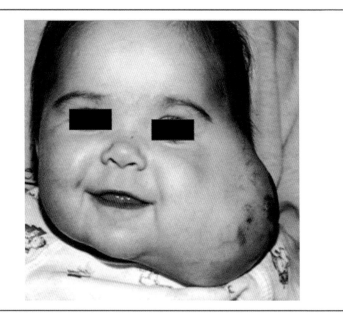

Figure 15-4. Infantile hemangioma of left parotid gland after proliferation phase.

Benign Tumors

Pleomorphic adenoma (benign mixed tumor) is the most common solid salivary gland tumor in children. It is composed of epithelial and myoepithelial cells. It generally occurs in the lateral aspect of the parotid gland and grows slowly, with a firm, lobulated appearance. Diagnosis is usually made by FNA biopsy. Treatment is complete surgical excision with avoidance of tumor spillage and facial nerve preservation. Recurrence can approach 20%.

Pleomorphic adenomas also may occur in minor salivary glands and can be confused with torus palatine when occurring in the palate. These lesions are smooth, with a rubbery consistency, and are not fixed to the overlying mucosa. Computed tomography or MRI can assist with surgical planning.

Other benign tumors include neurofibromas, Warthin tumors (papillary cystadenoma lymphomatosum), basal cell adenomas, and lipomas, all of which are rarely found in salivary glands.

Embryomas are rare benign epithelial tumors that present within the first year after birth. There is a fairly high potential for malignant transformation, and complete excision is the recommended treatment.

Most of these tumors exhibit slow growth and initially can be managed conservatively. Pleomorphic adenoma has a recurrence rate of up to 20%, especially in cases of tumor spillage, and a 4% risk of malignant transformation if untreated over 20 to 30 years. Embryomas also have a high rate of malignant transformation within the first years after birth, but complete excision is curative.

Options for imaging benign salivary lesions include MRI or CT. Magnetic resonance imaging usually demonstrates well-circumscribed T2 hyperintense enhancing masses. Computed tomography reveals a heterogenous signal and variable-sized cystic lesions that are usually well defined and well circumscribed. They can also differentiate deep lobe parotid lesions from other parapharyngeal masses. In general, a high T2 signal suggests benign salivary gland pathology.

Malignant Tumors

Rapid growth and facial nerve weakness are signs specifically concerning for malignancy. Treatment of salivary gland malignancies usually consists of surgical excision, with cervical lymphadenectomy if regional metastases are present, and adjunctive external beam radiation.

Epithelial tumors occur more often in older children and adolescents, whereas sarcomas are more frequently identified in early childhood. Cranial nerve involvement and regional adenopathy are more indicative of high-grade malignancy. These tumors are more likely to occur in younger children.

Mucoepidermoid carcinoma and acinic cell carcinoma are the most common low-grade malignant salivary gland tumors in children. Both of these lesions are slowly growing and painless. They are found more frequently in the parotid gland.

High-grade mucoepidermoid carcinoma, adenocarcinoma, and adenoid cystic carcinoma are most likely to cause involvement of the facial nerve and fixation to surrounding structures. In the submandibular gland, hypoglossal or marginal mandibular nerve (lower facial nerve branch) weakness is suggestive of a malignant process.

Rhabdomyosarcoma is the most common sarcoma affecting salivary glands in the pediatric population. These tumors can present in the area of the parotid gland and may initially be mistaken for a primary parotid tumor. Diagnosis is confirmed by biopsy, and, in this instance, incisional biopsy may be more diagnostic than FNA. Resection followed by irradiation and chemotherapy is generally the treatment of choice.

The parotid gland also can be a site for metastasis from facial or scalp primary tumors, including melanoma. The PCC should examine these areas if malignancy is suspected.

Low-grade malignancies, such as acinic cell carcinoma, and low-grade mucoepidermoid carcinoma both have an excellent 5-year survival rate of greater than 90%; however, the 20-year survival rate drops to around 50% because of late recurrences.

High-grade lesions, including adenoid cystic carcinoma, high-grade mucoepidermoid carcinoma, and adenocarcinoma, have a high rate of spread to regional lymph nodes, neural involvement, and hematogenous spread. The 5-year survival rate for patients with these lesions is around 80%, but long-term survival (>20 years) is significantly worse.

Rhabdomyosarcoma survival is directly related to the tumor stage, with 8-year survival rates ranging from 80% for stage 1 to 72% for stage 2 and 25% to 40% for stage 3.

Imaging for malignant salivary lesions includes CT, MRI, and fluorodeoxyglucose-positron emission tomography. Images can demonstrate local invasion, associated lymphadenopathy, and metastatic disease. Gland displacement or invasion may show on CT. On MRI, T1 images are often hypointense, whereas T2 images are frequently hyperintense. Both CT and MRI are used most frequently for treatment planning and follow-up purposes. Positron emission tomography/CT will reveal increased glucose uptake in the affected gland along with metastatic adenopathy.

> **Pearl:** Solid tumors of the salivary glands are more likely to be malignant in the pediatric population. Malignant salivary gland tumors present with rapid growth and cranial nerve involvement and require immediate subspecialty referral.

VASCULAR MALFORMATIONS

Lymphatic and Venous Malformations

Lymphatic malformations may develop within the parotid gland or affect the function of smaller salivary glands. They are soft, compressible, congenital lesions that present in the immediate perinatal period. They will increase in size in the setting of infection or trauma as a result of lymph accumulation within the lesion. Venous malformations have a propensity to occur in the masseteric and buccal spaces. Magnetic resonance imaging is the modality of choice to delineate these lesions.

Although small, asymptomatic lymphatic malformations require no therapy, treatment should be considered for large lesions or those causing inflammation, functional compromise, or cosmetic deformity. Macrocystic lesions may be amenable to intralesional sclerotherapy and/or surgery; microcystic lesions generally require surgical intervention. In these cases, treatment is usually performed in multiple stages, and up to 15% of lesions that have been excised surgically recur, with persistent cosmetic and functional deformity not uncommon. Because lymphatic malformations in or near the salivary glands typically approximate the facial nerve, protection of the nerve during treatment is of utmost importance. Venous malformations generally require sclerotherapy, with or without surgical resection, for definitive management.

■ Selected References

Al-Khafaji BM, Nestok BR, Katz RL. Fine-needle aspiration of 154 parotid masses with histologic correlation: ten-year experience at the University of Texas M. D. Anderson Cancer Center. *Cancer.* 1998;84(3):153–159

Bower CM, Dyleski RA. Diseases of the salivary glands. In: Bluestone CD, Stool SE, Alper CM, et al, eds. *Pediatric Otolaryngology.* 4th ed. New York, NY: Saunders; 2003:1251–1267

Buckmiller LM. Propranolol treatment for infantile hemangiomas. *Curr Opin Otolaryngol Head Neck Surg.* 2009;17(6):458–459

Casselman JW, Mancuso AA. Major salivary gland masses: comparison of MR imaging and CT. *Radiology.* 1987;165(1):183–189

Ericson S, Zetterlund B, Ohman J. Recurrent parotitis and sialectasis in childhood. Clinical, radiologic, immunologic, bacteriologic, and histologic study. *Ann Otol Rhinol Laryngol.* 1991;100(7):527–535

Erkul E, Gillespie MB. Sialendoscopy for non-stone disorders: the current evidence. *Laryngoscope Investig Otolaryngol.* 2016;1(5):140–145

Friedman E, Patiño MO, Udayasankar UK. Imaging of pediatric salivary glands. *Neuroimaging Clin N Am.* 2018;28(2):209–226

Garden AS, el-Naggar AK, Morrison WH, Callender DL, Ang KK, Peters LJ. Postoperative radiotherapy for malignant tumors of the parotid gland. *Int J Radiat Oncol Biol Phys.* 1997;37(1):79–85

Gayner SM, Kane WJ, McCaffrey TV. Infections of the salivary glands. In: Cummings CW, Fredrickson JM, Harker LA, et al, eds. *Otolaryngology-Head and Neck Surgery.* St. Louis, MO: Mosby-Yearbook; 1998:1234–1246

Gravello W, Redaelli M, Galluzzi F, Pignataro L. Juvenile recurrent parotitis: a systematic review of treatment studies. *Int J Pediatr Otorhinolaryngol.* 2018;112:151–157

Ibrahim HZ, Handler SD. Diseases of the salivary glands. In: Wetmore R, Muntz H, eds. *Pediatric Otolaryngology.* New York, NY: Thieme Medical Publishers; 2000:647–658

Leverstein H, van der Wal JE, Tiwari RM, et al. Malignant epithelial parotid gland tumours: analysis and results in 65 previously untreated patients. *Br J Surg.* 1998;85(9):1267–1272

Megerian CA, Maniglia AJ. Parotidectomy: a ten year experience with fine needle aspiration and frozen section biopsy correlation. *Ear Nose Throat J.* 1994;73(6):377–380

Morgan DW, Pearman K, Raafat F, Oates J, Campbell J. Salivary disease in childhood. *Ear Nose Throat J.* 1989;68(2):155–159

Morse E, Fujiwara RJT, Husain Z, Judson B, Mehra S. Pediatric salivary cancer: epidemiology, treatment trends, and association of treatment modality with survival. *Otolaryngol Head Neck Surg.* 2018;159(3):553–563

Myer C, Cotton RT. Salivary gland disease in children: a review, part 2—congenital lesions and neoplastic disease. *Clin Pediatr (Phila).* 1986;25(7):353–357

Nahlieli O, Shacham R, Shlesinger M, Eliav E. Juvenile recurrent parotitis: a new method of diagnosis and treatment. *Pediatrics.* 2004;114(1):9–12

Nozaki H, Harasawa A, Hara H, Kohno A, Shigeta A. Ultrasonographic features of recurrent parotitis in childhood. *Pediatr Radiol.* 1994;24(2):98–100

Rice DH. Non-neoplastic diseases of the salivary glands. In: Paparella MM, ed. *Otolaryngology.* Philadelphia, PA: Saunders; 1991

Roby BB, Mattingly J, Jensen EL, Gao D, Chan KH. Treatment of juvenile recurrent parotitis of childhood: an analysis of effectiveness. *JAMA Otolaryngol Head Neck Surg.* 2015;141(2):126–129

Salomão DR, Sigman JD, Greenebaum E, Cohen MB. Rhabdomyosarcoma presenting as a parotid gland mass in pediatric patients: fine-needle aspiration biopsy findings. *Cancer.* 1998;84(4):245–251

Schuller DE, McCabe BF. Salivary gland neoplasms in children. *Otolaryngol Clin North Am.* 1977;10(2):399–412

Schwarz Y, Bezdjian A, Daniel SJ. Sialendoscopy in treating pediatric salivary gland disorders: a systematic review. *Eur Arch Otorhinolaryngol.* 2018;275(2):347–356

Seibert RW, Seibert JJ. High resolution ultrasonography of the parotid gland in children. *Pediatr Radiol.* 1986;16(5):374–379

Shott SR. Salivary disease in children. In: Cotton RT, Meyer CM, eds. *Practical Pediatric Otolaryngology.* Philadelphia, PA: Lippincott-Raven Publishers; 1999:693–710

Smith RJH. Non-neoplastic salivary gland diseases. In: English GM, ed. *Otolaryngology.* Philadelphia, PA: JB Lippincott; 1994:1–29

Teresi LM, Kolin E, Lufkin RB, Hanafee WN. MR imaging of the intraparotid facial nerve: normal anatomy and pathology. *AJR Am J Roentgenol.* 1987;148(5):995–1000

Williams MA. Head and neck findings in pediatric acquired immune deficiency syndrome. *Laryngoscope.* 1987;97(6):713–716

Work WP. Cysts and congenital lesions of the parotid gland. *Otolaryngol Clin North Am.* 1977;10(2):339–343

Wotman S, Mercadante J, Mandel ID, Goldman RS, Denning C. The occurrence of calculus in normal children, children with cystic fibrosis, and children with asthma. *J Periodontol.* 1973;44(5):278–280

Wurster CF. Non-neoplastic salivary gland disorders. In: Gates GA, ed. *Current Therapy in Otolaryngology Head and Neck Surgery.* St. Louis, MO: Mosby-Yearbook; 1994:238–243

Yang WT, Ahuja A, Metreweli C. Sonographic features of head and neck hemangiomas and vascular malformations: review of 23 patients. *J Ultrasound Med.* 1997;16(1):39–44

Yeh S. The salivary glands. In: Ballenger JJ, ed. *Diseases of the Nose, Throat, Ear, Head & Neck.* Philadelphia, PA: Lea & Febiger; 1991:308–311

SECTION 5

Airway and Swallowing

CHAPTER 16

Stridor in Infants and Children

Steven Sobol, MD, MSc, and Conor M. Devine, MD

■ Introduction

Stridor is an abnormal sound produced by turbulent airflow through a partially obstructed supraglottis, glottis, or trachea. Stridor is a symptom, not a diagnosis or disease. The character of stridor and the respiratory phase in which it occurs will direct the workup and provide clues to the location and severity of anatomical or physiologic narrowing. Obstructing lesions or physiologic collapse in the supraglottis will result in high-pitched inspiratory stridor. The glottis and subglottis are fixed segments of the airway with little physiologic collapse. Noisy breathing generated by these lesions is appreciable in both phases of the respiratory cycle, resulting in biphasic stridor. The intra-thoracic trachea and main stem bronchi undergo physiologic narrowing during expiration. Obstructing lesions at this level will also cause expiratory stridor.

    The clinical history is key in directing the primary care clinician (PCC) to the cause of the stridor (**Box 16-1**). Identifying the precise

Box 16-1. Differential Diagnosis of Pediatric Stridor

Congenital
Laryngomalacia
Tracheomalacia
Laryngeal cleft
Vocal fold paralysis
Glottic stenosis
Subglottic stenosis
Subglottic cyst

Idiopathic
Vocal fold paralysis
Subglottic stenosis
Intubation trauma

Inflammatory
Gastroesophageal reflux disease
Eosinophilic esophagitis

Neoplastic
Airway hemangioma

Trauma/Toxin
Foreign body—tracheal or
esophageal
Caustic ingestion
Laryngotracheal trauma

Infectious
Recurrent respiratory papillomatosis
Croup (laryngotracheitis)
Epiglottitis
Tracheitis

underlying cause is imperative because appropriate management is dictated by an accurate diagnosis. The degree of respiratory distress and feeding difficulties on presentation determine the extent of the initial workup and urgency of intervention. Acute respiratory distress demands establishment of a secure airway regardless of the diagnosis, while patients in stable condition can undergo a more thorough history and physical examination.

Stridor in infants and children is most commonly congenital (85%). Laryngeal lesions such as laryngomalacia (LM), vocal fold paralysis (VFP), and subglottic stenosis (SGS) make up most diagnoses. Tracheal abnormalities tend to occur less frequently than laryngeal problems, with tracheomalacia (TM) and congenital vascular anomalies that result in external compression of the airway and subsequent stridor the anomalies most commonly seen.

■ History

A complete birth history is essential. This should include information about congenital anomalies or syndromes, respiratory distress at the time of birth, endotracheal intubation, birth weight, prematurity, meconium aspiration, prolonged or difficult delivery, and birth injury (**Box 16-2**). The history and length of neonatal intensive care stay or intubation during the neonatal period are critically important. Even a transient intubation for meconium aspiration can be relevant to future development of stridor.

Box 16-2. History for Children With Stridor

◆ **Onset** (acute, chronic, progressive)
◆ **Fluctuation** (positional changes that improve stridor)
◆ **Age at Onset**
◆ **Prior Respiratory Problems**
  — Recurrent croup
  — Aspiration
  — Pneumonia
  — Reactive airway disease
◆ **Birth History**
  — Extremely premature
  — NICU stay
◆ **Prior Intubation**
◆ **GERD Symptoms**
◆ **Sleep-Disordered Breathing**
  — Snoring
  — Nocturnal cough
  — Witnessed apneas
◆ **Wheezing Episodes**
◆ **Feeding Problems**
  — FTT, weight gain, choking episodes
◆ **Acute Changes in Clinical Status**
  — Fever
  — Respiratory distress
  — Cough
  — Drooling
  — Change in voice or cry
  — Decrease in oral intake
  — Body position

Abbreviations: FTT, failure to thrive; GERD, gastroesophageal reflux disease; NICU, neonatal intensive care unit.

The patient's age at symptom onset is important in guiding PCCs toward a diagnosis. Stridor that develops shortly after birth is likely to have a congenital etiology. Laryngomalacia, the most common laryngeal anomaly and source of congenital stridor, classically develops in the first 2 weeks after birth. Bilateral vocal fold paralysis (BVFP) or congenital SGS is present and usually symptomatic immediately after birth, whereas airway hemangiomas result in symptoms at least 1 month after birth. Acquired abnormalities usually develop later in infancy or during childhood and are most often associated with some form of airway trauma, manipulation, or intubation. Transient "acquired" causes of stridor, such as infectious croup, develop between ages 6 months and 6 years, with a peak incidence at around age 2 years. Transient stridor that develops shortly after extubation may be secondary to edema. Symptoms related to acquired SGS can develop weeks to months after intubation injury.

Symptom progression or fluctuation is also an important factor that helps make the diagnosis. The severity of stridor may progress in the case of airway hemangioma during its proliferative phase. In LM, the character of stridor will change with feeding, crying, and supine positioning, and the intensity will change with growth of the infant. Acute decompensation and prolonged respiratory illness may be seen in patients with infectious conditions and those with developing SGS.

The PCC should always document the quality of the voice or volume of the cry. A change in voice (dysphonia) usually suggests pathology involving the vocal folds. In unilateral vocal fold paralysis (UVFP), patients usually have a weak cry or "breathy" voice, while in BVFP, the cry is typically strong. Voice changes due to masses, such as granulomas or papillomas, are variable.

Parents should be questioned about feeding difficulties. For example, symptoms of choking, cough, regurgitation, or failure to thrive are present in severe LM. In UVFP, cough, aspiration, and recurrent pneumonia can be present until the mobile, contralateral vocal fold compensates for the gap left by the nonmobile side. Similar symptoms may be present in children with tracheoesophageal fistula, in which TM is the cause of the stridor, and with laryngeal clefts in which redundant arytenoid mucosa may cause noisy breathing.

Symptoms related to sleep help distinguish pharyngeal obstruction from laryngeal, tracheal, or bronchial obstruction. Pharyngeal obstruction (stertor) generally worsens during sleep; laryngotracheal obstruction (stridor) is usually worse while awake and with activity.

Comorbidities, such as gastroesophageal reflux, neuromuscular disorders, and congenital heart disease, are also important because they may exacerbate patient symptoms.

> **Pearl:** The parent or caregiver should hold the child to calm him or her and help ensure an accurate evaluation. This is especially helpful if the child is in respiratory distress.

■ Physical Examination

The physical examination begins with simple, direct observation of the patient. The PCC should always assess urgency based on signs of acute or progressive respiratory distress, such as tachypnea, nasal flaring, retractions, or cyanosis. Cyanosis is often a late sign of airway distress. These symptoms require immediate intervention to secure the airway independent of the underlying diagnosis. Once a stable airway is established, the child will undergo a more thorough examination.

Auscultation is the next step in evaluation. It provides information about symmetry and efficiency of breath sounds. In addition to the lungs, the PCC should sequentially listen over the nares, mouth, and neck. The latter is facilitated by using the rubber tubing from a stethoscope from which the diaphragm and head are removed. Attention to the character of stridor and its respiratory phase is paramount, because it allows the PCC to more accurately determine the site of the anatomical abnormality by identifying the location of maximal noise. For instance, inspiratory stridor suggests an extrathoracic etiology, while intrathoracic etiologies may present with wheezing and/or expiratory stridor. This, in turn, may direct the PCC to the underlying cause of the stridor. The patient also may be placed in various positions to assess the effect on stridor. For example, stridor associated with LM improves in the prone position. In patients with UVFP, lying down on the side of the normal vocal fold mobility may reduce the severity of the stridor.

> **Pearl:** *In*spiratory stridor suggests an extrathoracic etiology, while *ex*piratory stridor (wheezing) suggests an *in*trathoracic etiology.

■ Additional Evaluation

While the patient's history and physical examination findings may suggest the most likely diagnosis, further evaluation may be necessary. The PCC must determine his or her comfort level in directing this evaluation based on the characteristics and severity of the child's stridor. For example, children whose symptoms are classic for LM or croup and whose symptoms are minimal may reasonably be managed medically with close follow-up. In such cases, the PCC may choose to order studies that help confirm the diagnosis. However, when the stridor or associated symptoms do not suggest a particular pathology or symptoms are severe, otolaryngological consultation, including endoscopic assessment, should be the next step.

Radiographs, in certain cases, can contribute to the evaluation of a child with stridor. In children whose history and physical examination findings are highly suggestive of LM and whose stridor is of mild severity, radiographs of the airway and chest may be useful in assessing the likelihood of more distal causes of stridor. Posteroanterior and lateral neck radiographs also may be useful in evaluating laryngeal infection. In supraglottitis, the radiograph will show an enlarged epiglottis protruding from the anterior wall of the hypopharynx, a finding known as the "thumb sign" (**Figure 16-1**). In children with croup, imaging usually demonstrates a steeple sign reflecting inflammation of the subglottis (**Figure 16-2**). However, such films must be obtained using high kilovoltage and may be very technique-sensitive. When feeding difficulties are present, barium esophagography may reveal a vascular ring; radiographs and pH probe studies may also aid in diagnosing gastroesophageal reflux that may contribute to stridor.

The PCC also may decide to assess the severity of pathology based on objective data. Pulmonary function tests, pulse oximetry, and apnea monitoring may help identify those children whose stridor requires more immediate attention.

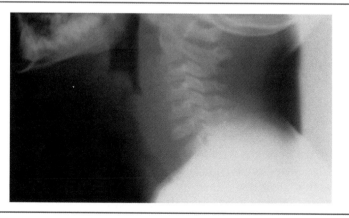

Figure 16-1. In acute supraglottitis, swelling of the epiglottis results in the "thumb sign" observed on lateral radiographs of the neck.

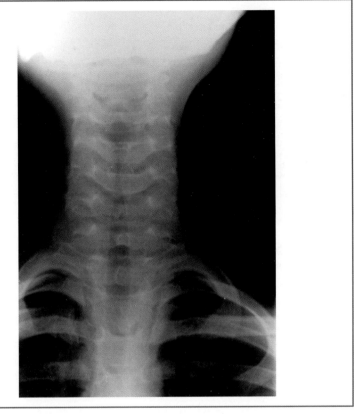

Figure 16-2. Anteroposterior radiograph of the upper airway demonstrating steeple sign, suggestive of subglottic narrowing.

▨ Endoscopy

In most cases, otolaryngologists will perform flexible fiberoptic endoscopy (**Figure 16-3**) during the initial clinical evaluation. Flexible fiberoptic endoscopy allows excellent assessment of the supraglottic and glottic larynx and is easy to perform. In neonates and young infants, endoscopy can often be performed transorally. Older infants and children may require topical nasal decongestion and local analgesia for transnasal laryngoscopy.

Flexible fiberoptic endoscopy facilitates assessment of the tongue base, vallecula, pyriform sinuses, and supraglottic and glottic larynx, with attention to the presence of secretions and vocal fold mobility. However, visualization of the glottis may occasionally be compromised by pathology, excess secretions, or overhanging epiglottis, and the subglottis and trachea are

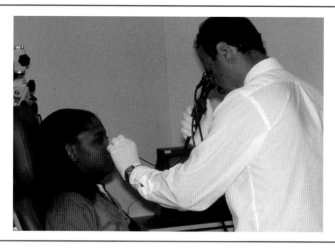

Figure 16-3. Flexible fiberoptic laryngoscopy is performed in most children without difficulty.

rarely well seen. Vocal fold mobility can also be difficult to assess in the neonate.

Operative microdirect laryngoscopy and bronchoscopy (MLB), the most definitive assessment, is routinely performed but may not be necessary for every child with stridor. There are multiple indications for MLB (**Box 16-3**). The role of endoscopy under anesthesia is to establish a diagnosis when stridor is not otherwise explained and to direct appropriate surgical intervention. Additionally, MLB is used to evaluate for synchronous lesions. In patients with chronic stridor, synchronous lesions have been reported to occur in anywhere from 7.5% to 60% of patients. Synchronous lesions are usually suspected when the clinical picture is not fully explained by the diagnosis provided by other means. Fortunately, the risks of endoscopy are rare and mostly related to the underlying pathology necessitating evaluation. These risks include postoperative edema, respiratory infection, possible need for extended treatment with steroids, lengthened hospitalization, airway injury causing SGS or glottic web, and voice changes.

The key limitation of operative endoscopy is that it may not assess the airway in its normal physiologic state, which can make evaluation of dynamic changes, such as vocal fold movement or TM, difficult. To accurately assess vocal fold mobility, the patient should be examined while fully awake and phonating (usually crying) immediately before operative endoscopy. Similarly, TM can be assessed

> ## Box 16-3. Direct Laryngoscopy and Bronchoscopy Indications
>
> ♦ To establish a diagnosis (when other measures fail)
> ♦ To evaluate for synchronous lesions (usually suspected when the clinical picture is not fully explained by the diagnosis established by other measures)
> ♦ Concern regarding subglottic lesion
> ♦ Severe or progressive stridor
> ♦ Cyanosis or apnea concerns
> ♦ Radiologic abnormalities
> ♦ Concern regarding foreign body
> ♦ Parental or physician anxiety

with spontaneous ventilation using a flexible bronchoscope or rigid telescope only.

■ Common Causes of Stridor

LARYNGOMALACIA

Laryngomalacia is the most common congenital laryngeal anomaly and cause of stridor in infants. It is generally a self-limited process, but when severe it may cause life-threatening airway obstruction or failure to thrive. Laryngomalacia is classically characterized by an omega-shaped epiglottis, short aryepiglottic folds, and cuneiform cartilage prolapse (**Figure 16-4**). Laryngomalacia is a clinical entity distinct from TM, which is far less common. The term *laryngotracheomalacia* has no clinical significance and should not be used in medical parlance. Multiple etiologic theories of LM exist, though it is still unclear whether neurologic or anatomical pathology, or both, play a role in the symptomatic child.

The classic presentation of LM is intermittent inspiratory staccato stridor with a musical quality that worsens with feeding, agitation, excitement, or supine positioning. Stridor usually develops during the first 2 weeks after birth, and most cases present by 4 months of age. The natural course of LM is for stridor to peak over 6 to 8 months, then spontaneously resolve by 12 to 24 months of age. Associated sequelae include respiratory symptoms, such as desaturations, tachypnea, retractions, and recurrent respiratory infection, as well as feeding difficulties. In the most severe cases of LM, apnea, cyanosis, or cor pulmonale can occur; fortunately, such cases are rare.

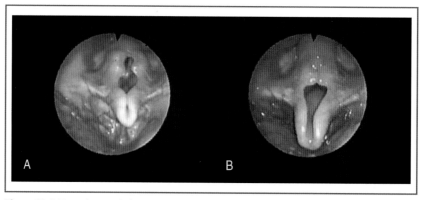

Figure 16-4. Two phases of obstruction in a patient with laryngomalacia. A, The epiglottis is curled tightly on itself, while the vocal folds and posterior laryngeal cartilages are open. B, The epiglottis has unfurled somewhat, while the posterior laryngeal cartilages have prolapsed over the vocal folds.

Feeding difficulties have been reported as the second most common symptom in LM. The most common signs of feeding difficulties include cough, choking, gastroesophageal regurgitation, nasal obstruction, nasopharyngeal reflux, and poor weight gain. Other signs include recurrent emesis, aspiration, oxygen desaturations with feeding, and slow and laborious feeding associated with failure to thrive. Though no causal effect has been established, gastroesophageal reflux disease (GERD) and laryngopharyngeal reflux are the most common comorbidities in LM.

Laryngomalacia can usually be diagnosed from the clinical history and presentation. The key anatomical findings of LM—an omega-shaped epiglottis, cuneiform prolapse, and shortened aryepiglottic folds—are confirmed on flexible fiberoptic laryngoscopy (FFL). It is important to note that the diagnosis of LM requires the anatomical findings and pattern of inspiratory collapse producing stridor.

Most infants have mild LM with intermittent stridor and occasional feeding symptoms such as cough, choking, or regurgitation. Fewer than 8% of infants have an associated comorbidity (eg, GERD, cardiac disease, neurologic disease, craniofacial syndrome). If indicated, following GERD precautions with or without acid suppression has been effective in controlling symptoms. Disease progression occurs in up to 30% of patients within 2 months after diagnosis. Therefore, these patients should be followed up for the development of respiratory sequelae or persistent feeding difficulties.

Patients with moderate LM typically present with stridor and have the highest rate of feeding symptoms. The most common feeding symptom is postprandial regurgitation. Acid suppression resolves most feeding symptoms, but these patients should be monitored closely for refractory symptoms. Most symptoms resolve within 12 months, but up to 28% of patients require surgical intervention for disease progression within 2 months. Half of these patients have an associated comorbidity. Common indications for intervention include aspiration, cyanosis with feeding, and failure to thrive unresponsive to acid suppression.

Severe LM presents with stridor, cyanosis, or apnea during feeding. Because of airway obstruction and a poorly coordinated suck-swallow-breathe mechanism, these patients may develop failure to thrive, aspiration, and frequent respiratory illnesses or pneumonia. Other respiratory sequelae include apparent life-threatening events, retractions, or, rarely, chronic hypoxia and cor pulmonale. Half will have a comorbidity, and up to 80% of these patients may have a secondary airway lesion. Management of GERD should be optimized because these patients may develop postoperative feeding issues related to scarring and surgical alteration to the complex neural pathways that provide tonicity to laryngeal cartilages. All of these patients undergo surgical intervention.

Most cases of LM are mild and treated expectantly with positioning and medical therapy for comorbidities such as gastroesophageal reflux. Authors have reported that between 11% and 22% of infants with LM require surgical intervention. Endoscopic techniques, most commonly supraglottoplasty, have now largely supplanted tracheostomy as the gold-standard operative treatment. Supraglottoplasty is designed to open the larynx by dividing shortened aryepiglottic folds or reducing redundant arytenoid mucosa. This procedure is routinely performed endoscopically with a microdebrider, a carbon dioxide (CO_2) laser, or cold-steel instrumentation, with successful outcomes in 38% to 100% of cases.

DISCOORDINATE PHARYNGOLARYNGOMALACIA

This entity was first described in the late 1990s. It is defined as severe LM with complete supraglottic collapse during inspiration, without shortened aryepiglottic folds or redundant mucosa, and with associated pharyngomalacia. Normal pharyngeal patency is maintained by pharyngeal muscle activity influenced by the cerebral cortex in response to neural and chemical inputs. An immature central nervous system (CNS) leads to depressed pharyngeal dilator muscle activity, resulting in pharyngolaryngomalacia. Children with neurologic abnormalities, such as cerebral palsy, may receive this diagnosis. In short, discoordinate pharyngolaryngomalacia is symptomatically similar to LM and physiologically neurologic in nature. Treatment options include continuous positive airway pressure (CPAP)/bilevel positive airway pressure (BiPAP) or tracheostomy. Surgical techniques traditionally used for LM (ie, aryepiglottic fold division) are not useful and may worsen airway obstruction.

TRACHEOMALACIA

The pathophysiology and natural history associated with TM are quite different from those of LM. While LM typically produces inspiratory stridor that resolves spontaneously with growth, stridor associated with TM is expiratory. It is often accompanied by a characteristic harsh "brassy" cough caused by an intrathoracic location of collapse. Other important respiratory features of TM include tracheal wheeze that does not respond to, and may even worsen with, bronchodilator therapy, neck hyperextension, dyspnea, and recurrent respiratory tract infections. Reflex apnea, or "dying spells," are vagally mediated neural reflexes occurring in the area of compression that cause total occlusion of the trachea and apnea that may progress to cardiac arrest. It can be associated with feeding. Recurrent respiratory infections result from respiratory obstruction and impaired clearance of secretions. Not infrequently, when these children present in the neonatal intensive care unit (NICU), they are difficult to ventilate because of tracheal collapse occurring distal to the end of the endotracheal tube. In addition, many children with TM have feeding difficulty, poor weight gain, and failure to thrive.

Primary TM results from a congenital deformity of the tracheal rings. The lack of mature cartilaginous support results in dynamic collapse. Increased intrathoracic pressure and flaccid cartilaginous rings decrease the anteroposterior diameter of the airway, causing a flattening of the normal trachea. This may be segmental in nature and can extend into the main bronchi. The cartilage-membranous ratio shifts from the normal 4:1 to 2:1 (**Figure 16-5**). Secondary TM usually has an appearance of asymmetric flattening on endoscopy and occurs as a result of extrinsic compression from congenital vascular anomalies. The most common cause of secondary TM is innominate artery compression (**Figure 16-6**). The diagnosis and type of TM are

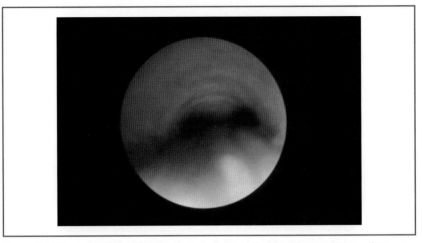

Figure 16-5. Tracheomalacia. Note the abnormally low ratio of cartilaginous to membranous trachea.

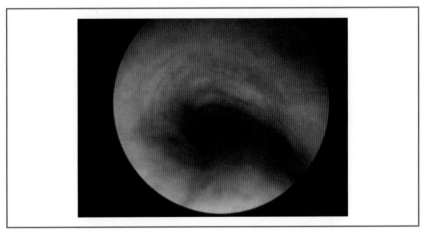

Figure 16-6. Asymmetric flattening of the trachea due to innominate artery compression.

confirmed by tracheoscopy in a spontaneously breathing patient so that the dynamic collapse is readily visible. Primary TM has more of a "fish-mouth" shape, while extrinsic compression causes asymmetric flattening of tracheal rings (**figures 16-6** and **16-7**). Patients with secondary TM should undergo a thorough cardiac workup, including computed tomographic (CT) angiography of the thorax to rule out any anatomical causes of external compression such as congenital vascular anomalies or mediastinal masses.

In most cases of primary TM, symptoms improve as the tracheobronchial tree grows. However, patients may be symptomatic for

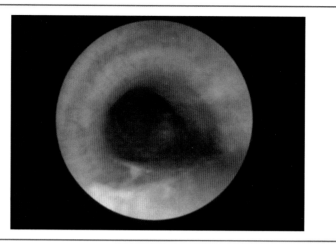

Figure 16-7. Compression of the trachea by vascular ring, including right-sided aortic arch.

years. Treatment involves observation, control of associated comorbidities (eg, GERD), and positive-pressure ventilation to stent airways open (CPAP/BiPAP). Severe cases associated with reflex apnea, airway obstruction, or frequent respiratory illnesses may require tracheostomy with custom-length tubes to bypass the distal collapse. Stents are primarily palliative because of considerable morbidity secondary to granulation formation or stent displacement. Secondary TM is treated with correction of the vascular anomaly, followed by conservative management similar to that in primary TM. In spite of surgical correction, stridor may be present for years because of residual TM. Gormley et al followed up patients for 9 years postoperatively and found that 75% experienced complete resolution of symptoms.

VOCAL FOLD PARALYSIS

True VFP is the second most common cause of stridor in the neonate after laryngomalacia. Vocal fold paralysis in children is classified as congenital or acquired, complete or partial, and unilateral or bilateral. Bilateral vocal fold paralysis often results in airway obstruction due to the inability to abduct the paralyzed vocal folds from a paramedian position. Congenital BVFP should be considered in cases of respiratory distress immediately after delivery, and, in severe cases, urgent intervention to secure the airway is necessary. Though the respiratory symptoms associated with BVFP can be quite profound, the aforementioned adducted position of the folds often allows for normal voice, cry, and feeding. Unilateral vocal fold paralysis, however, is typically marked by breathiness, dysphonia, and weak cry. Airway obstruction is less common in UVFP because the contralateral vocal fold is still able to abduct. These children are at higher risk of experiencing aspiration and may require thickening of feeds or nasogastric feeding.

Bilateral vocal fold paralysis and UVFP may be idiopathic, iatrogenic, or central (neurologic) in etiology. Iatrogenic causes include prolonged intubation and cardiac surgery, among others. The risk of developing VFP following cardiac surgery varies depending on the type of surgery. The incidence of left UVFP following patent ductus arteriosus ligation ranges from 20% to 60%, with increased risk for very-low-birth-weight infants. Because of the clear association between cardiac procedures and VFP, as well as the significant clinical implications of UVFP, some PCCs advocate routine screening with flexible laryngoscopy following cardiac surgery. Certainly, any child who displays symptoms of dysphonia, dysphagia, or voice changes after cardiac surgery should be evaluated for VFP.

Central nervous system anomalies are another cause of VFP. In particular, Chiari malformations should be considered in any patient with VFP. Various studies note that up to 50% of patients with Chiari malformations have some degree of vocal fold paresis. In particular, Chiari II malformations (Arnold-Chiari malformations) have a strong association with BVFP. For this reason, laryngological evaluation is recommended in patients with Chiari malformations, as development of symptoms of vocal fold impairment may help direct surgical timing. Surgical decompression may lead to recovery of vocal fold function.

The evaluation of VFP should include assessment of the entire course of the recurrent laryngeal nerve. This begins with a complete history, with particular attention paid to the type of delivery, any history of endotracheal intubation or previous surgery, and previous diagnosis of any neurologic disorders. The physical examination should include a complete neurologic assessment. Flexible fiberoptic laryngoscopy is the gold standard in evaluating vocal fold mobility, as it allows for dynamic examination. Occasionally, this will require more than 1 confirmatory FFL, as diagnosis can be complicated by movement and poor visualization of the infant's larynx. Imaging is useful to identify any cardiovascular anomalies, CNS anomalies, or lesions along the course of the recurrent laryngeal nerves. Assessment for Arnold-Chiari malformation is critical because VFP, usually bilateral, will often resolve with management of the CNS abnormality. The workup should also include a functional assessment of swallowing, such as a video fluoroscopic swallow study or an endoscopic evaluation of swallowing. For a large percentage of patients with unilateral and BVFP, no clear etiology will be identified.

Idiopathic cases of VFP have a higher rate of spontaneous recovery than iatrogenic or pathological cases. As a result, BVFP can sometimes be managed expectantly if the patient is in stable condition, with minimal symptoms or sequelae. Weight gain and feeding issues along with the status of the respiratory tract must be closely monitored in these instances. Surgical management is usually needed for more severe airway obstruction. Tracheostomy is the standard intervention for BVFP; however, endoscopic anterior and posterior cricoid split procedures have been used successfully in selected cases to improve patency of the airway and avoid tracheostomy while awaiting possible recovery of fold motion. Vocal cordotomy and arytenoidectomy may also be performed endoscopically, but these procedures result in permanent alterations of the glottis that may lead to complications such as dysphonia or aspiration.

Because of the high rate of spontaneous recovery, UVFP can often be managed expectantly while awaiting return of function. However, determining a child's candidacy for watchful waiting should include assessment by a speech and language pathologist for functional deficits. This assessment often includes a modified barium swallow (also known as a speech swallow or video swallow study) if there is concern for aspiration. Speech therapy is often an effective intervention for improving safe swallowing techniques. Voice therapy may be helpful for patients struggling with dysphonia. For older patients who struggle with aspiration and/or significant dysphonia, vocal fold injections with various temporary or semipermanent materials are common. The injected material medializes the paralyzed vocal fold, improving the glottis gap and leading to better voice and swallow. Patients who derive benefit from these injections and demonstrate no evidence of recovery of function may be candidates for thyroplasty, a surgical procedure in which an implant is used to more permanently medialize the paralyzed vocal fold. For certain patients following iatrogenic nerve injury, recurrent laryngeal nerve reinnervation procedures may lead to improved voice and swallow.

AIRWAY HEMANGIOMA

Infantile hemangiomas of the airway are an uncommon but important diagnosis to consider in any child with symptoms of stridor. Like most infantile hemangiomas, those of the airway are usually subclinical at birth, go through a proliferative phase during the first year after birth, and then gradually involute during childhood. It is during the proliferative phase, usually within the first 6 months after birth, that children often first exhibit symptoms.

Though airway hemangiomas may develop anywhere along the airway, they are most common in the subglottis. As such, the presentation is often similar to other infectious and inflammatory conditions that affect the subglottis, namely croup. Proliferation of the hemangioma results in a narrowing of the subglottic airway, which results in biphasic stridor and barky cough. The similarities between croup and airway hemangiomas, including the initial response to steroids and racemic epinephrine, often lead to a delay in diagnosis.

Airway hemangiomas may be focal or segmental. Up to 50% of patients with airway hemangiomas also have cutaneous lesions. The converse, however, is not true, as the vast majority of children with cutaneous hemangiomas do not have concurrent airway lesions. However, the presence of multiple cutaneous lesions in the "beard distribution," including the lips, chin, neck, and parotid glands, has a relatively high correlation with airway hemangiomas. In such cases, the hemangioma is likely segmental, and the airway is just one of the affected sites. Airway hemangioma also should be suspected in children without cutaneous lesions who present with persistent or multiple recurrent croup symptoms, especially in the absence of infection.

In children with suspected airway infantile hemangioma, evaluation often begins with flexible fiberoptic endoscopy and plain neck radiographs, which may demonstrate asymmetry of the airway suggestive of hemangioma. Though visualization of the subglottis is often not possible in infants without general anesthesia, airway hemangiomas often involve multiple subsites of the larynx, so bedside evaluation may elicit a diagnosis. The next step in making a diagnosis may be imaging of the airway or operative microlaryngoscopy and bronchoscopy. On endoscopy, airway hemangiomas often appear bluish or pink with a smooth surface, and are easily compressible (**Figure 16-8**). This compressible nature occasionally may lead PCCs to reach a mistaken diagnosis of soft subglottic stenosis. Both CT and MRI have been used to diagnose airway hemangiomas; however,

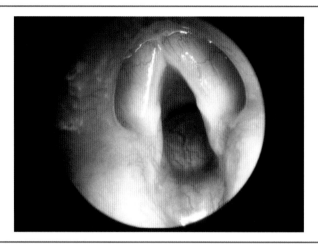

Figure 16-8. Airway hemangioma emanating from the posterior tracheal wall.

CT is often performed preferentially to avoid the need for general anesthesia.

Following diagnosis, management is determined by the clinical presentation and severity of symptoms. While systemic and intra-lesional steroids and partial laser resection traditionally were the mainstay of medical management, these treatments were largely supplanted by propranolol therapy in 2008 when its ability to inhibit hemangioma growth and induce involution was discovered. Standard propranolol therapy is initiated at 1 mg/kg/day and titrated up to 3 mg/kg/day. During initiation of therapy and when any subsequent increases in dosage are made, patients should be carefully monitored for bradycardia and hypoglycemia. Propranolol also may cause bron-chospasm, diarrhea, and sleep disorders. The exact mechanism of action of propranolol has not been fully elucidated, but it is hypothe-sized to work by blocking vascular endothelial growth factor or basic fibroblast growth factor.

For most cases, medical management will suffice; however, surgical excision remains an option for patients who do not respond fully to propranolol therapy or who have significant symptoms requiring more urgent intervention. Surgical management most commonly involves endoscopic partial resection with a laser or microdebrider or open surgical excision, often in combination with intralesional steroid injection. The most common lasers used for airway hemangiomas are potassium titanyl phosphate, CO_2, and yttrium aluminum garnet lasers. Though safe for endoscopic use, the resulting tissue destruction leads to subglottic stenosis in up to 25% of cases. Also, though intralesional steroids have exhibited success rates as high as 80%, if used in isolation, injections may need to be repeated every few months. Open surgical excision with or without cartilage grafting is rarely performed today because of the success of propranolol therapy. Tracheostomy is an option when other modalities fail or to establish an airway urgently when physicians who are experienced in hemangioma management are not readily available.

POSTINTUBATION INJURIES

Following intubation, infants and children are at risk for a wide variety of intubation-associated injuries. Given the frequency with which premature neonates require intubation and the small size of their airways, it is not surprising that this population is particularly affected. Risk factors for injury include NICU history, frequent and prolonged intubation, emergent intubations by less-experienced personnel, abnormal larynx, and recurrent self-extubation. Stridor, respiratory distress, history of recurrent or prolonged croup, and multiple comorbidities (eg, genetic syndrome, GERD) are factors that may lead to intubation and result in an injury. Symptoms may present months to years after the injury.

In 2018, Benjamin proposed a general classification system for describing postintubation changes that includes 5 primary categories: early nonspecific changes, edema, granulation tissue, ulceration, and miscellaneous. On endoscopic evaluation, the early nonspecific changes primarily consist of edema, hyperemia, and some patchy ulceration. Edema typically resolves after extubation, but it may persist and cause worsening airway obstruction following removal of the endotracheal tube. The edema may then lead to re-intubation. Periextubation steroids may be administered in an attempt to counteract this swelling. Granulation tissue may develop around an endotracheal tube within the first 48 hours of intubation. Again, this often resolves quickly without intervention once the tube has been removed, but granulation tissue may lead to formation of firm granulomas, interarytenoid adhesions, and stenosis of the posterior glottis. Airway ulceration from intubation may result in scarring and subsequent stenosis depending on the depth, location, and extent of ulceration. Finally, rare miscellaneous injuries to the airway include arytenoid dislocation, airway perforation (often related to endotracheal tube stylets), and vocal fold lacerations. It is not clear what percentage of patients with each of these postintubation injuries will go on to develop chronic airway damage. Additional postintubation injuries are detailed as follows.

Subglottic Cysts

Subglottic cysts (**Figure 16-9**) are relatively uncommon postintubation injuries. The vast majority occur in premature infants following intubation, irrespective of the duration of intubation. Cyst development begins with mucus gland hypertrophy and duct blockage. Cysts typically occur along the posterior lateral subglottic wall and can be multiple. They present with stridor and airway obstruction, which may increase with an upper respiratory infection. Because patients may not present for months following intubation, their symptoms— inspiratory stridor, cough, and initial response to steroids and racemic epinephrine—may initially be attributed to croup. Once cysts are diagnosed, they can be removed using a variety of endoscopic techniques, including microdebrider, cup forceps, and various lasers.

Posterior Glottic Injury/Interarytenoid Web

Intubation resulting in granulation tissue, deep ulceration over the arytenoids, or posterior glottis injury may result in scarring that progresses to posterior glottic stenosis (**Figure 16-10**). While the

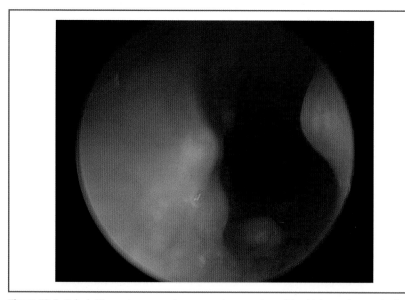

Figure 16-9. Subglottic cysts are most common in neonates with a history of prematurity and endotracheal intubation.

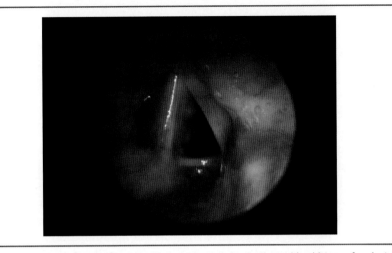

Figure 16-10. Posterior glottic scar and subglottic cysts in a patient with a history of perinatal intubation.

former requires only simple division, the latter is more serious and difficult to manage. Posterior glottic stenosis may be mistaken for BVFP because it results in bilateral true vocal fold immobility, which, in turn, can lead to acute respiratory distress and airway obstruction. To distinguish this entity from VFP, operative endoscopy and palpation of the arytenoid are required. Posterior glottic expansion, cordectomy, arytenoidectomy, or tracheostomy can be used to manage this injury.

Subglottic Stenosis

Acquired SGS has a reported incidence of as high as 17% after intubation in an intensive care setting, and is a problem with tremendous variation in its presentation and severity. The clinical picture may range from mild biphasic stridor and endoscopic findings of subglottic inflammation that respond to steroids and expectant management to severe stenosis that requires surgical intervention. The classic history is failed extubation in a premature neonate after prolonged ventilation. Fortunately, the incidence of this disease is decreasing with improved NICU ventilation techniques and awareness of the need to avoid large tubes for long durations in small airways. The typical progression to stenosis begins with edema, granulation, ulceration, perichondritis/chondritis, and scarring. The subglottis is most commonly involved because it is the only portion of the airway that is cartilaginous circumferentially (cricoid ring).

When SGS is suspected, complete airway endoscopy from the nasopharynx to carina is indicated. When stenosis is found, the endoscopist makes note of the length of the stenosis, location of the stenosis (ie, glottic, subglottic, or tracheal), character of the stenosis (soft and early or firm and mature), and grade of the stenosis based on the involved cross-sectional area.

Grade I (0%–50% obstruction) and asymptomatic grade II (50%–70% obstruction) stenoses can frequently be managed with medical therapy, including antibiotics, antireflux medications, and intermittent steroid bursts to manage acute inflammation. Symptomatic grade II and select mild grade III (70%–99% obstruction) stenoses are amenable to multiple endoscopic modalities, including balloon dilation with or without laser excision. Steroids and antibiotics are used in conjunction with endoscopic procedures to decrease inflammation and control granulation, and mitomycin C is occasionally applied topically to minimize scarring by inhibiting fibroblast proliferation.

More severe grade III and grade IV (no discernible lumen) stenoses, and those that fail to respond to endoscopic treatments, are candidates for open surgical procedures. The most common open surgical procedures are laryngotracheal reconstruction with rib cartilage augmentation and cricotracheal reconstruction. General medical status, comorbid conditions, and parental expectations will dictate the timing of surgery. Tracheotomy may be necessary to maintain the airway until these issues are addressed. Children with congenital or acquired SGS frequently have cardiac or pulmonary comorbidities as well as other sequelae of prematurity. Consequently, a multidisciplinary approach is imperative. These patients should receive complete pulmonary, cardiac, pediatric surgery, or gastroenterology consultations as deemed necessary.

CONGENITAL AIRWAY ANOMALIES

Several common congenital airway anomalies are briefly described as follows.

Congenital Subglottic Stenosis

In addition to acquired lesions of the subglottis that result from endotracheal injuries, SGS can be congenital. Endoscopically, the subglottis appears abnormally narrow and has an elliptical-shaped cricoid ring in the absence of scar (**Figure 16-11**). Congenital SGS has been reported to occur in up to 2% of neonates. The presentation of neonates with congenital SGS is very similar to that of neonates

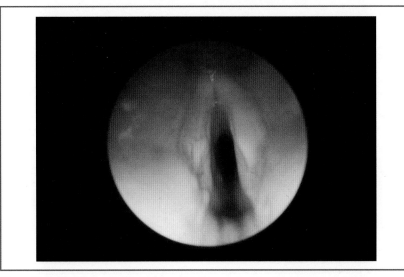

Figure 16-11. Elliptical cricoid causing subglottic narrowing and stridor in an infant.

with acquired SGS. Neonates with severe congenital SGS may require intubation secondary to respiratory distress, making the diagnosis of congenital SGS difficult. However, patients with mild congenital SGS have symptoms without a history of intubation. Mild cases of congenital SGS are often outgrown without any surgical intervention.

Anterior Glottic Web and Laryngeal Atresia

Anterior glottic webs (**Figure 16-12**) and laryngeal atresia are rare congenital airway anomalies that result from incomplete recanalization of the laryngeal airway in utero. Cases of complete laryngeal atresia are usually identified prenatally, allowing for a planned ex utero procedure to secure the airway with tracheotomy. If diagnosed at birth, the child will have airway obstruction, including aphonia, cyanosis, and rapid decompensation. Fortunately, this is an extremely rare anomaly. More commonly, children with anterior glottis webs have a weak hoarse cry, dysphonia, or stridor depending on the severity of the web. Acute respiratory distress is uncommon because the posterior glottis remains patent. Glottic webs are frequently associated with 22q11.2 deletion syndrome, and, as such, all patients diagnosed with glottis web merit an appropriate workup. Surgical management is challenging owing to the high rate of recurrence. When symptoms are not severe, it may be advisable to defer treatment until the child has grown and the airway is more amenable to surgical

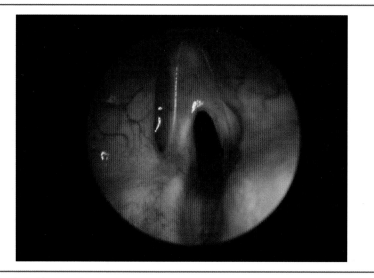

Figure 16-12. Glottic webs may be congenital or acquired. Anterior webs often cause dysphonia alone; with greater posterior involvement of the larynx, stridor becomes increasingly apparent.

intervention. While thin bands may be successfully divided with laser or cold instrumentation followed by a period of intubation to prevent re-scarring, thicker webs require more definitive surgery, often involving open or endoscopic division followed by keel stent placement. This may require tracheostomy to secure a safe airway.

Laryngeal Cleft

Laryngeal clefts (also called laryngotracheoesophageal clefts) are a midline defect representing failure of formation of the posterior laryngeal wall and the common wall separating the trachea and esophagus. Affected children may have stridor but are primarily symptomatic because of aspiration and an inability to handle their secretions. A cleft should be suspected whenever a child develops chronic cough with feeding, failure to thrive, recurrent aspiration pneumonia, and stridor early in life. Diagnosis is made by means of lateral distraction of the arytenoid cartilages during airway endoscopy. Clefts are classified as types I to IV based on the extent of laryngeal involvement. Type I clefts extend to the vocal folds; type II clefts extend into the subglottis but do not involve the entire cricoid; type III clefts involve the entire cricoid cartilage and extend into the cervical trachea; and type IV clefts extend deep into the thoracic trachea and are often fatal.

Treatment varies with the extent of the cleft. Type I clefts (**Figure 16-13**) are the most common yet often overlooked cause of cough and desaturation during feeding. When they cause symptoms, type I clefts are treated by endoscopic repair or injection of filler. Type II clefts also may be amenable to endoscopic repair but more commonly require open repair (laryngofissure) with posterior buttressing. Type III and IV clefts present immediately after birth and are life threatening, requiring immediate open surgical intervention. Type IV clefts must be approached via thoracotomy.

Patients with laryngeal clefts should be screened for cardiovascular defects and also require acid suppression. Dysphagia studies should be performed to determine the safety of swallowing and risk of aspiration. If oral feeding is unsafe, a feeding tube can be placed.

Vascular Rings/Slings

Children with cardiovascular anomalies often exhibit stridor and some degree of airway obstruction related to their abnormal mediastinal vasculature. The 3 most common anomalies are aberrant innominate artery (most common), double aortic arch, and aberrant right subclavian artery that may course posterior to the esophagus, otherwise called *dysphagia lusoria*. The presentation of these children is similar to that of children with TM. They have harsh expiratory stridor and characteristic cough and may experience "dying spells." Evaluation should include an esophagram and imaging of the thoracic vasculature via CT angiography. When identified on tracheobronchoscopy, a fish-mouth

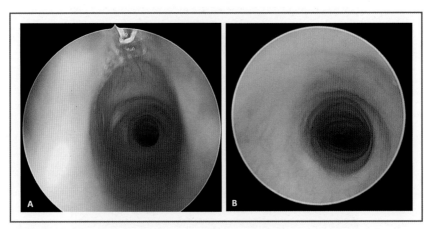

Figure 16-13. Endoscopic views of trachea with complete rings in a 4-month-old. A, Narrowing of midtrachea seen from level of vocal folds. B, Completeness of rings more apparent on close-up view.

appearance of the trachea is seen with pulsatile compression. If there is an aberrant innominate artery, compression will be anterior; if a double aortic arch or an aberrant right subclavian is present, compression (see **Figure 16-7**) will be from the posterior aspect of the trachea. Symptomatic children require open vascular decompression.

Congenital Tracheal Stenosis

Congenital tracheal stenosis (CTS) develops as a structural abnormality inherent to the trachea itself, resulting in a narrowing of the trachea that produces airway obstruction. In most cases, the narrowed segment of the trachea is characterized by complete cartilaginous rings that involve a segment of the trachea of variable length (**Figure 16-14**).

The spectrum of respiratory symptoms in CTS ranges from isolated intermittent stridor to acute life-threatening events requiring cardiopulmonary resuscitation. Rarely, air exchange may be so compromised that extracorporeal membrane oxygenation may be necessary. Symptoms generally appear within the first few weeks after birth. Patients are often misdiagnosed as having croup; however, croup is exceedingly rare among neonates. Failure to thrive results from the caloric demand of increased work of breathing combined with poor feeding. Congenital tracheal stenosis is frequently associated with other congenital malformations of the pulmonary, cardiovascular, and gastrointestinal systems. A pulmonary artery sling is present in 30% to 50% of patients and should be ruled out before a definitive management plan is established.

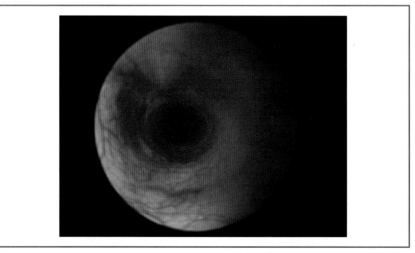

Figure 16-14. Congenital tracheal stenosis. Note the funnel shape of the trachea and absence of membranous trachea at narrowing.

The diagnosis of CTS is usually established via bronchoscopy performed to evaluate the etiology of the stridor. The trachea will appear funnel shaped, and passage of a telescope or bronchoscope will be restricted. Once identified, it is important not to cause inflammation in the narrowed segment from trauma from the scope or an endotracheal tube used to secure the airway. The airway is best secured with an endotracheal tube placed with the tip proximal to the narrowed segment; generally, neither intubation nor tracheotomy is useful because of the severity of the stenosis or the distal location of the obstruction. Following endoscopy, CT scanning with 3-dimensional reconstruction may be used to establish the length and diameter of the stenotic segment.

Management strategies include conservative measures and surgery. In milder cases, stridor may be tolerated and acute exacerbations treated with systemic and inhaled steroids. However, more severe cases require surgical intervention. In short-segment stenosis, it is often possible to resect the narrowed portion of the trachea and suture together the portions of normal caliber. Long-segment stenosis usually requires a slide tracheoplasty in which the stenosis is divided horizontally and the cut ends are slid over one another and sutured, widening and shortening the trachea.

RECURRENT RESPIRATORY PAPILLOMATOSIS

Recurrent respiratory papillomatosis (RRP) is the most common benign neoplasm of the larynx in children and the second most frequent cause of childhood hoarseness (after vocal fold nodules). It is caused by the human papillomavirus (HPV), most commonly serotypes 6 and 11. Human papillomavirus has a propensity for transitional zones in which squamous epithelium and respiratory epithelium meet. As a result, RRP often presents in the laryngeal ventricle and the undersurface of the vocal folds. The incidence of RRP is 4.3 per 100,000 children in the United States. The most common mode of transmission involves passage through the birth canal of an infected mother, with the presence of maternal anogenital lesions at the time of birth accounting for the highest rate of transmission. Fortunately, with the introduction of widespread HPV vaccination in various countries, the incidence of RRP appears to be declining.

Because most RRP cases involve the larynx, the most common presenting symptoms include chronic cough, dysphonia, or hoarseness. However, progression of the disease with increased disease burden of the glottis may result in stridor. Recurrent respiratory papilloma may also lead to dyspnea, and, in severe cases, respiratory distress and airway obstruction. Diagnosis is most often made at around 3 years of age, but it may be delayed while affected children are treated for asthma, chronic cough, bronchitis, or croup. Although RRP most commonly involves the larynx (**Figure 16-15**), it can occur anywhere within the aerodigestive tract. Spread of the disease beyond the larynx to the tracheobronchial airway occurs in up to 30% of cases. Malignant transformation is extremely rare.

Diagnosis often can be made by means of in-office flexible laryngoscopy revealing exophytic, cauliflower lesions on the larynx. Further workup and diagnosis usually involve bronchoscopy and, occasionally, imaging. Bronchoscopy allows for direct visualization of disease with evaluation of the upper airway and bronchi, as well as biopsy for confirmatory pathological diagnosis. A helical chest CT is recommended for complete evaluation of RRP suspected in the tracheobronchial tree and pulmonary parenchyma. Pulmonary RRP lesions usually appear as nodular single or multilobulated lesions, which often develop central cavitation.

Surgical management remains the mainstay for patients with RRP, especially for disease limited to the larynx. Goals of therapy include creating a safe and patent airway, avoiding tracheostomy, and reducing tumor burden while preserving voice quality. Most often, the microdebrider is used to remove bulky lesions. Managing RRP in children can be challenging because of the propensity for the disease to recur and require multiple surgeries, which leads to significant psychological

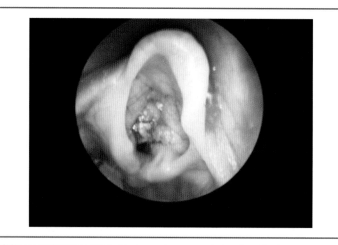

Figure 16-15. Respiratory papillomatosis most commonly involves the larynx.

and emotional effects on the child and family. In addition to the stress of frequent surgical interventions, patients struggle with the social effects of the resulting dysphonia. For the most severe cases of RRP resulting in tracheostomy or involving significant pulmonary disease, medical adjuvant therapy is available. These therapies should be considered when a patient requires more than 4 surgeries in a 12-month period or experiences airway obstruction despite complete surgical therapy. Intralesional, topical, or systemic cidofovir is a commonly used antiviral medication that has been shown to reduce the frequency of surgeries and result in lesion regression. Interferon therapy has also been used with some degree of success. However, more recently, the monoclonal antibody bevacizumab has shown tremendous promise for management of severe cases. In a small number of patients, systemic bevacizumab administered at 5 to 10 mg/kg every 2 to 4 weeks has been shown to lead to lesion regression and increase the interval between surgeries. The US Food and Drug Administration has approved use of the quadrivalent HPV vaccine (active against serotypes 6, 11, 16, and 18) for males and females to help prevent HPV infection and reduce the incidence of cervical cancer. While data are not yet available for the United States, a decreased incidence of RRP has been recorded since the introduction of HPV vaccination in Australia. In addition, the 9-valent HPV vaccine has been used to treat already infected children, with some success in increasing intervals between surgical management.

PARADOXICAL VOCAL FOLD MOVEMENT DISORDER

Paradoxical vocal fold movement disorder (PVFMD), formerly referred to as vocal fold dysfunction, is a disorder of the larynx characterized by paradoxical adduction of the vocal folds during inspiration. Affected patients experience frequent, episodic attacks of dyspnea, hoarseness, cough, wheezing, chest tightness, inspiratory stridor, and resulting anxiety. The disorder is often mistaken for poorly controlled asthma, leading to years of escalating medical therapy, emergency department visits, and expensive health care utilization. In certain communities, up to 30% of children with poorly controlled asthma have been found to have PVFMD. Although this condition traditionally has been considered largely psychogenic, our current understanding of PVFMD recognizes several contributing comorbidities, including gastroesophageal or laryngopharyngeal reflux, asthma, tobacco use, allergic laryngitis, viral illness, and even obstructive sleep apnea.

The typical patient with PVFMD presents with episodic symptoms of throat tightness and acute-onset dyspnea. Common triggers include stress, anxiety, inhaled irritants, and exercise. In fact, the disorder is commonly seen in high-performing athletes and is brought on by intense physical activity. Usually, symptoms resolve as quickly as they began, often with cessation of exercise.

Paradoxical vocal fold movement disorder often is a diagnosis of exclusion, as patients typically demonstrate no laryngoscopic abnormalities unless they are symptomatic at the time of the procedure. During symptomatic episodes, flexible laryngoscopy demonstrates adduction during inspiration, with severe cases exhibiting the pathognomonic anterior vocal fold closure with posterior chink on inspiration. This obstruction decreases laminar airflow through the glottis and produces an inspiratory wheeze or stridor similar to that heard in those with asthma, making the 2 entities difficult to differentiate symptomatically. In asthma alone, however, a posterior glottic chink is not seen. Some PCCs find it helpful to perform flexible laryngoscopy and/or obtain flow-volume loops after having the patient exercise vigorously to incite an episode. Patients typically demonstrate a limitation of inspiratory flow suggestive of variable extrathoracic obstruction (inspiratory loop flattening).

Once a diagnosis of PVFMD has been made, patients should be referred to a speech and language pathologist for laryngeal control therapy (LCT) or respiratory retraining therapy. These interventions involve a variety of controlled breathing techniques, including abdominal breathing, nasal inspiration, and breathing through a short straw. Laryngeal control therapy can be used both as a preventive measure as well as a measure to break active episodes. In addition to LCT, control of contributing comorbidities, including gastroesophageal reflux, allergies, and asthma, and management of stress and anxiety are critical in reducing PVFMD. Medical therapy for acute exacerbations of vocal cord dysfunction includes heliox, a gaseous mixture of oxygen and helium that is less dense than air and reduces turbulence in the airway, as well as topical lidocaine and anxiolytics to break the cycle of hyperactive laryngeal adduction and muscle contractions. Fortunately, with LCT, most patients are able to break acute episodes and avoid escalation of care.

■ Conclusion

Stridor in infants and children may have a varied presentation and clinical course. Acute respiratory distress should be addressed immediately by securing the airway. Patients in more stable condition can be evaluated more thoroughly. Because the differential diagnosis may be extensive, several historic facts should be considered in the initial assessment, including birth history, age at onset, intubations, progression, and feeding difficulties. The physical examination should begin with an observation of the patient and proceed systematically, by moving on to flexible fiberoptic laryngoscopy and operative endoscopy, as necessary. A multidisciplinary approach, including pediatric otolaryngology, pediatric surgery, speech pathology, occupational therapy, intensivists, pulmonology, anesthesiology, cardiology, and gastroenterology, may be taken to optimize care.

■ Selected References

Benjamin B. Prolonged intubation injuries of the larynx: endoscopic diagnosis, classification, and treatment. *Ann Otol Rhinol Laryngol.* 2018;127(8):492–507

Benjamin JR, Smith PB, Cotten CM, Jaggers J, Goldstein RF, Malcolm WF. Long-term morbidities associated with vocal cord paralysis after surgical closure of a patent ductus arteriosus in extremely low birth weight infants. *J Perinatol.* 2010;30(6):408–413

Best SR, Mohr M, Zur KB. Systemic bevacizumab for recurrent respiratory papillomatosis: a national survey. *Laryngoscope.* 2017;127(10):2225–2229

Buckmiller LM. Update on hemangiomas and vascular malformations. *Curr Opin Otolaryngol Head Neck Surg.* 2004;12(6):476–487

Buckmiller LM, Munson PD, Dyamenahalli U, Dai Y, Richter GT. Propranolol for infantile hemangiomas: early experience at a tertiary vascular anomalies center. *Laryngoscope.* 2010;120(4):676–681

Choi SS, Tran LP, Zalzal GH. Airway abnormalities in patients with Arnold-Chiari malformation. *Otolaryngol Head Neck Surg.* 1999;121(6):720–724

Choi SS, Zalzal GH. Changing trends in neonatal subglottic stenosis. *Otolaryngol Head Neck Surg.* 2000;122(1):61–63

Cotton RT. Management of subglottic stenosis. *Otolaryngol Clin North Am.* 2000;33(1): 111–130

Cotton RT, Myer CM. *Practical Pediatric Otolaryngology.* Philadelphia, PA: Lippincott-Raven; 1999:637–660

Darrow DH. Management of infantile hemangiomas of the airway. *Otolaryngol Clin North Am.* 2018;51(1):133–146

de Jong AL, Kuppersmith RB, Sulek M, Friedman EM. Vocal cord paralysis in infants and children. *Otolaryngol Clin North Am.* 2000;33(1):131–149

Denipah N, Dominguez CM, Kraai EP, Kraai TL, Leos P, Braude D. Acute management of paradoxical vocal fold motion (vocal cord dysfunction). *Ann Emerg Med.* 2017; 69(1):18–23

Derkay CS, Bluher AE. Recurrent respiratory papillomatosis: update 2018. *Curr Opin Otolaryngol Head Neck Surg.* 2018;26(6):421–425

Derkay CS, Wiatrak B. Recurrent respiratory papillomatosis: a review. *Laryngoscope*. 2008; 118(7):1236–1247

Dickson JM, Richter GT, Meinzen-Derr J, Rutter MJ, Thompson DM. Secondary airway lesions in infants with laryngomalacia. *Ann Otol Rhinol Laryngol*. 2009;118(1):37–43

Fortes HR, von Ranke FM, Escuissato DL, et al. Recurrent respiratory papillomatosis: a state-of-the-art review. *Respir Med*. 2017;126:116–121

Friedman EM, Vastola AP, McGill TJ, Healy GB. Chronic pediatric stridor: etiology and outcome. *Laryngoscope*. 1990;100(3):277–280

Froehlich P, Seid AB, Denoyelle F, et al. Discoordinate pharyngolaryngomalacia. *Int J Pediatr Otorhinolaryngol*. 1997;39(1):9–18

FUTURE I/II Study Group; Dillner J, Kjaer SK, Wheeler CM, et al. Four year efficacy of prophylactic human papillomavirus quadrivalent vaccine against low grade cervical, vulvar, and vaginal intraepithelial neoplasia and anogenital warts: randomised controlled trial. *BMJ*. 2010;341:c3493

Goldman J, Muers M. Vocal cord dysfunction and wheezing. *Thorax*. 1991;46(6):401–404

Gormley PK, Colreavy MP, Patil N, Woods AE. Congenital vascular anomalies and persistent respiratory symptoms in children. *Int J Pediatr Otorhinolaryngol*. 1999;51(1):23–31

Hartley BE, Cotton RT. Paediatric airway stenosis: laryngotracheal reconstruction or cricotracheal resection? *Clin Otolaryngol Allied Sci*. 2000;25(5):342–349

Hartzell LD, Richter GT, Glade RS, Bower CM. Accuracy and safety of tracheoscopy for infants in a tertiary care clinic. *Arch Otolaryngol Head Neck Surg*. 2010;136(1):66–69

Ho AS, Koltai PJ. Pediatric tracheal stenosis. *Otolaryngol Clin North Am*. 2008;41(5): 999–1021, x

Hoff SR, Schroeder JW Jr, Rastatter JC, Holinger LD. Supraglottoplasty outcomes in relation to age and comorbid conditions. *Int J Pediatr Otorhinolaryngol*. 2010;74(3): 245–249

Husain S, Sadoughi B, Mor N, Sulica L. Time course of recovery of iatrogenic vocal fold paralysis. *Laryngoscope*. 2019;129(5):1159-1163

Jabbour J, North LM, Bougie D, Robey T. Vocal fold immobility due to birth trauma: a systematic review and pooled analysis. *Otolaryngol Head Neck Surg*. 2017;157(6):948–954

Jephson CG, Manunza F, Syed S, Mills NA, Harper J, Hartley BE. Successful treatment of isolated subglottic haemangioma with propranolol alone. *Int J Pediatr Otorhinolaryngol*. 2009;73(12):1821–1823

Jomah M, Jeffery C, Campbell S, Krajacic A, El-Hakim H. Spontaneous recovery of bilateral congenital idiopathic laryngeal paralysis: systematic non-meta-analytical review. *Int J Pediatr Otorhinolaryngol*. 2015;79(2):202–209

Landry AM, Rutter MJ. Airway anomalies. *Clin Perinatol*. 2018;45(4):597–607

Léauté-Labrèze C, Dumas de la Roque E, Hubiche T, Boralevi F, Thambo JB, Taïeb A. Propranolol for severe hemangiomas of infancy. *N Engl J Med*. 2008;358(24): 2649–2651

Lim J, Hellier W, Harcourt J, Leighton S, Albert D. Subglottic cysts: the Great Ormond Street experience. *Int J Pediatr Otorhinolaryngol*. 2003;67(5):461–465

Linder A, Lindholm CE. Laryngologic management of infants with the Chiari II syndrome. *Int J Pediatr Otorhinolaryngol*. 1997;39(3):187–197

Lindstrom DR III, Book DT, Conley SF, Flanary VA, Kerschner JE. Office-based lower airway endoscopy in pediatric patients. *Arch Otolaryngol Head Neck Surg.* 2003; 129(8):847–853

Maschka DA, Bauman NM, McCray PB Jr, Hoffman HT, Karnell MP, Smith RJ. A classification scheme for paradoxical vocal cord motion. *Laryngoscope.* 1997;107(11 Pt 1):1429–1435

Matrka L. Paradoxic vocal fold movement disorder. *Otolaryngol Clin North Am.* 2014; 47(1):135–146

Milczuk HA, Smith JD, Everts EC. Congenital laryngeal webs: surgical management and clinical embryology. *Int J Pediatr Otorhinolaryngol.* 2000;52(1):1–9

Moungthong G, Holinger LD. Laryngotracheoesophageal clefts. *Ann Otol Rhinol Laryngol.* 1997;106(12):1002–1011

Myer CM III, O'Connor DM, Cotton RT. Proposed grading system for subglottic stenosis based on endotracheal tube sizes. *Ann Otol Rhinol Laryngol.* 1994;103(4 Pt 1):319–323

Newman KB, Mason UG III, Schmaling KB. Clinical features of vocal cord dysfunction. *Am J Respir Crit Care Med.* 1995;152(4 Pt 1):1382–1386

Pezzettigotta SM, Leboulanger N, Roger G, Denoyelle F, Garabédian EN. Laryngeal cleft. *Otolaryngol Clin North Am.* 2008;41(5):913–933

Rameau A, Foltz RS, Wagner K, Zur KB. Multidisciplinary approach to vocal cord dysfunction diagnosis and treatment in one session: a single institutional outcome study. *Int J Pediatr Otorhinolaryngol.* 2012;76(1):31–35

Richter AL, Ongkasuwan J, Ocampo EC. Long-term follow-up of vocal fold movement impairment and feeding after neonatal cardiac surgery. *Int J Pediatr Otorhinolaryngol.* 2016;83:211–214

Richter GT, Thompson DM. The surgical management of laryngomalacia. *Otolaryngol Clin North Am.* 2008;41(5):837–864, vii

Richter GT, Wootten CT, Rutter MJ, Thompson DM. Impact of supraglottoplasty on aspiration in severe laryngomalacia. *Ann Otol Rhinol Laryngol.* 2009;118(4):259–266

Rutter MJ, Cohen AP, de Alarcon A. Endoscopic airway management in children. *Curr Opin Otolaryngol Head Neck Surg.* 2008;16(6):525–529

Rutter MJ, Hart CK, Alarcon A, et al. Endoscopic anterior-posterior cricoid split for pediatric bilateral vocal fold paralysis. *Laryngoscope.* 2018;128(1):257–263

Sakakura K, Chikamatsu K, Toyoda M, Kaai M, Yasuoka Y, Furuya N. Congenital laryngeal anomalies presenting as chronic stridor: a retrospective study of 55 patients. *Auris Nasus Larynx.* 2008;35(4):527–533

Schroeder JW Jr, Bhandarkar ND, Holinger LD. Synchronous airway lesions and outcomes in infants with severe laryngomalacia requiring supraglottoplasty. *Arch Otolaryngol Head Neck Surg.* 2009;135(7):647–651

Schweiger C, Manica D, Kuhl G, Sekine L, Marostica PJ. Post-intubation acute laryngeal injuries in infants and children: a new classification system. *Int J Pediatr Otorhinolaryngol.* 2016;86:177–182

Stern Y, Cotton RT. Evaluation of the noisy infant. In: Cotton RT, Myer CM, eds. *Practical Pediatric Otolaryngology.* Philadelphia, PA: Lippincott-Raven Publishers; 1999:471–476

Tadié JM, Behm E, Lecuyer L, et al. Post-intubation laryngeal injuries and extubation failure: a fiberoptic endoscopic study. *Intensive Care Med.* 2010;36(6):991–998

Thompson DM. Abnormal sensorimotor integrative function of the larynx in congenital laryngomalacia: a new theory of etiology. *Laryngoscope.* 2007;117(6 Pt 2 Suppl 114): 1–33

Thompson DM. Laryngomalacia: factors that influence disease severity and outcomes of management. *Curr Opin Otolaryngol Head Neck Surg.* 2010;18(6):564–570

Zoumalan R, Maddalozzo J, Holinger LD. Etiology of stridor in infants. *Ann Otol Rhinol Laryngol.* 2007;116(5):329–334

Feeding Disorders and Ankyloglossia in Infants and Children

Joan C. Arvedson, PhD, CCC-SLP, BCS-S,
and Lisa Ann Brock, RN, BSN, CBS, IBCLC-RLC

Pediatric Feeding Disorders

▇ Introduction

Feeding is a complex process that involves multiple systems that function in interactive ways. Feeding is much broader than swallowing and includes not only the central and peripheral nervous system but also oropharyngeal and esophageal swallowing, the cardiopulmonary system, and the gastrointestinal (GI) tract. *Dysphagia* is the term that describes swallowing deficits. Not all children with feeding disorders have dysphagia, but children with dysphagia fit into the broad category of feeding disorders. The act of feeding is a dyadic process that requires interaction between feeders, usually mothers, and newborns, infants, and children. From the beginning, feeding should be neonate/infant led with emphasis on the quality of feeding, and not on the volume consumed. When major efforts are made to increase the volume consumed, it is not surprising that stressful feedings and potentially reduced volume and refusals become evident. The pleasure of eating extends beyond the feeling of satiety to the pleasure gained through food ingestion—taste, texture, and temperature of foods. The interaction between newborn and primary caregiver is the first such relationship for every neonate. It serves as a foundation for normal development, somatic growth, communication skills, and psychosocial well-being. When feeding is disrupted, the sequelae can include undernutrition/malnutrition, behavioral abnormalities, and severe distress for the newborn, infant, or child and family, which may result in irreversible arrested growth and development.

Epidemiology

Annually, more than 100,000 newborns and infants are given diagnoses of feeding problems after being discharged from acute care hospitals, and more than one-half million children between ages 3 and 17 years in the United States are diagnosed with dysphagia. Among preterm newborns and infants, approximately 40% have feeding or swallowing disorders. Medical and technological advances have improved survival of newborns, infants, and children born preterm, but many of these patients have complex medical problems, including, but not limited to, genetic, cardiac, pulmonary, GI, and neurologic abnormalities. Sequelae exacerbate, or may be exacerbated by, feeding disorders.

> **Pearl:** Feeding and swallowing disorders are present in about 40% of preterm newborns and infants and often complicate their already compromised medical status. Early referral to feeding and swallowing specialists may reduce the medical effect of these disorders.

■ Medical History

A *whole-child* approach to intervention is advocated. Thus, a thorough history is taken to identify underlying disorders that may affect oral feeding. Medical history is gathered from parents and caregivers, other health care professionals, and medical charts or records. A prenatal history of maternal infection, drug use, or polyhydramnios suggests a child is at increased risk for dysphagia because of neurologic compromise. A birth history of cervical trauma, anoxia, prolonged resuscitation, low Apgar scores, and technology dependence also suggests a poor prognosis. Congenital anatomical anomalies causing dysphagia include palatal clefts, laryngotracheal clefts, and vocal cord paralysis. Most older children with dysphagia are compromised neurologically, although disorders such as gastroesophageal reflux, eosinophilic esophagitis, cardiac and pulmonary diagnoses, and food allergies or sensitivities may contribute as well.

It takes a team to evaluate and manage children who are at high risk of experiencing multiple complications across a wide range of medical, surgical, neurodevelopmental, cognitive/communicative, and behavioral factors. Findings from all evaluations must be communicated clearly as a basis for appropriate coordinated recommendations. Physician input is of utmost importance in development of management plans for most children, including children who on first impression may appear to have "simple" sensorimotor or behavioral problems related to feeding. Determination of contributing medical factors provides the basis for optimal treatment.

■ Presenting Signs and Symptoms

Newborns, infants, and children present with swallowing and feeding disorders in multiple ways and at various ages and stages of development. As a result, it is important that primary care clinicians (PCCs) ask pertinent questions of parents and other caregivers at every encounter. These key questions, or red flags, can aid in determining whether referral for a clinical feeding and swallowing assessment is indicated (**Table 17-1**). Parents or caregivers should be asked to describe a child's feeding routine, including route and types of alimentation, feeding frequency, and duration of feedings, among other factors (**Box 17-1**). Children typically do not gain weight or grow well in a grazing pattern. Children with upper airway obstruction (eg, hyperplastic tonsils) or neuromuscular diagnoses (eg, muscular dystrophy, spinal muscular atrophy) often have more difficulty swallowing solid

Table 17-1. Red Flags/Key Questions to Aid in Decisions for Referral to Clinical Feeding and Swallowing Assessment

Questions	Examples of Parental Reports and Observations
Airway: Does your child cough or have gurgly voice when eating/drinking? Frequent respiratory infections?	◆ Gurgly voice, coughing, and multiple swallows are best predictors of dysphagia. ◆ Repeated chest infections and hospitalizations are common signs of unsafe swallowing.
Feeding duration: How long does it take to feed your child?	◆ Longer than 30 minutes frequently or longer than $2\frac{1}{2}$ hours per day. ◆ Feeding duration of longer than 45 to 60 minutes can lead to malnutrition.
Weight/growth: Is there a lack of weight gain in 2 to 3 months for infants and children younger than 2 years? How about weight loss in older children?	◆ Lack of weight gain over 2 to 3 months in infants and children younger than 2 years is like weight loss in older children and adults. ◆ Oral sensorimotor impairment may affect functional capacity of children and health quality of life.
Gastrointestinal: Does your child vomit or show other signs of reflux related to eating or drinking?	◆ Up to 77% of children undergoing PEG placement have histories of vomiting or retching indicative of gastroesophageal reflux. ◆ PEG insertion does not lead to increased reflux in children with cerebral palsy.
Stress: Are mealtimes stressful?	◆ Battles are not likely to get the child to eat more. ◆ Poor feeding ability is a major stress for parents. ◆ Stress may be more prominent in parents, the child, or both.

Abbreviation: PEG, percutaneous endoscopic gastrostomy.

food because of residue in the pharynx caused by reduced pharyngeal muscle strength. Children with central nervous system etiologies or vocal cord paralysis or paresis typically are at risk of aspiration from thin liquids. Slow, inefficient feeding is often a reason for inadequate weight gain or undernutrition. Odynophagia and emesis may be associated with pharyngeal and/or esophageal dysphagia.

> ## Box 17-1. Common Presentations That May Result in Referral for Feeding and Swallowing Evaluation
>
> ◆ Infants may present with 1 or more of the following:
> — Sucking and swallowing incoordination
> — Weak suck
> — Breathing disruptions or apnea during feeding
> ◆ Excessive gagging or recurrent coughing during feeds
> ◆ New onset of feeding difficulty
> ◆ Diagnosis of disorders associated with dysphagia or undernutrition
> ◆ Weight loss or lack of weight gain for 2 to 3 months, especially in the first 2 years after birth (ie, undernutrition)
> ◆ Severe irritability or behavior problems during feeds
> ◆ History of recurrent pneumonia and feeding difficulty
> ◆ Concern for possible aspiration during oral feeds
> ◆ Lethargy or decreased arousal during feeds
> ◆ Feeding periods longer than 30 to 40 minutes on a regular basis
> ◆ Unexplained food refusal and undernutrition (better term than failure to thrive)
> ◆ Drooling persisting beyond age 5 years
> ◆ Nasopharyngeal reflux with feeding
> ◆ Delay in feeding developmental milestones
> ◆ Children with craniofacial anomalies

Used with permission from Arvedson JC, Lefton-Greif MA, Reigstad DJ. Clinical swallowing and feeding assessment. In: Arvedson JC, Brodsky L, Lefton-Greif MA. *Pediatric Swallowing and Feeding: Assessment and Management.* 3rd ed. San Diego, CA: Plural Publishing; 2019:261–330. Copyright ©2020 Plural Publishing, Inc. All rights reserved.

Dysphagia may be classified as oral, oropharyngeal, pharyngeal, and/or esophageal. Oropharyngeal deficits are common, as oral inefficiencies affect timing and coordination of initiating pharyngeal swallows. Oral and oropharyngeal deficits are often seen in children with delayed oral skill development that may be related to more global neurologic deficits (**Table 17-2**). Infants may demonstrate weak or inefficient sucking at the breast and/or bottle, characterized by reduced coordination of tongue, lips, and jaw with spillage out of the corners of the mouth. Infants may have difficulty sequencing sucking, swallowing, and breathing for nipple feeding, resulting in diminished endurance. Infants may demonstrate poor labial seal for sucking, while older children may not get lip closure with spoon-feeding. Parents and caregivers may describe messy eating and food residue in the mouth following meals. Other patterns in infants and children with neurologic deficits may include jaw and tongue thrust on presentation of food, jaw retraction, clenching, and tonic bite, all of

Constructs	Considerations for Pediatric Swallowing and Feeding Disorders
Body functions and structures	*Functions:* Sucking, swallowing, biting, chewing; sensorimotor skills; positioning; cognitive/communication; physiological stability *Structures:* Anatomy, physiology, neurophysiology of oral, pharyngeal, and upper esophageal structures; also laryngeal and other airway structures; gastrointestinal tract
Activity and participation	Activities involved in drinking from bottle or cup, eating age-appropriate food; use of utensils; body positioning Need to determine whether adaptations/modifications are needed in areas of self-help to include positioning alterations, special utensils, limited textures in diet; modifications in strategies to optimize levels of activity. Participation includes family mealtimes, social situations, and educational settings. Need to determine strategies to promote inclusiveness in all environments with adaptations as needed; examples include children on tube feedings and those who need additional assistance in getting food and liquid to the mouth.
Environmental and personal factors	Consideration of caregiver/family understanding of the newborn's, infant's, or child's feeding/swallowing disorder; access to appropriate food, liquids, utensils, and seating/positioning equipment. Determine caregivers' willingness and ability to prepare food and liquid in modified forms, use special utensils and seating systems, and apply special strategies to help the child eat and drink safely. Consider cultural and societal judgments of the family with a newborn, infant, or child having feeding and/or swallowing disorder.

Table 17-2. *International Classification of Functioning, Disability and Health* **Model to Describe Constructs and Considerations for Newborns, Infants, and Children With Swallowing and Feeding Disorders**

which interfere with the expected ability to chew and swallow food. Reduced oral sensation is common in infants and children with reduced sensorimotor skills.

> **Pearl:** Oropharyngeal dysphagia is seen commonly in children with neurodevelopmental disorders.

Parents and caregivers often describe coughing, gagging, and choking with foods and liquids. However, it is estimated that 70% to 90% of children with oropharyngeal dysphagia are silent aspirators; that is, there is no cough or any other overt signs, most commonly with thin liquid. Some of these children may have a history of pneumonia or acquire recurrent upper respiratory infections. Other findings with pharyngeal dysfunction may include liquid and/or food in the valleculae and pyriform sinuses because of delayed initiation of a pharyngeal swallow. These children are at risk for laryngeal penetration and aspiration before swallowing. A less common basis for material in the pyriform sinuses and high risk for aspiration is reduced opening of the upper esophageal sphincter (ie, cricopharyngeal muscle). Absent swallow initiation is uncommon but may occur as a result of neurologic injury, such as hypoxia or closed head injury, resulting in laryngeal penetration and aspiration.

If possible, observation of a feeding interaction is encouraged for all health care professionals who come into contact with infants and children and their families in whom there may be even the smallest question or concern about feeding. Not all children will end up needing a full interdisciplinary or multidisciplinary team approach, but they are likely to need input from more than 1 professional discipline. Some common presentations that may result in referral for a clinical feeding evaluation are shown in **Box 17-1.**

> **Pearl:** Simple key questions posed by the PCC can aid in determining which newborns, infants, and children may need a referral for a clinical evaluation with a feeding and swallowing specialist.

Physical Examination

The physical examination begins with a general assessment of the patient's level of alertness and interaction with caregivers, breathing patterns (eg, rate, quiet or noisy, lips closed or open as a possible sign of mouth breathing), neuromuscular tone, and head and trunk control. Inspection of the oral cavity may reveal anatomical factors that may interfere with oral feeding (eg, poor lip closure, ankyloglossia, macroglossia, cleft palate). Children with neuromuscular disorders may exhibit hypotonia, dystonic activity, or excessive salivation, to name a few possibilities. Responses to sensory stimulation, including tactile, visual, auditory, and olfactory, are noted, along with self-regulation and self-calming abilities.

Clinical Evaluation of Feeding and Swallowing

The clinical feeding and swallowing evaluation with a feeding and swallowing specialist focuses on identification and description of attributes that are observable while infants and children are drinking and eating (to whatever extent is possible for them). Clinical evaluations are usually performed in person; however, telehealth may be an option for families with limited availability of health care professionals. It is not possible to evaluate pharyngeal swallowing function by clinical observation; such function can only be *inferred* during a clinical feeding evaluation. A video fluoroscopic swallow study (VFSS), or modified barium swallowing examination, defines oropharyngeal, pharyngeal, and upper esophageal function. A fiber-optic endoscopic evaluation of swallowing (FEES) defines some aspects of pharyngeal function, but no information is obtained for oral or esophageal function.

The clinical evaluation is an important routine component of feeding and swallowing investigations for infants and children. The approaches to evaluation may vary by the setting, age of the patient, and the patient's presenting problems. In newborns and infants, the oral sensorimotor assessment begins with evaluation of reflexive rooting and nonnutritive sucking. The infant with a normal rooting response may turn his or her head in response to stroking or may search for the breast or bottle nipple if hungry without external stimulation. During nonnutritive sucking on a gloved finger, a physician can note lingual tone, bite force, and respiratory patterns, including rate and effort (eg, noisy breathing). Inspiratory stridor may indicate upper airway obstruction (eg, laryngomalacia). Stertor (snore) may indicate nasal obstruction (eg, deviated septum, choanal stenosis).

Nutritive sucking may be assessed, providing the newborn or infant has no prominent respiratory or GI difficulties, which could interfere with the evaluation. Patients on nasogastric tube feedings may or may not have their tubes removed prior to the examination. If an infant or a child is receiving primary nutrition and hydration via tube feedings, and there are questions related to the potential for advancing oral feeding safely and efficiently, a clinical feeding observation with the tube in place is most logical because the tube will likely continue to be used for some time.

Infants who are bottle-feeding usually suck in bursts of 10 to 30 sucks at a rate of 1 suck per second, with each suck followed by a swallow and a breath. They should be capable of maintaining this pattern over feedings of 15 to 20 minutes in order to meet nutritional needs. Failure to initiate sucking and weak lip seal may suggest cranial neuropathies. Tongue thrust, tonic bite, and lip retraction in older children on presentation of a nipple or spoon may be caused by neurologic deficits. Children may gag, but this represents a sensory response rather than a swallowing problem. A gurgly voice quality may raise suspicions that saliva and secretions are at the level of the vocal folds.

Older children who follow verbal directions and imitate movements can demonstrate range of motion of the lips, tongue, and jaw prior to feeding. The physician also assesses gag reflex (although there is no direct relationship between presence or absence of a gag reflex and swallowing function), spontaneous and reflexive cough, and spontaneous swallowing of secretions or saliva. Velar function may be noted for speech by phonation of "ah," but there is no direct correlation to swallowing function. Oral feeding is assessed initially with the infant or child in a customary feeding position, which may be altered to an optimal position as the session proceeds. The patient is given a variety of textures and volumes depending on developmental levels and concerns noted by parents or other guardians, usually beginning with preferred or "easy" foods and progressing to challenging foods or liquid. It is most important to be systematic in determining what the patient takes appropriately without stress and then changing in very small steps in 1 dimension at a time, with demonstration for parents who are actively participating. In that way, the parents will be able to follow guidelines at home. Observe the child taking liquids in whatever way is usual at home, with the awareness that thin liquids pose the greatest risk of aspiration. Oral skills are noted with spoon-feeding and any solid, chewable foods the child is consuming at home. Avoidance behaviors may include turning the head, closing the mouth or lips tightly, or spitting food out of the mouth. Infants and children with oral skill deficits, such as poor lip closure and limited chewing, may be exhibiting signs of deficits of cranial nerves V and VII. Delayed pharyngeal swallow initiation and nasopharyngeal backflow may be associated with impairment of cranial nerves IX and/or X. Lingual dysfunction can be seen with cranial nerve XII neuropathies.

The clinical or bedside evaluation is often sufficient to allow the feeding and swallowing specialist, a speech-language pathologist (SLP), and the referring physician to formulate a treatment plan. The SLP and primary caregivers determine the best positioning for oral feeding efficiency and safety, as well as the optimal textures of food and liquid for oral intake. The SLP makes recommendations for placement of food in the mouth and strategies to facilitate developmentally appropriate oral skills. When pharyngeal phase disorders are suspected or the child is at high risk of aspiration, additional examinations may be needed, particularly an instrumental swallowing study.

▦ Instrumental Evaluation of Feeding and Swallowing

The VFSS is the most frequently used instrumental examination for infants and children with suspected pharyngeal dysphagia. The FEES is often used when there are upper airway concerns along with swallowing problems. Decisions about the need for an instrumental assessment of swallowing are not taken lightly given the exposure to radiation with VFSS and the passing of a flexible endoscope through nasal passages to the level of the larynx with FEES. The VFSS is designed to define anatomy and physiology of the oral, pharyngeal, and upper esophageal swallowing function. The VFSS is not a study to determine presence or absence of aspiration, but if aspiration does occur, texture specificity and the reason(s) for the aspiration must be stated to make appropriate treatment recommendations. The SLP or feeding and swallowing specialist should also report whether aspiration events are texture specific and when in the swallowing process aspiration occurs, as well as whether the child made a response (eg, cough) to the aspiration event. Silent aspiration is reported to be far more common than an immediate or a delayed cough response in children with a neurologic basis for their dysphagia. Objective, quantifiable measures during VFSS are needed for more understanding of the underlying swallowing physiologic patterns (this topic is beyond the scope of this chapter).

The FEES procedures used with newborns, infants, and children were adapted from protocols established for adults. Flexible fiber-optic laryngoscopy is a minimally invasive procedure used by pediatric otolaryngologists to examine the upper airway in children of all ages, including newborns and infants in the neonatal intensive care unit (NICU). This procedure is an integral part of the dysphagia evaluation and is necessary to establish normal vocal fold function. Examination of swallowing in bottle-feeding and breastfeeding newborns and infants can be performed at the bedside, which provides valuable information for management decisions about advance of oral feeding. A team approach with an otolaryngologist and SLP is advocated.

> **Pearl:** Instrumental examination of swallowing may be needed when pharyngeal swallowing disorders are suspected because pharyngeal function can only be inferred by clinical feeding observation.

▨ Treatment Options

Treatment decisions for newborns, infants, and children with feeding and swallowing disorders are based on knowledge of and goals for adequate nutrition and GI function, stable pulmonary function, and developmentally appropriate oral sensorimotor and feeding skills. Medical, surgical, and nutritional considerations are all critical for identifying optimal treatment strategies. Maximal participation of children in the social and communication activities associated with family mealtimes is a higher-priority global goal than advancement of oral skills and increasing volume. Some children are exclusively oral feeders. However, when children cannot meet their nutritional needs safely by oral feeding alone, supplemental nutrition routes are needed. Nonoral feeding should not be viewed as a failure or last resort but should be considered a tool for maximizing safety, growth, and development. Underlying condition(s), chronological and developmental age of the child, social and environmental arena, and psychological and behavioral factors will all influence treatment recommendations. Therapeutic interventions may be addressed in early intervention programs, schools, and rehabilitation programs. Regardless of the setting, treatment decision-making and adjustments in therapeutic interventions occur during every evaluation and examination, just as all intervention sessions include evaluation of status. Thus, it is not possible to separate evaluation and management, given the integrated functions within each newborn, infant, and child.

In considering treatment approaches, basic principles recognized by many pediatric feeding and swallowing specialists include the following:

● The relationships between children and caregivers are important considerations of feeding evaluations and subsequent follow-up treatment plans.
● Children and families should be included in treatment planning and implementation.
● Oral, respiratory, and neurologic systems should be examined carefully.
● Tone and movement patterns throughout the entire body must be optimized before making specific changes to the oral sensorimotor system.
● Tone and movement patterns in the jaw, tongue, lips, and palate must be improved when necessary to reduce the effect of oral reflexes that may interfere with feeding.
● Normal patterns of movement must be facilitated and replace abnormal movement patterns that interfere with function.
● The functional ability to accept and integrate visual, auditory, tactile, vestibular, proprioceptive, taste, and temperature information is necessary before direct facilitation of new oral feeding pattern attempts can be made.
● Oral sensorimotor treatment may be included during children's typical daily activities such as play, meals, toothbrushing, and vocal play/communication.

The acquisition of functional motor skills is achieved to a great extent through appropriate sensory input. When children have reduced sensory input or a disordered response to sensory input, the consequences may be evident with decreased motor function. Thus, it is helpful to consider sensorimotor skills in a generic sense to appreciate the interrelationship of sensory input and motor function.

Optimal treatment options should reflect neurophysiological sensorimotor learning principles. The process of skill acquisition for advancing oral feeding appears related to sensorimotor learning approaches in school-aged children and likely in infants and young children, as well. Deficiencies in swallowing and feeding may encompass eating, saliva control, swallowing during oral hygiene, and swallowing medications. Physicians are reminded that increases in oral skills tend to correlate closely with global acquisition of motor skills. A basic tenet of sensorimotor learning is the concept of training to the task as directly as possible.

For children in whom oral feeding seems appropriate, even if tube fed for primary nutrition and hydration needs, modifications may include, but are not limited to

- Posture and position alterations
- Texture, taste, and temperature changes of food and/or liquid
- Broad-based sensorimotor interventions
- Scheduling mealtimes and snack times to facilitate hunger (ie, nothing between those scheduled mealtimes and snack times, except water if a child is thirsty and it is safe for the child to ingest thin liquids)
- Structure and routines at mealtimes that minimize stress to improve parent-child interactions and behavioral responses of the child

Clinically, evidence-based practice is an indispensable safeguard against pseudoscience and the potential use of harmful assessment and treatment methods. Even interventions that seem plausible can be ineffective or exert iatrogenic consequences. All interventions are associated with costs (ie, time, money, and/or energy). Unfortunately, objective data supporting treatment in pediatric feeding and swallowing disorders are limited and often devoid of information that identifies efficacious treatments. Physicians are encouraged to review information pertinent to their specific patient populations from credible sources including, but not limited to, prospective research, Cochrane reviews, consensus statements, white papers, and, with caution, trustworthy websites.

Oral sensorimotor intervention is often performed with newborns, infants, and children in a variety of ways, typically based on clinical experience, rather than evidence-based research. The range of approaches include stretching and stroking, passive range of motion, vibratory oral tools, and neuromuscular electrical stimulation. Oral sensorimotor stimulation in preterm newborns and infants seems to be more effective with pacifier-facilitated nonnutritive sucking than direct oral stimulation to attain earlier total oral feeding by nipple. However, most studies have found that discharge from the NICU did not occur earlier in the study groups despite the newborns or infants achieving total oral feeding about 1 week earlier than those not in the experimental groups. Thus, there is a need for high-quality, properly conducted, and clearly defined evidenced-based research studies on which to base optimal recommendations relating to all types of interventions, particularly oral sensorimotor interventions for children with dysphagia.

Intervention for children with feeding and swallowing deficits must be based on an accurate diagnosis of the underlying etiologies and not be just a series of imprecise or ill-defined oral sensorimotor techniques in response to specific signs that children exhibit. For example, a child who demonstrates open mouth posture may be harmed by exercises aimed at lip closure when the underlying reason the child has his or her mouth open is to assist breathing. A subtle upper airway obstruction may be manifested only by the open mouth posture. In this instance, the medical examination and follow-up treatment must be undertaken before one could expect results with oral sensorimotor intervention. On the other hand, if the underlying etiology is a neuromuscular diagnosis without airway obstruction, oral sensorimotor exercises may facilitate lip closure that could aid posterior tongue propulsion to produce a timely swallow. The extent and degree of a child's neuromuscular weakness may be a limiting factor for achieving functional lip closure.

> **Pearl:** Objective data supporting treatment in pediatric feeding and swallowing disorders are limited and often devoid of information that identifies efficacious treatments. Physicians are encouraged to review information pertinent to their specific patient populations from credible sources, including, but not limited to, prospective research, Cochrane reviews, consensus statements, white papers, and (with caution) trustworthy websites.

Evidence-Based Outcomes

Limited reports of therapeutic outcomes are available, with a few related to tube weaning procedures. A report in the United States by Silverman et al revealed that 51% of 77 children in a 2-week intensive inpatient program were completely weaned from gastrostomy tube feedings, with an additional 12% completely weaned within 1 year of outpatient follow-up; nutrition stability was maintained at the 1-year follow-up. A 3-week program in Israel with both inpatient and out-patient approaches reported that at the 6-month follow-up, 24 of 26 children maintained or improved target goals of complete or partial tube weaning and nutrition diversity for selective eaters (Shalem et al, 2016). Anecdotal reports abound about children weaned off gastrostomy tube feedings by gradual reduction in tube feedings as oral feeding increases, often requiring that children tolerate bolus tube feedings to facilitate hunger and tolerance of larger volumes than if they had required slow, continuous feedings. The highest priority for all children is adequacy of nutrition and hydration along with global well-being, whether they are fed orally, by a combination of tube and oral feeding, or by total tube feeding with minimal oral tastes.

Ankyloglossia

▥ Introduction

Ankyloglossia (tongue-tie) can be described as a congenital abnormal-ity that limits the range of motion of the tongue and may interfere with feeding or speech. In many cases, the restriction is caused by a short, anteriorly attached lingual frenulum (anterior ankyloglossia). Less commonly, a more posteriorly attached frenulum or submucosal band (posterior ankyloglossia) may cause restricted tongue mobility. However, there are no universally accepted definitions or criteria for diagnosis; nor is there consensus about how ankyloglossia should be managed. Controversies about whether a newborn or an infant has ankyloglossia and if treatment is needed are reflected in wide varia-tions in medical practice, and there is a lack of high-quality clinical studies to provide guidance.

In recent years, with increased emphasis on facilitation of breastfeeding, greater attention has been paid to the possible implications of anterior and posterior ankyloglossia, as well as teth-ering of the upper lip. In some newborns and infants, ankyloglos-sia may impair the anteroposterior movement of the tongue that is necessary for the patient to achieve transfer of milk without causing pain to the mother during breastfeeding. Similarly, tethering of the upper lip caused by a tight frenulum may limit the flaring of the upper lip that is required for feeding at the breast and with the bottle. The ideal study of the effect of ankyloglossia in new-borns and infants will need to include objective assessment of feeding, evaluation of oral anatomy and function, recognition of medical factors that affect feeding, randomization to standardized surgical (frenotomy/frenectomy) procedures and observation, and precise measures of changes in feeding, with an adequate follow-up period. Evidence-based data are needed to develop a standard of care.

▓ Epidemiology

A 2007 methodological review of studies on various aspects of ankyloglossia noted that the prevalence of restricted lingual frenu-lum is not well documented because of lack of a standard definition and a reliable clinical method of classification. With different diag-nostic criteria, the review found 5 studies reporting a prevalence of ankyloglossia between 4% and 11%. Some studies reported a mild male predominance. Diagnosis and intervention have increased exponentially in recent years. A 2018 report from Australia noted that frenotomy rates increased 420% from 2006 to 2016 with dif-ferences among states and territories in the magnitude of the change. An American study found that the diagnosis of ankylo-glossia among inpatients increased each year from 1997 to 2012. Ankyloglossia was diagnosed more frequently in firstborn neonates and infants and in newborns and infants from families of higher socioeconomic levels. Some authors have suggested that advocacy for breastfeeding by the American Academy of Pediatrics (AAP) may, in part, be resulting in increased detection of ankyloglossia among newborns and infants whose parents follow the organiza-tional guidelines.

▓ Presenting Signs and Symptoms

Most newborns and infants with ankyloglossia are asymptomatic, without feeding issues for the baby or discomfort for the mother. However, when parents are concerned about the possibility of ankylo-glossia, they usually report issues that relate to feeding, with studies demonstrating that breastfeeding problems are more frequent among neonates and infants with ankyloglossia than in those without (25% versus 3%). Such problems include, but are not limited to, poor latch, latch easily lost, clicking noises when feeding, poor weight gain, and maternal discomfort. It is important for PCCs to recognize that only some breastfeeding difficulties are related to ankyloglossia and that some neonates and infants with restrictive ankyloglossia can breastfeed quite well. Thus, careful and thorough examination must be performed with each breastfeeding neonate or infant and mother, so that multiple interrelating factors are taken into account, and not just the structural limitations of the tongue. An interdisciplinary breastfeeding clinic is desirable for comprehensive, coordinated examination. A multidisciplinary team may include SLPs, lactation consultants, otolaryngologists, nurses, and, in some instances, pediatricians and occupational therapists or other personnel as needed.

> **Pearl:** Only some breastfeeding difficulties are related to ankyloglossia. Some neonates and infants with restrictive ankyloglossia can breastfeed quite well.

The most common sign of ankyloglossia in newborns and infants is an abnormally short lingual frenulum that is visible on physical examination. As a newborn or an infant attempts to bring the tongue forward, a heart-shaped indentation may be noted. The newborn or infant may not protrude the tongue beyond the lower lip. On occasion, there may be no visible anatomical restriction at tongue tip, but a submucosal band is palpable. Anteroposterior tongue mobility is likely reduced. This restriction is described as a posterior ankyloglossia. Varying degrees of decreased tongue mobility may be observed with a tight frenulum. Tethering of the upper lip may be present. The upper lip may be manipulated into a flared position, but the patient cannot maintain that position during active sucking at the breast or bottle.

> **Pearl:** Some newborns and infants with anterior and/or posterior ankyloglossia present with feeding difficulties at the breast and bottle, with greater difficulty of breastfeeding.

The older child with ankyloglossia often demonstrates restricted tongue mobility and may have a diastema (space) between the lower central incisors created by chronic pressure exerted by the frenulum during function. It is critical to note that children's failure to vocalize or develop language skills is not related to a restricted lingual frenulum. Moreover, ankyloglossia rarely has an effect on articulation because most lingual-alveolar sounds (eg, t, d, n, l, s, z), which are typically generated by contact of the tongue tip to the anterior palate, require only minimal tongue elevation or can be made alternatively using the blade of the tongue.

Preteens and adolescents with ankyloglossia may present with mechanical problems caused by tongue mobility deficit. This may include difficulty with oral hygiene, licking ice cream, kissing, licking lips, local discomfort, and playing a wind instrument.

> **Pearl:** Ankyloglossia rarely has an effect on articulation because most lingual-alveolar sounds (eg, t, d, n, l, s, z), which are typically generated by contact of the tongue tip to the anterior palate, require only minimal tongue elevation or can be made alternatively using the blade of the tongue.

Physical Examination

The physical examination of newborns and infants suspected of having congenital ankyloglossia begins with observation of tongue function while the patient is calm and when fussing or crying. A notched or indented heart shape observed when the patient is not trying to protrude the tongue while calm is a sign of marked restriction of anteroposterior tongue motion. As the patient moves the tongue anteriorly, if it cannot be protruded past the lower gum ridge, a shortened frenulum is a likely cause of the restricted movement. Examination of the tongue is best performed with the physician and parent facing each other, knees touching. The patient can be laid on the parent's lap with his or her head toward the physician, which allows the physician the best visualization of the patient's mouth; best visualization cannot be achieved when the patient is sitting upright on a parent's lap. The frenulum can be visualized by lifting the tongue (varied techniques are described anecdotally). A tight frenulum often inserts at or near the tip of the tongue (**Figure 17-1**). The newborn or infant with ankyloglossia also cannot voluntarily elevate the tongue to the anterior palate, nor can the physician elevate it easily. The latter findings in the absence of a visible band of tissue suggest a posterior ankyloglossia that likely represents abnormality of the genioglossus muscle. The band, in these cases, is often palpable in the floor of the mouth. Placement of a finger in the mouth may be useful in testing the patient's strength of latch and to observe the pattern of tongue movement during nonnutritive sucking, which is in an

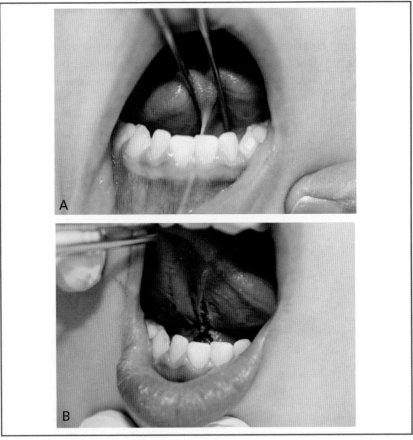

Figure 17-1. A, Ankyloglossia with tethered anterior lingual frenulum. B, Following division and suture closure (frenoplasty).

anteroposterior direction with lateral grooving for nonnutritive and nutritive sucking.

Tethering of the upper lip may be noted in isolation or with a restricted lingual frenulum. The upper labial frenulum can be assessed by gently using fingers to lift the upper lip. However, although there are published classifications to describe the appearance of the frenulum, there is no definite correlation between the anatomy of the frenulum and the likelihood of feeding issues. As a result, the tethered lip is, as previously described, most reliably diagnosed based on the failure of the lip to remain flared while breastfeeding. This observation suggests that the newborn or infant will not maintain an adequate seal around the nipple at the breast and during bottle-feeding. The newborn or infant may take in air while feeding or demonstrate spillage of milk from the mouth. In such cases, the mother may report more nipple pain with breastfeeding.

Direct observation of the breastfeeding newborn or infant is part of the physical examination. This evaluation should be performed by an International Board Certified Lactation Consultant (IBCLC), an SLP with extensive knowledge and experience in infant feeding, or, preferably, both. The assessment focuses on the patient's ability to latch adequately to the breast, to transfer milk for needed intake, and to feed without causing maternal discomfort. The AAP suggests the top 10 ways busy pediatricians can support breastfeeding (Thomas and Ware, 2019).

In older children, tethering of the tongue is diagnosed based on a visually and palpably tight lingual frenulum. Observation typically reveals reduced tongue mobility in elevation, protrusion, and lateral excursion.

> **Pearl:** The frenulum is best visualized by lifting the tongue while the newborn or infant is supine with his or her head toward the physician.

Several diagnostic tools have been described, although they are often difficult to apply and rely on subjective assessment that may result in poor interrater reliability. The efficacy of these tools for measurement of therapeutic and surgical outcomes is not well established. Tools include, but are not limited to, the Hazelbaker Assessment Tool for Lingual Frenulum Function (HATLFF), the Bristol Tongue Assessment Tool (BTAT), the LATCH (*l*atch, *a*udible swallowing, *t*ype of nipple, *c*omfort, *h*old) tool, the Infant Breastfeeding Assessment Tool (IBFAT), the Mother-Baby Assessment score, the Mother-Infant Breastfeeding Progress Tool, and the Systematic Assessment of the Infant at Breast (SAIB). Although these tools have objective measures, there is still some subjectivity in observations and designations. Thus, visualization of the restricted tongue movement may define ankyloglossia based on the anatomical findings of a shortened and tethered lingual frenulum.

> **Pearl:** Diagnostic tools have been described, although they are often difficult to apply and rely on subjective assessment, often resulting in poor interrater reliability. Furthermore, the efficacy of these tools for measurement of therapeutic and surgical outcomes is not established. Evidence-based research is needed.

■ Treatment Options

As described in this chapter, more research is needed to provide a standardized approach to the definition, classification, examination, diagnosis, and treatment of ankyloglossia. Opinions and practice related to ankyloglossia vary among and within professional groups. This lack of consensus is related to the absence of a uniformly accepted standard for diagnosis. However, because this disorder most likely comes to light in newborns or infants struggling to breastfeed efficiently, intervention is often sought by parents and PCCs. Before any consideration of surgical intervention, the mother and the newborn or infant should have undergone a thorough evaluation by an IBCLC and/or a feeding and swallowing specialist (usually an SLP). Interventions such as alterations in positioning of the neonate or infant, implementation of relaxation techniques for the mother, and alterations in the infant's intake volume and frequency of feeding may improve breastfeeding and obviate the need to consider surgery.

Surgical intervention for the lingual frenulum may be a consideration in refractory cases in which a poor latch or significant maternal discomfort is present. However, the procedure should be recommended with caution. Reports of outcomes following lingual frenotomy and maxillary labial frenotomy are variable because of limitations that include small sample size, lack of long-term follow-up, multiple frenotomy techniques with and without anesthesia, absence of randomized controlled trials, and absence of universally accepted diagnostic criteria. A 2017 Cochrane review found that frenotomy reduced nipple pain in breastfeeding mothers in the short term but failed to find a consistent positive effect on infant breastfeeding. Evidence quality was rated "low to moderate."

The procedure to release the lingual frenulum in an infant younger than 6 months is typically performed in an ambulatory setting; however, complete release of a posterior ankyloglossia or any ankyloglossia in an older child may be more safely performed in a surgery suite. To date, there are no data to suggest that a single technique or instrument used to perform the procedure is superior to another. Use of topical anesthesia seems to add little benefit and is generally not recommended. Potential complications include prolonged bleeding and excessive scarring at the surgical site. Use of laser or cautery reduces the likelihood of prolonged bleeding but may be more likely to cause excessive scarring. Injury to the submandibular ducts is possible but should be easily avoided. There are no data to suggest that stretching exercises after the procedure reduce contractures, but there is little risk to this additional intervention. These exercises may be stressful to the patient, which could contribute to increased risk of feeding disorders. In all instances, following release of ankyloglossia, infants and mothers are encouraged to follow up with an IBCLC, as modifications in positioning of the infant at the breast may be necessary once the tongue has been released.

> **Pearl:** A 2017 Cochrane review found that frenotomy reduced nipple pain in breastfeeding mothers in the short term but failed to find a consistent positive effect of the procedure on infant breastfeeding. The study characterized the evidence quality as "low to moderate."

▧ Natural History and Prognosis

Many newborns and infants with ankyloglossia have mild restriction of tongue function that goes unnoticed and does not interfere with nipple feeding at the breast or with the bottle. However, in instances in which there are clinically significant problems that are clearly caused by the tongue restriction, spontaneous resolution is not likely, at least in the short term. The diagnosis of ankyloglossia has risen in recent years with the increasing numbers of mothers who are breastfeeding. Caution is urged by health care professionals who are involved with assessment and management of newborns and infants with feeding issues. Some breastfeeding difficulties are caused by ankyloglossia, but some newborns and infants with anatomical restriction of tongue movement can breastfeed successfully without pain and discomfort experienced by their mothers, whereas mothers may experience pain and discomfort when breastfeeding newborns and infants who have no anatomical restrictions. These mothers are urged to seek lactation consultation with an IBCLC. Finally, while older children with mechanical signs or symptoms or social embarrassment related to tongue mobility impairment may experience improved function following frenoplasty, children with articulation errors rarely experience improved speech production with frenulum release alone.

▧ Selected References

Arvedson JC. Assessment of pediatric dysphagia and feeding disorders: clinical and instrumental approaches. *Dev Disabil Res Rev.* 2008;14(2):118–127

Arvedson JC, Lefton-Greif MA. Instrumental assessment of pediatric dysphagia. *Semin Speech Lang.* 2017;38(2):135–146

Arvedson J, Rogers B, Buck G, Smart P, Msall M. Silent aspiration prominent in children with dysphagia. *Int J Pediatr Otorhinolaryngol.* 1994;28(2-3):173–181

Billington J, Yardley I, Upadhyaya M. Long-term efficacy of a tongue tie service in improving breast feeding rates: a prospective study. *J Pediatr Surg.* 2018;53(2):286–288. Published online November 13, 2017

Cawse-Lucas J, Waterman S, St Anna L. Clinical inquiry: does frenotomy help infants with tongue-tie overcome breastfeeding difficulties? *J Fam Pract.* 2015;64(2):126–127

Douglas PS. Rethinking "posterior" tongue-tie. *Breastfeed Med.* 2013;8(6):503–506

Geddes DT, Kent JC, McClellan HL, Garbin CP, Chadwick LM, Hartmann PE. Sucking characteristics of successfully breastfeeding infants with ankyloglossia: a case series. *Acta Paediatr.* 2010;99(2):301–303. Published online November 4, 2009

Gosa M, Dodrill P. Pediatric dysphagia rehabilitation: considering the evidence to support common strategies. *Perspect ASHA Spec Interest Groups.* 2017;2(13):27–35

Hazelbaker AK. *Tongue-tie: Morphogenesis, Impact, Assessment and Treatment.* Columbus, OH: Aidan and Eva Press; 2010

Hogan M, Westcott C, Griffiths M. Randomized, controlled trial of division of tongue-tie in infants with feeding problems. *J Paediatr Child Health.* 2005;41(5-6):246–250

Ingram J, Johnson D, Copeland M, Churchill C, Taylor H, Emond A. The development of a tongue assessment tool to assist with tongue-tie identification. *Arch Dis Child Fetal Neonatal Ed.* 2015;100(4):F344–F348

Kapoor V, Douglas PS, Hill PS, Walsh LJ, Tennant M. Frenotomy for tongue-tie in Australian children, 2006-2016: an increasing problem. *Med J Aust.* 2018;208(2):88–89

Kleim JA, Jones TA. Principles of experience-dependent neural plasticity: implications for rehabilitation after brain damage. *J Speech Lang Hear Res.* 2008;51(1):S225–S239

Manipon C. Ankyloglossia and the breastfeeding infant: assessment and intervention. *Adv Neonatal Care.* 2016;16(2):108–113

O'Shea JE, Foster JP, O'Donnell CP, et al. Frenotomy for tongue-tie in newborn infants. *Cochrane Database Syst Rev.* 2017;(3):CD011065

Reynolds J, Carroll S, Sturdivant C. Fiberoptic endoscopic evaluation of swallowing: a multidisciplinary alternative for assessment of infants with dysphagia in the neonatal intensive care unit. *Adv Neonatal Care.* 2016;16(1):37–43

Shalem T, Fradkin A, Dunitz-Scheer M, et al. Gastrostomy tube weaning and treatment of severe selective eating in childhood: experience in Israel using an intensive three week program. *Isr Med Assoc J.* 2016;18(6):331–335

Sheppard JJ. Using motor learning approaches for treating swallowing and feeding disorders: a review. *Lang Speech Hear Serv Sch.* 2008;39(2):227–236

Silverman AH, Kirby M, Clifford LM, et al. Nutritional and psychosocial outcomes of gastrostomy tube-dependent children completing an intensive inpatient behavioral treatment program. *J Pediatr Gastroenterol Nutr.* 2013;57(5):668–672

Srinivasan A, Al Khoury A, Puzhko S, et al. Frenotomy in infants with tongue-tie and breastfeeding problems. *J Hum Lact.* 2019;35(4):706–712

Thomas J, Ware JL. Top 10 ways busy pediatricians can support breastfeeding. AAP News. https://www.aappublications.org/news/2019/10/24/focus102419. Published October 24, 2019. Accessed November 20, 2019

Walsh J, Tunkel DE. Tongue-tie and frenotomy: what evidence do we have and what do we need? *Med J Aust.* 2018;208(2):67–68

Webb AN, Hao W, Hong P. The effect of tongue-tie division on breastfeeding and speech articulation: a systematic review. *Int J Pediatr Otorhinolaryngol.* 2013;77(5):635–646

World Health Organization. *International Classification of Functioning, Disability and Health for Children and Youth.* http://www.who.int/classifications/icf/en. Accessed November 21, 2019

CHAPTER 18

Gastroesophageal and Laryngopharyngeal Reflux

Karen B. Zur, MD

Introduction
Gastroesophageal Reflux
   and Airway
Diagnosis of Gastroesopha-
   geal Reflux Disease
   Esophageal pH
    Monitoring
   Combined Multiple Intra-
    luminal Impedance
    With pH Monitoring

Contrast Studies
Scintigraphy
Endoscopy With Biopsy
Eosinophilic Esophagitis
Motility Studies
Treatment of Gastroesopha-
   geal Reflux

■ Introduction

Gastroesophageal reflux (GER) occurs when gastric contents pass from the stomach into the esophagus. Physiologic reflux occurs in healthy individuals, with episodes occurring infrequently and associated with rapid clearance of refluxed material from the esophagus. Physiologic reflux causes no irritation to esophageal mucosa. However, when esophageal mucosa is chronically exposed to an increasing frequency of reflux events, or the duration of acid exposure within the esophagus increases with each reflux event, the mucosa becomes inflamed. Chronic inflammation of esophageal mucosa by reflux is a hallmark of gastroesophageal reflux disease (GERD). In children, GERD may manifest with irritability, failure to thrive, food refusal, cough, dysphagia, stridor, hoarseness, bronchospasm, recurrent croup, recurrent pneumonia, and apnea. Episodes of obvious regurgitation need not be present with GERD.

Laryngopharyngeal reflux (LPR), otherwise known as *silent reflux* or *respiratory reflux*, has the hallmarks of endoscopic findings of extraesophageal regurgitation, however without the obvious symptoms of GERD, such as abdominal or chest pain or emesis. The results of an esophagogastroduodenoscopy (EGD) may be normal owing to end-organ damage. The clinical results, however, are consistent with regurgitation of acid and non–acid refluxate that ultimately leads to inflammation and irritation of the pharynx, and may even lead to congestion and irritation of the nasal passages, ears, larynx, and airway.

> **Pearl:** Gastroesophageal reflux occurs commonly in children. Gastroesophageal reflux disease only occurs when secondary problems develop, such as the development of esophagitis, failure to thrive, food refusal, and airway symptoms. In laryngopharyngeal reflux, classic symptoms of pain and emesis are usually absent.

Several physiologic mechanisms protect against GERD. The lower esophageal sphincter (LES) is a tonic high-pressure zone at the level of the diaphragm that prevents reflux events. It is composed of involuntary smooth muscle fibers and must allow a bolus transiting the esophagus from above into the stomach. The LES also relaxes for belching and vomiting. The upper esophageal sphincter is another high-pressure zone at the level of the cricoid cartilage. It is composed of a combination of smooth and striated muscle fibers that limit the transfer of reflux material into the hypopharynx, where it may be aspirated.

When reflux events do occur, they are normally cleared from the esophagus. Saliva and secretions produced by mucous glands within the esophagus neutralize gastric acid. Peristaltic action within the esophagus clears gastric secretions from the esophagus, protecting the lining of the esophagus from inflammatory actions of the reflux material.

Reflux is commonly seen in infants because of the immature neuromuscular mechanisms at that age. As the child matures and as the diet advances, fewer episodes of reflux are typically seen. However, if a child experiences chronic constipation or consumes a diet that is rich in acid, grease, peppermint, citrus, spice, or other irritants, inflammation of the laryngopharyngeal mucosa may increase and more regurgitation of secretions from the gastrointestinal (GI) tract may occur.

Gastroesophageal Reflux and Airway

Reflux contributes to the development of a variety of symptoms associated with the upper aerodigestive tract. Gastric acid or activated digestive enzyme-containing fluid (pepsin) may ascend up the esophagus from the stomach and enter the hypopharynx. Refluxate may then bathe the laryngeal structures, causing edema, erythema, and pain. It may penetrate into the larynx through the interarytenoid notch and irritate the vocal folds, causing hoarseness or trigging a cough response. Refluxate may also be aspirated, causing tracheal or bronchial irritation and symptoms of recurrent croup. In cases of chronic aspiration, areas of consolidation in lung fields may develop.

> **Pearl:** Extraesophageal reflux episodes can irritate the airway. Symptoms related to the airway may be the only outward sign of gastroesophageal reflux. This is the essence of laryngopharyngeal, or respiratory, reflux.

Chronic exposure of the supraglottic larynx to refluxed materials induces chronic throat clearing and cough behaviors. Bronchospasm has also been linked to GER. Aspiration of gastric contents or stimulation of vagally mediated reflexes from the irritation of receptors in the esophageal mucosa may be responsible for this phenomenon.

Globus pharyngeus (sensation of a mass or foreign body in the throat) is often linked to LPR. Chronic pharyngitis may be caused by reflux as well. Pharyngeal pain, worse in the morning, may be caused by increased frequency of reflux events occurring when in a supine or recumbent position. This is especially true for children who eat and snack immediately before bedtime. It is important to increase the interval between food and beverage consumption and avoid eating 1.5 to 2 hours before bedtime. This should allow enough time for the food and beverages to transit down the GI tract and minimize overnight regurgitation. Children with delayed gastric and esophageal motility may need to stop eating more than 2 hours before bedtime to minimize this phenomenon.

In patients with recurrent croup, a component of their symptoms or the actual trigger may be related to reflux. A couple of possibilities may explain these symptoms of recurrent croup or a recurrent croupy cough. Baseline edema found in the airway of patients with reflux may predispose to airway compromise due to heightened irritability of the larynx from chronic acid and non–acid refluxate exposure. When a child with LPR is exposed to a concomitant viral infection, the chronically inflamed airway may contribute to more acute symptoms that mimic subglottic stenosis, but actually are caused by effective narrowing caused by edema. The other possibility is that the stridor, or a barky cough that parents often relay when recounting a history of "recurrent croup," is likely related to a spasm of the vocal folds leading to inspiratory noises and a barky cough. Parents often recount their healthy child going to sleep with no fever or viral prodrome but wakening in the middle of the night with a barky cough and inspiratory noises. In between episodes, the child has no airway symptoms and no dyspnea or exercise limitation. In the past, the author recommended a bronchoscopy under anesthesia and an EGD with biopsy and possible impedance probe testing with the gastroenterologists. In those cases, the bronchoscopies were normal and the GI evaluation often revealed underlying issues, such as eosinophilic esophagitis (EoE), celiac disease, or GERD. For this reason, in the setting of episodic recurrent croup with no intervening airway issues and in the context of additional symptoms suggestive of regurgitation and a diet rich in acidic meals, bronchoscopies in the operating room are rarely recommended. Instead, it is useful to perform an in-office laryngoscopy, as well as a nasal/nasopharyngeal examination, to assess the upper aerodigestive tract.

Clinical examination findings suggestive of LPR include mucoid secretions in the nose that are not related to a cold or allergies, cobblestoning and edema of the nasopharynx, cobblestoning of the hypopharynx, vallecular cobblestoning, postcricoid mucosal edema, hyperemia and edema of the arytenoid cartilages, interarytenoid inflammation (pachydermia), and possible vocal fold edema. Quite often, it is possible to visualize the subglottic region during this office examination and rule out an obvious subglottic pathology (such as hemangioma, cyst, or stenosis). In the context of the history and office examination findings, it is prudent to discuss LPR risks with the child and family and make adjustments in the diet. If dietary modification fails, a GI evaluation alone or a possible joint procedure with a bronchoscopy may be pursued.

Reflux has been implicated in the etiology and pathogenesis of subglottic stenosis. Active acidic reflux increases the inflammation and swelling in an already compromised airway, serving as a fuel for airway stenosis and affecting mucosal healing after injury. For patients undergoing an evaluation for an airway reconstruction, the aerodigestive teams diligently work to rule out active LPR, GERD, and EoE, as active disease has been associated with failed airway reconstruction.

Extraesophageal reflux may also worsen symptoms of laryngomalacia. Edema of the supraglottic structures worsens symptoms of laryngomalacia, increasing the degree of airway collapse and increasing the work associated with breathing. This increased work of breathing increases negative pressure within the thoracic cavity. The pressure differential across the LES is thus raised, increasing the incompetence of the LES and producing more reflux events of increasing volume. Studies have shown that the supraglottic/glottic sensation of patients with reflux is diminished because of the reflux exposure, making these infants more likely to aspirate and experience feeding difficulties.

■ Diagnosis of Gastroesophageal Reflux Disease

No single symptom or symptom complex is diagnostic of GERD. Clinical suspicion may lead to specific tests to determine the presence and severity of GER. The most basic and important method to diagnose reflux is to obtain a thorough history that includes age at onset of symptoms, a thorough feeding and dietary history, patterns of regurgitation (overnight, during meals, long after feeds), a family history of reflux or allergies, growth history, prior medical therapy, and evaluations and presence of red flag signs such as bloody emesis, persistent forceful vomiting, rectal bleeding, chronic diarrhea, bilious vomiting, neurologic symptoms, failure to thrive, fever, and lethargy. The diagnosis of GERD is based primarily on clinical suspicion, and the choice of additional studies should be individualized to each child. In addition, the risk-benefit ratio of each study should be addressed. To date, no gold standard diagnostic tool exists for the diagnosis of GERD in infants and children.

ESOPHAGEAL pH MONITORING

In intraluminal esophageal monitoring, pH is recorded continuously for 24 hours. A probe is positioned within 3 cm of the LES for accurate recordings. To increase the sensitivity of the study, a second sensor can be positioned at the upper esophageal sphincter to assess the number of reflux events ascending to the level of the pharynx. The length of time the esophagus is exposed to a pH less than 4, number of episodes of acidic reflux, and number of reflux episodes lasting more than 5 minutes are determined. pH monitoring can detect only acidic events reaching the level of the sensor. The volume of reflux cannot be determined. Gastric contents that have been buffered to a neutral pH by foods, bile, or medications do not trigger the sensor as an event. Esophageal pH monitoring is useful in evaluating the effectiveness of antacid and antisecretory therapies for GER in the complex cases that fail to respond to typical therapies.

> **Pearl:** Combined multiple intraluminal impedance with pH monitoring is the best method of evaluating acid and nonacid regurgitation. It provides the most complete assessment of reflux episodes available to date.

COMBINED MULTIPLE INTRALUMINAL IMPEDANCE WITH pH MONITORING

A probe that measures a change in impedance between pairs of electrodes allows a determination of the presence of liquid, air, or solids in the esophagus passing the probe. Multiple pairs of electrodes allow a reflux event to be followed as it ascends the esophagus and, again, as it is cleared from the esophagus. A pH sensor is incorporated into the sleeve of the sensor to allow a determination of the acidic or neutral nature of the reflux event.

Impedance monitoring provides significantly more information about reflux events than does a pH probe study. Anterograde and retrograde flow through the esophagus can be measured. Acidic and neutral events can be identified. The height of a single event can be followed and the rate of clearance from the esophagus can be defined. This testing should be considered for correlation of persistent troublesome symptoms with acid and non–acid reflux events.

CONTRAST STUDIES

The upper GI study (barium contrast study) is useful in determining anatomical abnormalities of the upper GI tract, but it is not a useful study for the diagnosis of GERD. Reflux may be seen during the study, but the lack of identified reflux events does not rule out the diagnosis of GERD. Conversely, reflux events may be seen in healthy individuals without disease.

SCINTIGRAPHY

Food materials labeled with radionuclides are ingested, and prolonged imaging is performed to provide a means of determining the rate of gastric emptying and identifying reflux events. On these "milk scans," pulmonary aspiration of a reflux material may be recorded by the presence of label within the lung fields. A negative test result does not rule out the possibility of pulmonary aspiration of reflux materials because of the episodic nature of the events. These nuclear medicine scans are not recommended for routine evaluation of children suspected of having GER.

ENDOSCOPY WITH BIOPSY

Esophagogastroduodenoscopy allows visualization of the esophageal mucosa and permits biopsy specimens to be obtained from the proximal and distal esophagus. The stomach and duodenum are also examined. Breaks in the distal esophageal mucosa are the most reliable sign of reflux esophagitis. Mucosal erythema, pallor, and altered vascular patterns are suggestive of, but not specific findings for, reflux.

Histologic findings suggestive of GER are eosinophilia, elongation of the rete pegs, vascular hyperplasia, and dilation of intercellular spaces. The correlation between impedance monitoring and the results of esophageal biopsies is only moderate in pediatric populations.

EOSINOPHILIC ESOPHAGITIS

Eosinophilic esophagitis is an important pathological condition that is often seen in the pediatric aerodigestive practice. The symptoms of EoE can mimic those of reflux, and this entity should be considered if a child is not responding to typical reflux management. A history of allergies, eczema, multiple formula changes as an infant, or food impaction and/or a family history of reflux symptoms should lead the primary care clinician (PCC) to consider an EGD or a biopsy to rule out EoE. The visual inspection during a GI endoscopy may reveal a normal-appearing esophageal mucosa, and, therefore, multiple random esophageal biopsies are important. Skip lesions are often seen in EoE and so randomly performed biopsies are essential. When the disease is more advanced, the endoscopy may reveal esophageal findings of edema and longitudinal furrowing in the esophageal mucosa, and sometimes the esophagus may look like the rings of a trachea in a process called *trachealization*. This is an end-stage change of the esophageal mucosa related to deposits of inflammation in the basement membrane of the esophagus. Whitish streaks mimicking *Candida* may be seen, and biopsies of these are needed as well.

The distinction between reflux and EoE is important as the treatment strategies are different. The following section will address this in more detail.

MOTILITY STUDIES

Although rarely indicated in an evaluation of GER, esophageal manometry findings may be abnormal in patients with GERD and EoE. Manometry is best suited to confirm the diagnosis of achalasia, but it is not sufficiently sensitive or specific to diagnose GERD. These studies should be considered when a motility disorder is suspected. Patients with poor motility often regurgitate gastroesophageal content into the laryngopharyngeal airway and require therapies that are more complex than antacid medications alone.

Additional Testing

In an academic setting, some other testing could be considered, but no test has become a gold standard or necessarily diagnostic. Follicular tracheitis (cobblestoning of the trachea) is often noted in bronchoscopies of patients with aerodigestive disorders. This is a nonspecific finding revealing chronic inflammation, which often raises suspicion for a possible associated GI pathology. A recent retrospective study of 117 children with recurrent croup revealed that 41% of the patients had follicular tracheitis on bronchoscopy. Follicular tracheitis has the appearance of bumps in the tracheal mucosa, thus the term *cobblestoning* because of the similarity to cobblestones on the road. In this cohort, 59% of the children were diagnosed with GERD in at least 1 investigation; EoE was diagnosed in 9 of 117 patients; half of the patients who underwent a pH probe study for recurrent croup had evidence of reflux; and biopsies conducted in a few patients revealed chronic inflammation. Because this is a nonspecific but suggestive finding, we do not typically perform biopsies of these mucosal changes.

Pepsin is an exogenous protein that has been implicated in LPR. Studies are underway to evaluate its diagnostic potential, correlation with LPR, and response to treatment, as well as its impact on other aerodigestive symptoms such as adenoiditis, chronic cough, chronic vocal fold disease, and persistent airway inflammation. Reports of pepsin levels in saliva, on biopsy specimens, and in bronchoalveolar lavage specimens can be found; however, the clinical utility and specificity of such testing have yet to be determined.

■ Treatment of Gastroesophageal Reflux

Treatment of reflux should be approached in stages. First, attention should be directed toward the dietary habits of the child and the family. These considerations depend on the child's age. Infants who are breastfed may have an intolerance to human milk protein and may reflux as a result of constipation or allergy. Some infants are affected by the breastfeeding mother's diet, and the PCC should have a discussion with the family about keeping a diary of the mother's food and beverage intake to determine whether her diet may impact the infant's reflux. If this dietary modification does not help and the diary does not reveal any inciting factors, then trying a formula might be helpful, and some infants need more hypoallergenic or hydrolytic formulas to improve their tolerance. For some, thickened formula can lead to a reduction in the incidence of reflux events reaching the hypopharynx; however, there is no evidence that this modification has a significant impact on reflux in infants. Modifications of feeding volumes and feeding intervals are low-risk maneuvers, and a 2-week trial is recommended to determine if these changes help the regurgitation.

For older patients, it is essential to ensure that the child is not consuming highly acidic and allergenic meals. Baby food purchased in a store that is intended to have a long shelf life is acidified to reduce the risk of botulinum. The Food and Drug Administration regulates such premade meals and requires that the pH be <4.6. This means that, by definition, baby food that is purchased in a store, be it organic or not, is acidic. Applesauce is the most acidic of the store-bought baby food (and the most commonly seen in our patient population). The pH of applesauce hovers around 3.6, which is in the same range as seltzer water and somewhat better than the pH of vinegar, lemon/lime juice, and other soda products. Identifying and eliminating these acidic triggers in children can help reduce the inflammation of the hypopharynx and larynx and help resolve illnesses such as recurrent croup, chronic nasal congestion, persistent asthma, vocal cord dysfunction, dysphonia, and the like.

Alteration in positioning affects reflux. Upright positioning and the prone position have not been shown to treat symptoms of reflux in sleeping infants, and the current recommendation is *not* to use positional therapy for management of reflux in infants. Children may benefit from such positioning, but the evidence is too weak to support this notion. Conversely, a seated or semirecumbent position tends to increase pressure on the infant's abdomen and promote reflux events.

Medical treatment of reflux is reserved for individuals with excessive emesis episodes, irritability related to GER, failure to thrive, or recurrent respiratory symptoms. It should not be used to reduce crying or regurgitation in otherwise healthy infants.

Antacids neutralize gastric acid. High doses of aluminum medications may reach toxic levels in children, causing neutropenia, anemia, and neurotoxicity. According to the latest pediatric GER clinical practice guidelines (2018), use of antacids/alginates for long-term therapy of infants and children with reflux is not recommended.

Prokinetic agents increase the resting tone of the LES, increasing esophageal peristalsis and accelerating gastric emptying. These mechanisms reduce reflux events. Erythromycin or bethanechol have been used in complex cases involving delayed motility. Patients with aerodigestive disorders may derive benefits from these medications, as well as from azithromycin given in higher anti-inflammatory/ prokinetic doses, to reduce lung and airway inflammation.

Metoclopramide facilitates gastric emptying; however, it is associated with lethargy and irritability and may cause irreversible tardive dyskinesia. It is not recommended for use in children and infants with GERD.

Sucralfate adheres to the surface of gastric ulcers and protects esophageal mucosa from the corrosive effects of gastric acid. Because it contains aluminum, care must be taken in children.

Histamine receptor antagonists (H_2 blockers) ranitidine and cimetidine suppress gastric acid production. They reduce symptoms of GER and promote healing of the histologic changes associated with esophagitis.

Proton pump inhibitors (PPIs) are the most effective acid suppressants. However, there is concern about the safety of PPI use. Increased rates of community-acquired pneumonia, gastroenteritis, and *Candida* infections have been associated with prolonged use of PPIs. Proton pump inhibitors are recommended as a first-line treatment of reflux-related erosive esophagitis in children and infants with GERD.

> **Pearl:** Proton pump inhibitors are the most effective medication for the treatment of gastroesophageal reflux disease. However, prolonged use of proton pump inhibitors can lead to a decline in bone health and should be reserved for use when other nonmedical therapies have failed to resolve significant reflux.

Surgical treatment is reserved for patients with severe, medically unmanageable GER. A fundoplication procedure, of which there are many types, attempts to re-create a functional LES by wrapping a portion of the greater curvature of the stomach around the esophagus. The primary complications associated with this procedure are gas bloat, gas-bloat syndrome, retching, gagging, dumping syndrome, and recurrent reflux symptoms.

■ Selected References

Ali T, Roberts DN, Tierney WM. Long-term safety concerns with proton pump inhibitors. *Am J Med*. 2009;122(10):896–903

Dalby K, Nielsen RG, Markoew S, Kruse-Andersen S, Husby S. Reproducibility of 24-hour combined multiple intraluminal impedance (MII) and pH measurements in infants and children. Evaluation of a diagnostic procedure for gastroesophageal reflux disease. *Dig Dis Sci*. 2007;52(9):2159–2165

Duval M, Meier J, Asfour F, et al. Association between follicular tracheitis and gastroesophageal reflux. *Int J Pediatr Otorhinolaryngol*. 2016;82:8–11

Euler AR, Byrne WJ. Twenty-four-hour esophageal intraluminal pH probe testing: a comparative analysis. *Gastroenterology*. 1981;80(5 Pt 1):957–961

Gong X, Wang XY, Yang L, Sun MJ, Du J, Zhang W. Detecting laryngopharyngeal reflux by immunohistochemistry of pepsin in the biopsies of vocal fold leukoplakia. *J Voice*. 2018;32(3):352–355

Hart CK, de Alarcon A, Tabangin ME, et al. Impedance probe testing prior to pediatric airway reconstruction. *Ann Otol Rhinol Laryngol*. 2014;123(9):641–646

Kaul A, Rudolph CD. Gastrointestinal manometry studies in children. *J Clin Gastroenterol.* 1998;27(3):187–191

Koufman J, Wei JL, Zur KB. *Acid Reflux in Children: How Healthy Eating Can Fix Your Child's Asthma, Allergies, Obesity, Nasal Congestion, Cough & Croup.* New York, NY: Katalitix; 2018

Little FB, Koufman JA, Kohut RI, Marshall RB. Effect of gastric acid on the pathogenesis of subglottic stenosis. *Ann Otol Rhinol Laryngol.* 1985;94(5):516–519

McMurray JS, Gerber M, Stern Y, et al. Role of laryngoscopy, dual pH probe monitoring, and laryngeal mucosal biopsy in the diagnosis of pharyngoesophageal reflux. *Ann Otol Rhinol Laryngol.* 2001;110(4):299–304

Piquette RK. Torsade de pointes induced by cisapride/clarithromycin interaction. *Ann Pharmacother.* 1999;33(1):22–26

Putnam PE. Gastroesophageal reflux disease and dysphagia in children. *Semin Speech Lang.* 1997;18(1):25–338

Rosbe KW, Kenna MA, Auerbach AD. Extraesophageal reflux in pediatric patients with upper respiratory symptoms. *Arch Otolaryngol Head Neck Surg.* 2003;129(11):1213–1220

Rosen R, Vandenplas Y, Singendonk M, et al. Pediatric gastroesophageal reflux clinical practice guidelines: joint recommendations of the North American Society for Pediatric Gastroenterology, Hepatology, and Nutrition and the European Society for Pediatric Gastroenterology, Hepatology, and Nutrition. *J Pediatr Gastroenterol Nutr.* 2018;66(3):516–554

Sondheimer JM. Continuous monitoring of distal esophageal pH: a diagnostic test for gastroesophageal reflux in infants. *J Pediatr.* 1980;96(5):804–807

Suskind DL, Thompson DM, Gulati M, Huddleston P, Liu DC, Baroody FM. Improved infant swallowing after gastroesophageal reflux disease treatment: a function of improved laryngeal sensation? *Laryngoscope.* 2006;116(8):1397–1403

Tsou VM, Young RM, Hart MH, Vanderhoof JA. Elevated plasma aluminum levels in normal infants receiving antacids containing aluminum. *Pediatrics.* 1991;87(2):148–151

Tutuian R, Vela MF, Shay SS, Castell DO. Multichannel intraluminal impedance in esophageal function testing and gastroesophageal reflux monitoring. *J Clin Gastroenterol.* 2003;37(3):206–215

Wang CP, Wang CC, Lien HC, et al. Saliva pepsin detection and proton pump inhibitor response in suspected laryngopharyngeal reflux. *Laryngoscope.* 2019;129(3):709–714

Yellon RF, Szeremeta W, Grandis JR, Diguisseppe P, Dickman PS. Subglottic injury, gastric juice, corticosteroids, and peptide growth factors in a porcine model. *Laryngoscope.* 1998;108(6):854–862

CHAPTER 19

Speech and Voice Disorders

Stephen Maturo, MD, Christen Caloway, MD,
and Christopher Hartnick, MD

Introduction
Epidemiology
Presenting Symptoms
Physical Examination

Differential Diagnosis
Natural History and Treatment
Options

▉ Introduction

The development of speech and voice in children has a significant effect on social and educational development. The inability to communicate clearly affects the psychological and emotional well-being of the growing child. Children with speech and language disorders are more likely to have psychiatric disorders and become incarcerated. The effect on society also stretches to adulthood, during which 70% of adults who have speech disorders or reduced intelligibility are unemployed, and adults with speech problems have been found to be in a lower income group at a rate 1.5 times greater than that of controls. In a highly verbally communicative society, it is unacceptable to adopt an attitude of benign neglect of childhood speech and voice disorders given the potential lifelong effect on future personal interactions and vocation choices.

Speech and voice disorders encompass a broad category of diagnoses and are often confused as being a single disorder. Before diagnosing a voice or speech disorder, basic definitions of each should be provided. *Voice* is the sound produced by the larynx, whereas *speech* is the sound created by modification of the voice as it travels through the oropharynx, nasopharynx, and oral cavity (**Figure 19-1**). Articulation and resonance issues are considered speech disorders.

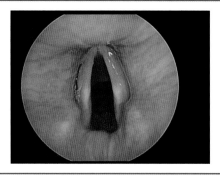

Figure 19-1. Normal-appearing vocal folds. The vocal folds make up a portion of the larynx or voice box.

Voice and speech are complicated processes that begin with a column of air generated from within the lungs and expressed through the vocal folds to the pharynx, oral cavity, and nasopharynx. Alterations at the level of the larynx lead to a *voice problem,* while changes after the air column has passed through the larynx are *speech problems.* Voice and speech are highly complicated processes that also require voluntary and involuntary neural inputs.

Most children with speech and voice disorders can be helped with a multidisciplinary team approach that includes pediatricians, otolaryngologists, pulmonologists, gastroenterologists, speech-language pathologists, teachers, and psychologists. Although most speech and voice disorders are benign processes, they can have a lasting effect on the overall development of the growing child if left untreated.

> **Pearl:** *Voice* is the sound produced by the larynx, whereas *speech* is the sound created by modification of the voice as it travels through the oropharynx, nasopharynx, and oral cavity. Alterations at the level of the larynx lead to a *voice problem*, while changes after the air column has passed through the larynx are *speech problems.*
> Although most speech and voice disorders are benign processes, they can have a lasting effect on the overall development of the growing child if left untreated.

■ Epidemiology

The prevalence of voice disorders in the pediatric population ranges between 3% and 10%. Studies have shown a slightly higher incidence in boys (7.5%) than girls (4.6%). One-third of all patients (including adults) experiencing speech or voice problems are of kindergarten age. The incidence of a specific diagnosis is age dependent, and other risk factors (besides gender) for childhood dysphonia are having older siblings and spending long days in large groups.

In the newborn, the most common "voice" concern is a weak or hoarse cry. One of the more common causes of hoarseness in a neonate is vocal fold paresis. While reports in the literature address both unilateral and bilateral paralysis, the incidence of bilateral vocal fold paralysis has been estimated at 0.75 cases per million births per year. Laryngomalacia can also cause a hoarse or weak cry, although most often these infants present with stridor as the hallmark feature of this disease. Finally, cleft lip and palate represents a congenital abnormality that can be problematic for speech development. Cleft lip with or without cleft palate is a prevalent disease throughout the world, affecting from 1:300 to 1:1,000 newborns. It is common in all populations, ranging from 1:1,000 in European populations to 1:300 to 1:500 in Asian and Hispanic populations, making this disease an important concern in every country.

The most common voice condition in children of preschool and elementary school age is vocal nodules (**Figure 19-2**). Approximately 50% of children with chronic hoarseness have vocal nodules; they are seen more commonly in boys—by a 2:1 ratio—until the teenage years,

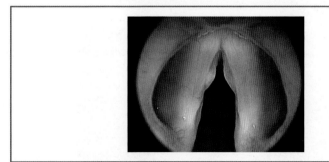

Figure 19-2. Bilateral vocal fold nodules in the classic area of the anterior third of the vocal folds. These nodules will improve with voice therapy; surgery is rarely, if ever, necessary.

when girls are more affected. The most common benign tumor of the larynx in children is juvenile-onset recurrent respiratory papilloma (JORRP) (**Figure 19-3**). Other, more common laryngeal abnormalities causing altered voice or speech in preadolescent children include vocal fold cysts and polyps.

In adolescents and teenagers, functional voice disorders, rather than organic pathology, are most common. Functional dysphonia and puberphonia are the most common disorders; however, their prevalence is largely unknown. Functional dysphonia, or muscle tension dysphonia, presents with an altered voice or, in some cases, aphonia with normal laryngeal and neurologic evaluation findings. Most often there is a significant emotional component to this disorder, but it may also be brought on by an organic disorder such as vocal nodules or a recent upper respiratory tract infection that causes laryngeal and extralaryngeal muscle hyperfunctioning. Puberphonia is the continued presence of the preadolescent voice in the child who has completed puberty. Most often, these conditions have a significant psychological component that is responsive to voice and behavioral therapy.

Another common concern of parents with young children is impairment of speech fluency, the most common example being stuttering. The age at which most children begin to stutter is around 3 years, with boys affected more than girls. Mild dysfluency is common, but further evaluation is warranted when children are struggling to talk and episodes are frequent.

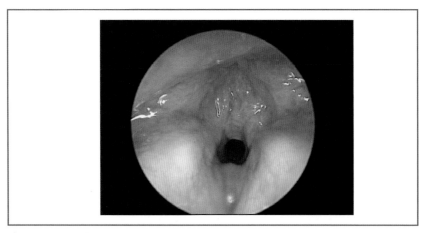

Figure 19-3. Papilloma obstructing most of the airway. Vocal folds are not visible.

> **Pearl:** In the newborn, the most common voice concern is a weak or hoarse cry, often due to vocal fold paralysis or paresis. In children of preschool and elementary school age, the most common voice condition is hoarseness due to vocal nodules. In adolescents and teenagers, functional voice disorders, such as muscle tension dysphonia and puberphonia, are most common.

■ Presenting Symptoms

A voice problem exists when the quality of the voice is not appropriate for the age or sex of the child. Limited data are in the pediatric literature regarding what constitutes a normal voice, but concerns about pitch, loudness, or quality may be the presenting complaint. The most common presenting voice or speech symptom is persistent hoarseness, but other complaints include hypernasality or hyponasality, cough, throat clearing, and snoring.

Although determining a voice or speech disorder usually is not difficult, the challenge for the primary care clinician (PCC) is to determine those that warrant further evaluation (**Box 19-1**) management. As with any medical evaluation, the key factors of the history include the characteristics of the disorder, time at onset, duration, aggravating factors, progression, and effect on the child. The PCC should also inquire about troublesome symptoms accompanying changes in voice or speech, including breathing difficulties, stridor, cyanotic episodes, hemoptysis, dysphagia, odynophagia, and nasal regurgitation during

---

Box 19-1. Indications for More Urgent Referral to an Otolaryngologist

♦ Shortness of breath
♦ Stridor
♦ Hemoptysis
♦ Aspiration
♦ Odynophagia
♦ Dysphagia
♦ Failure to thrive
♦ Cyanotic episodes
♦ Apparent life-threatening events

---

feeding. A history of trauma to the neck with voice changes is a concerning presentation and suggests disruption of normal laryngeal anatomy and the potential for airway embarrassment.

Infants with impairment of vocal fold mobility typically present with a breathy or hoarse cry, but vocal changes may be subtle. Occasionally, choking or coughing during feeds will be the presenting symptom in such children. When vocal fold paralysis or paresis in a neonate or an infant is suspected, otolaryngology consultation with endoscopic assessment of the larynx is indicated.

As mentioned earlier, hoarseness in toddlers and children of school age is usually due to vocal nodules caused by vocal abuse or strain. The typical history of a child with vocal fold nodules is a hoarse voice that worsens with increased use and improves with rest. The hoarseness may become more frequent, yet it is unlikely that airway or swallowing difficulties are ever associated with it. The PCC should inquire about opportunities for voice abuse such as competitive sports, cheerleading, choral singing, chronic cough or throat clearing, and competing to be heard in a household with older siblings. When hoarseness is also associated with stridor, a more significant mass of the vocal folds should be suspected. The most common such lesion is the respiratory papilloma, which is known to recur after surgical removal (recurrent respiratory papillomatosis [RRP]). This disorder may initially present with hoarseness in the absence of vocal abuse, with stridor becoming more apparent as the lesions grow in size or number. Although RRPs are benign tumors, left untreated they can lead to airway obstruction, thus underscoring the importance of a thorough evaluation of children with voice concerns lasting more than a few weeks or with any concerns associated with breathing problems. The average child diagnosed with RRP has symptoms for at least 1 year before receiving a definitive diagnosis.

> **Pearl:** In a child with hoarseness, the presence of stridor suggests a mass lesion of the vocal folds rather than vocal nodules.

While most cases of cleft palate are identified at birth or shortly thereafter, submucous cleft palate often goes unrecognized because the palatal mucosa is intact and only the palatal musculature and bone are maldeveloped. Affected children may present as infants with nasal regurgitation during feeding or emesis through the nose. Once speech develops, they will have difficulty because of nasal air emission while producing certain sounds, such as /s/, /sh/, /z/, /p/, /b/, /f/, and /v/. Occasionally, the disorder may be phoneme-specific, affecting, for example, only /s/, /sh/, and /z/. Suspected nasal air emission should be assessed by a speech pathologist and, if present, by an otolaryngologist.

Children who stutter have speech characterized by repetition of words, prolongation of words, and inability to start words. Secondary signs of stuttering may be the development of facial or body tics as a response to the tension of stuttering. The child may become withdrawn and less socially outgoing out of fear or embarrassment. The underlying cause of stuttering is likely a combination of genetic and environmental factors. There have been rare case reports of children developing stuttering after beginning treatment with stimulant and asthma medications; in such cases, the stuttering resolved after discontinuation of the medication. The optimal treatment for stuttering is debated, but involvement of a speech pathologist with behavioral therapists can provide relief to children who stutter.

Finally, the PCC should gauge the significance of voice and speech concerns to the affected child and caregiver. Children may manifest their concerns as shyness and avoidance of speaking, and many children, as well as their parents, may be embarrassed by the sound of their voice. A useful tool used by pediatric otolaryngologists who treat children with voice disorders is a validated survey to determine the effect of the vocal disorder on the child's quality of life (**Figure 19-4**). Although the specifics of this survey may not be as important to the PCC, it may serve as a useful screening document prior to the first visit for the family to determine their concerns regarding the voice complaints.

■ Physical Examination

To accurately identify a speech or voice disorder, a thorough head and neck examination is of utmost importance. Initially, a general assessment of the overall health of the child must be made. Rapid or difficult breathing may be perceived as a voice problem, but more often reflects a pulmonary or an airway issue requiring a more urgent evaluation by a specialist and, on occasion, securing of the airway. Urgent evaluations also may be needed in the setting of recent trauma

Please answer these questions based on what your child's voice (your own voice, if you are the teenage respondent) has been like over the past 2 weeks. Considering how severe the problem is and how frequently it happens, please rate each item below on how "bad" it is (that is, the amount of each problem that you have). Use the following rating scale:

1 = None, not a problem

2 = A small amount

3 = A moderate amount

4 = A lot

5 = Problem is "as bad as it can be"

6 = Not applicable

Because of my voice. . .	How much of a problem is this?
My child has trouble speaking loudly or being heard in noisy situations.	1 2 3 4 5
My child runs out of air and needs to take frequent breaths when talking.	1 2 3 4 5
My child sometimes does not know what will come out when he or she begins speaking.	1 2 3 4 5
My child is sometimes anxious or frustrated (because of his or her voice).	1 2 3 4 5
My child sometimes gets depressed (because of his or her voice).	1 2 3 4 5
My child has trouble using the telephone or speaking with friends in person (because of his or her voice).	1 2 3 4 5
My child has trouble doing his or her job or schoolwork (because of his or her voice).	1 2 3 4 5
My child avoids going out socially (because of his or her voice).	1 2 3 4 5
My child has to repeat himself or herself to be understood.	1 2 3 4 5
My child has become less outgoing (because of his or her voice).	1 2 3 4 5

Figure 19-4. Pediatric voice-related quality-of-life survey.

Reproduced with permission from *Archives of Otolaryngology-Head & Neck Surgery,* 2006; 132(7):717–720. Copyright ©2006 American Medical Association. All Rights Reserved.

in which an injury to the head or neck may have resulted in voice or speech alterations and point to more life-threatening injuries to the airway or neurovascular system.

Because the larynx cannot be directly examined by most PCCs, the physical examination of children with voice disorders focuses on recognition of the abnormality. The examination includes accurate characterization of the problem, including dysfunction of volume, pitch, resonance, fluency, and/or variability. The PCC also should identify physical findings that are associated with voice disorders, such as craniofacial and other syndromes. Many such children have laryngeal manifestations that may not be readily apparent, but vocal quality may be a parental concern that is not addressed because of multiple other medical issues of these children. Gross sensory or motor delay, whether it is readily apparent or picked up on a physical examination, may be associated with speech and voice disorders.

Evaluation of the nose, oral cavity, and pharynx can identify anatomical lesions that usually result in resonance or articulation disorders. Examination of the anterior nares could reveal enlarged turbinates or obstructive masses causing a change in airflow. Within the oral cavity, the palate should be examined to ensure there is no cleft and that the soft palate does not appear foreshortened. Mobility of the tongue and size of the tonsils also should be noted. In addition, the PCC should examine the neck and palpate for masses that could be compressing the laryngeal structures or causing dysfunction of the recurrent laryngeal nerve. Particular attention should be focused on the thyroid gland, especially in teenaged girls, in whom the incidence of thyroid disease and cancer becomes more common. A general neurologic examination that focuses on the cranial nerves is also important. Although this examination is sometimes difficult in the young child, the PCC can conduct a general neurologic assessment including most of the cranial nerves by observing the child. Any abnormalities should be further investigated with appropriate imaging, such as a computed tomography or magnetic resonance imaging.

Hearing is often overlooked in evaluating the child with speech or voice disorders. A common complaint among families is that their child speaks too loudly or is hard to understand. A thorough evaluation of the ears along with formal audiologic testing are recommended to rule out a hearing problem. Even children who have passed their newborn hearing screens may have an undiagnosed sensorineural hearing loss. Common middle-ear conditions in children younger than 7 years are chronic otitis media with effusion and recurrent ear infections, both of which are very familiar to PCCs, as is referral to an otolaryngologist for possible surgical management.

A complete evaluation of the nasal cavity, nasopharynx, oropharynx, and larynx is only available through the use of flexible nasopharyngoscopy. The nasopharyngoscope is a tool that is not typically present in a general primary care office, but it is an essential component of the physical examination for which the child with dysphonia should be referred to an otolaryngologist. This examination is relatively painless and is tolerated by most children when a gentle approach is used. The techniques and possible findings are beyond the scope of this chapter, but nasopharyngoscopy can be performed in most children in the office setting, avoiding the need for an evaluation in the operating room or endoscopy suite.

The need for further investigation, such as audiometry, pulmonary function tests, and pH probe studies, will be elucidated through answers from a thorough history. More pediatric centers have established airway and swallowing clinics in which there is collaboration among pediatric otolaryngologists, pulmonologists, and gastroenterologists, along with pediatric audiologists and speech-language pathologists. This multidisciplinary collaboration is not only a convenience for families but a truly comprehensive approach to speech and voice disorders.

> **Pearl:** The goal of the general physical examination in the pediatric patient with a speech or voice disorder is to identify a condition that may require a more urgent evaluation.

■ Differential Diagnosis

The differential diagnosis for children with voice or speech disorders is vast, and most anatomical abnormalities are impossible to diagnosis without direct visualization with a nasopharyngoscope or evaluation in the operating room. The key is to always consider any possible airway pathology that is affecting the voice. As with many diagnoses in children, age plays an important factor in determining an appropriate differential diagnosis.

Most evaluations of newborns are conducted out of concern for airway or breathing abnormalities, but a hoarse cry is suggestive of an anatomical disorder that warrants further evaluation. The differential diagnosis for voice complaints or hoarseness in a newborn must include vocal cord paralysis. Hoarseness with stridor is concerning for bilateral vocal fold paralysis, whereas unilateral vocal fold immobility may present with hoarseness or a weak cry alone. Unilateral vocal fold immobility is most likely iatrogenic because of cardiothoracic surgeries or idiopathic, but in the absence of surgery, an evaluation of the brain stem anatomy should be performed to rule out anatomical anomalies, such as Arnold-Chiari malformation. Other, less common causes of a hoarse cry in newborns include laryngeal webs (**figures 19-5** and **19-6**), transglottic hemangiomas (**figures 19-7** and **19-8**), and laryngeal clefts.

Velopharyngeal insufficiency (VPI) is often caused by a cleft palate, which can present with varying severity. Cleft palates can be complete, incomplete, and submucosal. Recognition of the more subtle types of this defect can be challenging, but suspicion should always prompt a referral to a craniofacial specialist to ensure that the child receives optimal treatment to develop the best possible speech as he or she grows older (see Chapter 12, Cleft Lip and Palate, for an in-depth discussion) (**figures 19-9** and **19-10**). Children who undergo repair of their cleft palate at a younger age often have some form of

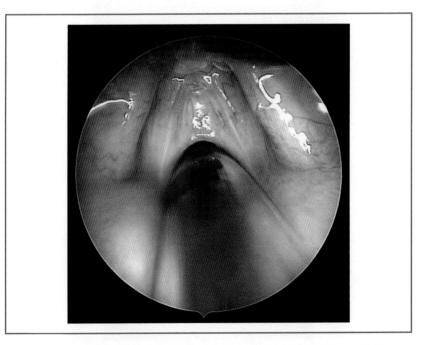

Figure 19-5. Two-week-old infant with weak cry and stridor due to laryngeal web, giving an appearance that the vocal folds are fused. An endotracheal tube is in place.

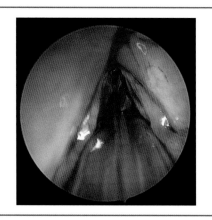

Figure 19-6. Laryngeal web divide with the anterior commissure of the glottis now open.

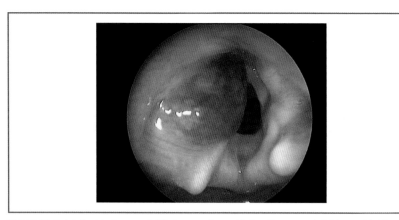

Figure 19-7. A left-sided supraglottic hemangioma. Notice the normal right vocal fold.

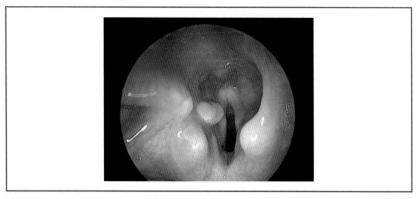

Figure 19-8. Six weeks after oral propranolol therapy and laser excision of supraglottic hemangioma.

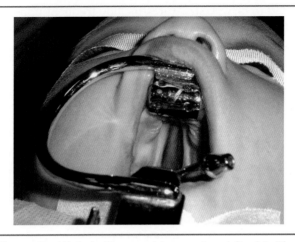

Figure 19-9. Ten-month-old infant with a complete secondary cleft palate. The structure in the middle of the cleft is the vomer.

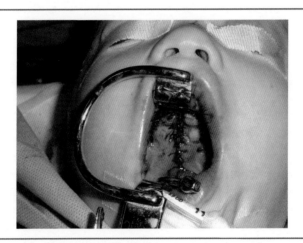

Figure 19-10. Completion of cleft palate repair. The child will be followed up closely for the next 5 to 10 years to ensure proper speech development.

VPI characterized by a hypernasal voice in which air escapes through the nose. This becomes apparent as the child begins to develop speech and as his or her vocabulary expands.

It must be noted, though, that not all voice and speech disorders are caused by the structures of the larynx and upper airway. A thorough history is important to identify the more common afflictions that can affect the voice and speech. Some of the more common diagnoses not directly related to airway structures include frequent upper respiratory tract infections, gastroesophageal reflux, and allergies. Most PCCs are comfortable diagnosing these more common entities, but close follow-up is warranted and further evaluation is needed if the child's voice or speech is not improving after treatment. Inflammatory voice disorders are the most common cause of dysphonia in children. Following an upper respiratory infection, dysphonia should resolve within 3 weeks. Chronic dysphonia warrants an evaluation by an otolaryngologist for nasopharyngoscopy to investigate alternate etiologies.

Box 19-2 lists the most common diagnoses according to newborn/infant, child, and adolescent categories. As has been stressed throughout this chapter, troubling symptoms include airway and swallowing findings. Newborns have not developed a speech or voice, but any report of hoarseness should prompt an otolaryngological evaluation. Also, many conditions in the newborn are not diagnosed until he or she begins developing vocalization.

> **Pearl:** Age is the most important consideration when formulating a differential diagnosis in the pediatric patient with a voice or speech disorder.

Natural History and Treatment Options

The natural history and prognosis of speech and voice disorders in children are best described in general terms based on specific diagnoses. Overall, most children with dysphonia caused by vocal fold nodules will experience improvement by the time they reach puberty, but at least 10% will not. It is this subset of children who may require surgery or, at the very least, a thorough multidisciplinary approach to their voice pathology. Similarly, newborns with idiopathic unilateral vocal fold paresis usually experience improvement with time and without any intervention. Children with a vocal fold paralysis caused by iatrogenic injury tend to compensate well and have minimal voice and speech deficits. For the child with vocal fold paralysis, temporary and permanent procedures are available that have been demonstrated to achieve good results when applied to the appropriate patient. Juvenile-onset recurrent respiratory papilloma (JORRP) is a challenging disease, especially in children with severe disease who require

Box 19-2. Common Diagnoses That Cause Speech and Voice Disorders

Newborn/Infant

♦ Vocal fold immobility (caused by paresis/paralysis)
♦ Gastroesophageal reflux disease
♦ Laryngomalacia
♦ Laryngeal hemangioma
♦ Laryngeal web
♦ Laryngeal cysts
♦ Laryngeal cleft
♦ Juvenile-onset recurrent respiratory papilloma
♦ Cleft lip/palate
♦ Velopharyngeal insufficiency
♦ Ankyloglossia (tongue-tie)

Child

♦ Voice abuse/misuse
♦ Vocal fold nodules
♦ Upper respiratory infections
♦ Juvenile-onset recurrent respiratory papilloma
♦ Vocal fold cysts/polyps
♦ Stuttering
♦ Velopharyngeal insufficiency
♦ Tonsil/adenoid hypertrophy
♦ Laryngeal web
♦ Vocal fold granuloma
♦ Vocal fold immobility (caused by paresis/paralysis)
♦ Ankyloglossia
♦ Muscle tension dysphonia

Adolescent

♦ Voice abuse/misuse
♦ Vocal fold nodules
♦ Muscle tension dysphonia
♦ Puberphonia
♦ Paradoxic vocal fold motion
♦ Laryngitides due to smoking
♦ Gastroesophageal reflux disease
♦ Thyroid disease

multiple visits to the operating room and consideration for adjuvant medical therapy. In most children, the disease burden runs its course by the teenage years, but in a small minority of children, JORRP progresses to the lungs, ultimately resulting in death. Adolescents with functional voice disorders are usually treated successfully with speech and behavioral therapy. In the adolescent with a recalcitrant voice disorder, consultation with a child psychiatrist may be worthwhile to investigate any ongoing issues.

Treatment options for voice and speech disorders depend on the specific diagnosis and include behavioral, medical, and surgical therapy. Most childhood speech and voice disorders are treated with speech therapy. The decision to proceed with surgery is not one to be taken lightly because interventions on the growing vocal fold can have lifelong effects that may be worse than the initial presenting symptom. One underlying theme in the evaluation and treatment of children with speech or voice disorders is the importance of a team approach in which various behavioral, medical, and surgical skill sets are combined and applied in an individualized manner.

Voice therapy is the most common management approach in children with voice disorders resulting from voice abuse or misuse or from hyperfunctional states. Of course, successful therapy depends on the commitment and cooperation of the child and family; therefore, there is debate about the efficacy of voice therapy in children. In those who have undergone surgical interventions for the larynx, voice therapy also plays a major role, both in the perioperative period and in secondary prevention strategies. Voice therapy programs vary according to training and experience of the speech-language pathologist, but certain underlying facets are demonstrated in most programs. The approach to a child with a speech or voice disorder is not the same as the approach taken with an adult. Family and school involvement is necessary, and age-appropriate activities with an emphasis on behavioral changes lead to successful results.

Behavioral therapy most often is used in conjunction with speech therapy. Children with paradoxic vocal fold motion or chronic cough or throat clearing are most likely to experience improvement with treatment by an experienced speech-language pathologist. In children in whom there is a psychological component such as anxiety, treatment may be supplemented by counseling with child psychologists or psychiatrists. We have found that first acknowledging the voice or speech component of these disorders makes the child and caregivers more responsive to seeking psychological counseling along with speech therapy.

Medical therapy most commonly includes treatment of gastroesophageal reflux disease and allergy if symptoms are present. Most PCCs are familiar with the signs and symptoms of allergy, and it would be the unique child who presented with hoarseness as the sole manifestation of allergy. Treatment with antihistamines and intranasal steroid medications usually results in success, but further evaluation by an allergist for persistent symptoms may be necessary. Empirical treatment with proton pump inhibitors for benign laryngeal disease, such as vocal fold nodules or mild to moderate laryngopharyngeal reflux, is controversial, as no prospective studies have demonstrated efficacy, but the relative safety profile of this medication makes it a common choice among otolaryngologists for children. The role of medical management for most other laryngeal disorders in children is limited but should be considered. For example, adjuvant antiviral and other medical therapies in RRP may reduce the frequency of surgical intervention, but results are variable; the search continues for a medication that provides relief with limited side effects.

The role of surgery depends on the specific diagnosis. As mentioned earlier, the most common diagnosis, vocal fold nodules, is not a surgical disease because voice therapy and medical management are usually successful. Microscopic laryngoscopy in the operating room may be necessary to establish the diagnosis in a child with presumed nodules who is refractory to speech therapy, but manipulation of the growing vocal fold likely will result in more harm than good. Specific phonosurgical procedures for such conditions as unilateral vocal fold paresis, laryngeal webs, respiratory papillomas, and vocal fold granulomas are beyond the scope of this chapter. For children with speech disorders, surgeries involving the tonsils, adenoid, and soft palate are common. A child with hyponasal speech (ie, decreased nasal airflow, sounding chronically nasally congested) or recurrent postnasal drip affecting voicing may be a candidate for adenoidectomy. A tonsillectomy is rarely performed for speech disorders but may be done in instances in which children with VPI are candidates for palate procedures. Finally, palate lengthening and augmenting procedures have been shown to improve voicing outcomes in patients with VPI.

> **Pearl:** Most children with speech or voice disorders are treated successfully with speech therapy. Adjuvant medical and surgical therapy may be required depending on the underlying cause of the disorder.

■ Selected References

Baker BM, Blackwell PB. Identification and remediation of pediatric fluency and voice disorders. *J Pediatr Health Care.* 2004;18(2):87–94

Blumin JH, Keppel KL, Braun NM, Kerschner JE, Merati AL. The impact of gender and age on voice related quality of life in children: normative data. *Int J Pediatr Otorhinolaryngol.* 2008;72(2):229–234

Boseley ME, Cunningham MJ, Volk MS, Hartnick CJ. Validation of the pediatric voice-related quality-of-life survey. *Arch Otolaryngol Head Neck Surg.* 2006;132(7):717–720

Carding PN, Roulstone S, Northstone K; ALSPAC Study Team. The prevalence of childhood dysphonia: a cross-sectional study. *J Voice.* 2006;20(4):623–630

Daya H, Hosni A, Bejar-Solar I, Evans JN, Bailey CM. Pediatric vocal fold paralysis: a long-term retrospective study. *Arch Otolaryngol Head Neck Surg.* 2000;126(1):21–25

Gray SD, Smith ME, Schneider H. Voice disorders in children. *Pediatr Clin North Am.* 1996;43(6):1357–1384

Hirschberg J, Dejonckere PH, Hirano M, Mori K, Schultz-Coulon HJ, Vrticka K. Voice disorders in children. *Int J Pediatr Otorhinolaryngol.* 1995;32(Suppl):S109–S125

Hooper CR. Treatment of voice disorders in children. *Lang Speech Hear Serv Sch.* 2004;35(4):320–326

Mori K. Vocal fold nodules in children: preferable therapy. *Int J Pediatr Otorhinolaryngol.* 1999;49(Suppl 1):S303–S306

Newman KB, Mason UG III, Schmaling KB. Clinical features of vocal cord dysfunction. *Am J Respir Crit Care Med.* 1995;152(4 Pt 1):1382–1386

Ruben RJ. Valedictory: why pediatric otorhinolaryngology is important. *Int J Pediatr Otorhinolaryngol.* 2003;67(Suppl 1):S53–S61

St. Louis KO, Hansen GR, Buch JL, Oliver TL. Voice deviations in coexisting communication disorders. *Lang Speech Hear Serv Sch.* 1992;23(1):82–87

CHAPTER 20

Drooling and Salivary Aspiration

Corrie E. Roehm, MD, and Scott R. Schoem, MD, MBA

Introduction	**Management**
Salivation	**Medication**
Etiology	**Other Types of Treatment**
Assessment	**Conclusion**

▓ Introduction

Sialorrhea, or drooling, is defined as an inability to control oral secretions and is a common difficulty in pediatric patients with neuromuscular disorders. Pathological sialorrhea is defined as saliva beyond the margin of the lip in patients older than 4 to 5 years who are in an alert state. This condition is not necessarily caused by an increased volume of saliva (hypersalivation) but by a lack of coordinated control of saliva by the oropharyngeal and tongue musculature that controls the voluntary oral phase of swallowing. An inability to direct saliva into the posterior oropharynx for swallowing leads to anterior pooling of secretions, with eventual spilling. Similarly, pooling in the posterior oropharynx with decreased swallowing may lead to laryngeal spilling and aspiration of secretions. Major causes of sialorrhea in pediatric patients include cerebral palsy, intellectual disability, and other causes of neurologic or neuromuscular dysfunction. Drooling has a broad effect on the patient, family, and caregivers, increasing daily care needs of cleaning, clothing, and bib changes. This requires a higher level of care at more time and cost, and often restricts the activities of patients and their caregivers. Many patients have lip and facial chapping that can lead to skin maceration, bleeding, and secondary infections. Visible drool detracts from the patient's physical appearance and can impair speech and social interactions, often reducing normal physical contact. Most importantly, sialorrhea involves an increased risk of aspiration and secondary pneumonia or pneumonitis, with potentially devastating morbidity.

■ Salivation

Normal salivation involves production of 1 to 1.5 L daily, requiring approximately 600 swallows a day, with the potential for up to 10 times more volume with salivary stimulation. Ninety percent of saliva is made by the submandibular, parotid, and sublingual glands, with a 10% contribution from minor salivary glands. Saliva consists of mucus and serous fluid in varying proportions based on the producing gland. The serous component has a lower calcium content and contains amylase for carbohydrate digestion of starch into maltose, while the more viscous mucous component provides lubrication and contains higher calcium levels. Saliva functions include enzymatic digestion of carbohydrates, lubrication of mucosal membranes, cleansing food debris, immune function with secretory IgA, protection of dentition with calcium and phosphate mineralization, and breaking down bacterial cell walls with lysozyme. The parotid gland produces thinner, more serous saliva, while the submandibular and sublingual glands secrete a thicker mixture of mucous and serous saliva. Salivation is stimulated by a reflex arch in the autonomic nervous system ultimately signaling through acetylcholine-driven muscarinic M_3 receptors of the cholinergic system. Cranial nerves V, VII, IX, and X bring afferent stimulation from chemoreceptors and mechanoreceptors in the oropharynx and upper gastrointestinal tract to the inferior and superior salivary nuclei in the medulla oblongata. The parotid gland is innervated by the ninth cranial nerve traveling from the inferior salivatory nucleus through the tympanic cavity on the tympanic segment of the glossopharyngeal nerve (Jacobson nerve), then through the lesser petrosal nerve, the otic ganglion, and along the auriculotemporal nerve to the gland. The submandibular, sublingual, and minor salivary glands are innervated by the seventh cranial nerve from the superior salivatory nucleus, with fibers traveling with chorda tympani along lingual nerves to the submandibular ganglion, finally terminating in the gland. Parasympathetic signaling stimulates saliva production within all of the glands, while the sympathetic system prompts contraction of the smooth muscle in salivary ducts for expulsion of saliva from the glands and specific production of the submandibular gland's thicker saliva.

Etiology

Sialorrhea is affected by a number of physical and anatomical factors, including oral motor dysfunction or oral sphincter deficiency, inadequate swallowing capacity, poor posture, hypoglossia, dental malocclusion, impaired nasal airway, and general hypotonicity. Altered concentration and diminished oral sensation can decrease a patient's awareness of the need to swallow and also lead to sialorrhea. Potential etiologies can be categorized as causes of decreased swallowing or increased saliva production (**Box 20-1**). Cerebral palsy is one of the main diagnoses associated with decreased swallowing, with 10% to 37% of pediatric patients with this disorder affected. Other common causes of decreased swallowing are intellectual disability and orthognathic abnormalities such as anterior open bite and macroglossia. Increased saliva production (hypersalivation) can

---

Box 20-1. Causes of Sialorrhea

Decreased Swallowing

♦ Cerebral palsy
♦ Causes of intellectual disability—Down syndrome
♦ Facial paralysis (Bell palsy)
♦ Encephalopathy
♦ Heavy metal neurotoxicity—mercury, thallium, copper, arsenic, antimony
♦ Wilson disease
♦ Angelman syndrome
♦ Pseudobulbar palsy
♦ Bulbar palsy

Decreased Ability to Swallow

♦ Anatomical abnormalities—macroglossia
♦ Orthodontic problems—anterior open bite, lip seal incompetence
♦ TMJ ankylosis
♦ Surgical defects following major head and neck resections

Increased Saliva Production

♦ Oral irritation—ulcerations, infection, trauma, dental appliances
♦ Medication adverse effects—cholinergic effects from anticonvulsants, clozapine, risperidone, nitrazepam, bethanechol
♦ Gastroesophageal reflux disease
♦ Organophosphate toxicity

Abbreviation: TMJ, temporomandibular joint.

---

be triggered by oral irritation, mouth breathing from a nasal airway obstruction, gastroesophageal reflux disease (GERD), or cholinergic stimulation from medication side effects (eg, anticonvulsants; antipsychotics, particularly clozapine and risperidone; nitrazepam; bethanechol) or organophosphate and heavy metal (eg, mercury, thallium) toxicity.

■ Assessment

Assessing a patient with sialorrhea and deciding on appropriate management involve an evaluation of the severity of drooling and the chronicity and progression of any underlying etiology. The amount of drooling can be quantified with direct measurement of saliva volume or with multiple grading methods to assess its relative frequency, severity, and associated complications. Examples of these scales include the Teacher Drooling Scale and Drooling Impact Scale (**Table 20-1** and **Figure 20-1**). Immediate visual evaluation can show active drooling, perioral skin irritation, or maceration. A complete examination includes a nasal examination for potential nasal airway obstruction, evaluation of dentition for caries and malocclusion, evaluation of tongue size and any active thrusting, and assessment of head

Table 20-1. Drooling Scales

Teacher Drooling Scale[a]		Drooling Frequency and Severity Scale[b]	
Grade	Symptom	Severity	Frequency
1	No drooling	1—Dry (never drools)	1—Never drools
2	Infrequent drooling, small amount	2—Mild (only wet lips)	2—Occasional drooling
3	Occasional drooling, on and off all day	3— Moderate (lips and chin)	3—Frequent drooling
4	Frequent drooling but not profuse	4—Severe (clothing)	4—Constant drooling
5	Constant drooling, always wet	5—Profuse (clothing, hands, tray, objects)	—

[a] Reprinted with permission from Camp-Bruno JA, Winsberg BG, Green-Parsons AR, Abrams JP. Efficacy of benztropine therapy for drooling. *Dev Med Child Neurol.* 1989; 31(3):309–319.

[b] Reprinted with permission from Thomas-Stonell N, Greenberg J. Three treatment approaches and clinical factors in the reduction of drooling. *Dysphagia.* 1988;3(2): 73–78.

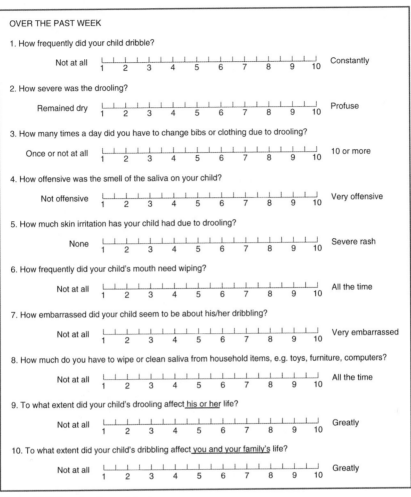

Figure 20-1. Drooling Impact Scale.

From Reid SM, Johnson HM, Reddihough DS. The Drooling Impact Scale: a measure of the impact of drooling in children with developmental disabilities. *Dev Med Child Neurol.* 2010;52(2):e23–e28, with permission from John Wiley & Sons.

posture and position. Answering a number of questions pertaining to the patient's history is useful in identifying treatable causes of sialorrhea and helping direct treatment decisions (**Box 20-2**).

The first step is to address immediately treatable underlying conditions (ie, GERD, nasal obstruction from adenoid hypertrophy, allergic rhinitis) and eliminate seizure medications such as clonazepam and schizophrenia medications such as clozapine, which have known hypersalivation side effects. Changes in the sialorrhea can be

> ### Box 20-2. Questions to Ask to Direct Treatment Decisions
>
> - How frequent/severe is the drooling?
> - Is the underlying cause of sialorrhea temporary?
> - Will the patient outgrow the problem, or will it likely remain the same or worsen?
> - Does the patient eat orally or through nonoral means (eg, gastric feeding tube)?
> - Does the patient have functional oral communication?
> - Is there any history of possible aspirations (eg, choking or coughing on saliva, particularly at night; prior pneumonia)?
> - Does the patient have any evidence of gastroesophageal reflux disease that could stimulate salivation?
> - Could any current medications cause hypersalivation or have cholinergic effects?
> - Is the patient's nasal airway obstructed, leading to mouth breathing and open mouth?

tracked through serial evaluations and scaling of its severity. If drooling is persistent or moderate or severe on initial evaluation, it may be managed more effectively with multidisciplinary input from a speech therapist, a neurologist, and an otolaryngologist. Often, the neurologist or speech therapist performs the assessment and refers the patient to the otolaryngologist for potential botulinum toxin injections or surgery when medical therapy is ineffective or insufficient.

■ Management

Treatment of sialorrhea depends on the severity of the problem and temporary versus permanent underlying etiologies and age, with the goal of eliminating excessive saliva and spilling while maintaining a moistened, healthy oral cavity. In patients younger than 5 years who are otherwise healthy, reassurance is appropriate because drooling tends to resolve with time. Other patients can be treated in a progressive manner to maximize conservative measures before considering more aggressive options in unresponsive cases (**Box 20-3**). These measures include oral stimulation programs with speech therapy to improve oromotor coordination and proprioception, decrease tongue thrusting, and prompt jaw and lip closure. Behavior modification can be useful in patients who are aware and cooperative enough to participate in posture training and positioning to improve oral closure and posterior salivary flow. Swallowing prompts with auditory signals or other cues, teaching oral motor skills and oral awareness, or palatal

---

Box 20-3. Progressive Management of Drooling

♦ Oral stimulation programs
♦ Behavior modifications
♦ Medication
♦ Botulinum toxin injections or surgical treatment

---

training appliances can guide the patient to better control lip and jaw closure and tongue movements and decrease drooling.

MEDICATION

Medications to reduce saliva production are the next therapeutic option in patients whose conditions do not improve with behavior modification and speech therapy. One key pharmacologic target to control drooling is the postganglionic muscarinic M_3 receptor, where parasympathetic action of acetylcholine normally stimulates salivary glands to increase saliva production. Several antimuscarinics that block this action have been shown to inhibit salivation. They include benztropine, benzhexol hydrochloride (trihexyphenidyl), glycopyrrolate, and scopolamine (**Table 20-2**). However, the action of antimuscarinic pharmacologics is not selective. Their effects on extrasalivary muscarinic receptors and on smooth muscles that are responsive to acetylcholine may cause systemic effects, including dilation of pupils, increased heart rate, decreased gut motility, urinary retention, and reduced sweating. Headache, irritability, confusion, nausea, tachycardia, blurred vision, xerostomia, and decreased taste are several of the most common side effects, and these anticholinergics are contraindicated in patients with glaucoma, obstructive uropathy, gastrointestinal obstruction, myasthenia gravis, or asthma to prevent exacerbations. Studies in the literature showing the effectiveness of scopolamine, benztropine, and glycopyrrolate as pharmacologic options for sialorrhea often are limited by small sample sizes and nonstandardized outcome measurements, but glycopyrrolate may have an advantage over the others because it has fewer side effects. Benztropine is a synthetic compound structurally similar to atropine that was shown to be effective in approximately 65% of 20 patients in a study by Camp-Bruno et al, with 15% (3 patients) discontinuing the medication because of significant systemic side effects. Long-term data on effect duration and adverse effects were not collected. Scopolamine has been shown to reduce drooling in patients with developmental delays and with

---

Table 20-2. Medications to Reduce Saliva Production			
Medication	**Doses Available**	**Dosage**	**Adverse Effects**
Glycopyrrolate	1- or 2-mg tablets	Adults: start 0.5 mg orally 1 to 3 times daily; titrate as needed (maximum dose, 8 mg/d) Children: 0.04 mg/kg per dose 2 to 3 times a day; titrate as needed	Xerostomia, blurred vision, hyperactivity, irritability, constipation, urinary retention
Scopolamine	1.5-mg transdermal patch	1 patch every 3 days	Xerostomia, blurred vision, irritability, dizziness, constipation, urinary retention
Benztropine	0.5-, 1-, or 2-mg tablets, 1 mg/mL injection	Average 3.8 mg daily[a]	Xerostomia, blurred vision, constipation, tachycardia, urinary retention, disorientation, rash
Benzhexol hydrochloride	2- or 5-mg tablets, 2 mg/5 mL elixir	2 to 3 mg twice daily[b]	Blurred vision, dizziness, urinary retention

[a] Camp-Bruno JA, Winsberg BG, Green-Parsons AR, Abrams JP. Efficacy of benztropine therapy for drooling. *Dev Med Child Neurol.* 1989;31(3):309–319.

[b] Reddihough D, Johnson H, Staples M, Hudson I, Exarchos H. Use of benzhexol hydrochloride to control drooling of children with cerebral palsy. *Dev Med Child Neurol.* 1990;32(11):985–989.

cerebral palsy, specifically, with a more than 50% reduction in drooling volume in 53% of patients.

Scopolamine has not been studied for long-term use. It also causes systemic effects, with unique side effects, including temporary toxic psychosis, in addition to classic antimuscarinic effects. Using a separate mechanism, clonidine patches also have been shown to be effective at reducing hypersalivation from antipsychotic medications by increasing adrenergic activity. Glycopyrrolate is a quaternary ammonium antimuscarinic structurally related to atropine that does not easily cross the blood-brain barrier, decreasing central side effects but maintaining the ability to decrease drooling scores by approximately 50% in a study by Bachrach et al. Blasco and Stansbury reported a

90% reduction in drooling, with a 28% rate of side effects, leading to discontinuation of treatment in 11 patients. The final effective dose ranged from 0.01 to 0.82 mg/kg/day in a pediatric study population. Dosing of antimuscarinic medications must be balanced to control drooling while avoiding adverse effects, if possible, and may be variable over time as drooling volumes change. Decreasing saliva production to the point of xerostomia is often uncomfortable for patients, can make speech and eating more difficult, and can lead to long-term complications, including dental caries.

OTHER TYPES OF TREATMENT

For patients with severe sialorrhea or poor responses to more conservative measures, therapies aimed at more prolonged reduction or elimination of salivary gland function should be considered, including botulinum toxin injections and surgery. Radiation therapy has been used to treat sialorrhea in geriatric patients with the aim of rendering the salivary glands nonfunctional with damage to serous acinic cells. However, this modality is not practically applicable in pediatric sialorrhea because of potential alteration of midface growth and increased malignancy risk 10 to 15 years after exposure.

Botulinum toxin injections are a more recent addition to the treatment options for pediatric sialorrhea; they use the action of a neurotoxin produced by *Clostridium botulinum* bacterium to decrease salivation. This toxin causes proteolytic cleavage of SNAP-25, an enzyme involved in vesicle fusion and acetylcholine release at the presynaptic membrane. Inhibition of acetylcholine action at the synapse establishes a temporary functional denervation of the salivary glands and prevents salivary stimulation for several weeks to months following injection.

Although injection sites can be estimated based on knowledge of salivary gland anatomy, ultrasound guidance is preferable, especially when injecting the submandibular gland. The procedure usually requires general anesthesia for pediatric patients. Various injection methods and dosing regimens have been reported, including single 5-U botulinum toxin A doses into the superficial parotid glands bilaterally, with 55% of patients exhibiting perceived benefit. Wilken et al administered 2 injections of approximately 15 U botulinum toxin A or B into the anterior and posterior parotid glands and approximately 15 U into the submandibular gland. The results showed an 83% reduction in Teacher Drooling Scale scores at 4 weeks and sustained reduction in drooling with 2- to 6-month injection intervals. One controlled trial evaluating the efficacy of botulinum toxin and scopolamine in pediatric patients with sialorrhea used weight categories for dosing of submandibular gland injections (15 U/gland for patients weighing less than 15 kg; 20 U/gland for those weighing 15 to 25 kg; 25 U/gland for those heavier than 25 kg). The study findings showed a 61% response rate 2 weeks after botulinum toxin injections, which caused fewer side effects than scopolamine treatment in the same study group. Comparisons of botulinum toxin A to toxin B show no significant difference in efficacy; however, more research is needed to determine optimal pediatric dosing for maximal efficacy and minimal risk of complications. These studies further defined the side effect profile of botulinum toxin injections as rare, mild complications including mild xerostomia, thickened saliva, transient flu-like symptoms, and short-lived injection-site tenderness. Thickened saliva is likely from preferential injection of the parotid gland, eliminating its thin serous saliva production, instead of the submandibular gland, which produces thicker, mucous saliva. More serious adverse effects reported were facial nerve weakness, oral closure, and chewing difficulty from masseter muscle weakness, likely the result of toxin diffusion from parotid injection sites, and dysphagia from systemic botulinum toxin effects on pharyngeal musculature. Patients responding to botulinum toxin injections can avoid more invasive surgical procedures, but injections still require general anesthesia in most pediatric patients as well as recurring injections for prolonged effect. Therefore, parents need to be prepared for botulinum injections under general anesthesia every 4 to 6 months versus the longer-lasting effects of surgical procedures.

Surgery

Surgery is often considered when less invasive or nonpermanent treatments fail to decrease drooling after 6 months of treatment in patients older than 5 to 6 years, to allow for full maturity of oropharyngeal motor coordination. Surgery is also more useful in patients unable to engage in behavioral or postural therapies or when aspiration, pneumonia, and other serious sequelae of drooling occur. One important factor to consider when choosing a surgical procedure for a drooling patient is the presence of aspiration, in which posterior ductal rerouting may be less beneficial, with its potential for posterior salivary pooling, theoretically increasing the risk of aspiration.

Historically, a variety of surgical procedures have been used in the treatment of sialorrhea to interrupt innervation or gland ductal drainage, redirect ductal drainage, or remove glands entirely.

Techniques have evolved over time in an attempt to improve postoperative results and avoid the risk of additional complications. These procedures can be categorized as salivary reduction or salivary diversion procedures (**Table 20-3**). One procedure no longer used is transtympanic nerve sectioning to interrupt fibers carrying salivary stimuli, including bilateral tympanic neurectomy transecting the Jacobson nerve of the glossopharyngeal nerve (cranial nerve [CN] IX) and the chorda tympani nerve section of the facial nerve (CN VII). The procedure has been abandoned because of the risks of loss of taste in the anterior two-thirds of the tongue innervated by facial nerve fibers within chorda tympani, tympanic membrane perforations, otitis media, and recurrence of drooling from nerve regeneration.

Salivary duct surgery for sialorrhea was introduced in 1967 by Theodore Wilkie, with parotid duct relocation to the tonsillar fossa to

Table 20-3. Surgical Options for Sialorrhea		
Surgical Option	**Advantages**	**Disadvantages**
Salivary Reduction		
Nerve sectioning	Fast procedure, under local anesthesia	Nerve regrowth can result in need for repeated sectioning; poor results, procedure abandoned
Ductal ligation	Simple procedure, decreases flow predictably	Temporary gland swelling, potential for sialocele or sialoliths
Gland excisions	Excellent reduction in salivary volume	Increased procedure complexity and risk to surrounding structures (eg, facial nerve branches, hypoglossal and lingual nerves), external scar, higher risk of xerostomia, dental caries
Salivary Diversion		
Submandibular duct rerouting	No external scar, reduces anterior pooling/spillage	Risk of anterior caries, ranula if sublingual gland is not excised, duct obstruction, potential aspiration risk
Parotid duct rerouting	No external scar, reduces anterior pooling/spillage of thin saliva	Risk of sialocele, potential aspiration risk, duct obstruction, parotid and facial swelling, parotitis

redirect salivary flow to the posterior oropharynx. This method was modified by Wilkie and Brody several years later to include bilateral submandibulectomy (removal of both submandibular glands), resulting in an 85% reduction in drooling but an associated 35% rate of adverse effects. Bilateral submandibulectomy became a logical surgical target because the submandibular glands produce approximately 70% of saliva volume, and excision of the glands reliably and dramatically reduced salivary volume. However, gland removal procedures, particularly those involving the parotid gland, involve an external scar, as well as risks of irreversible xerostomia and injury to the facial nerve trunk or branches.

Subsequently, salivary ductal ligation became popular because the ducts could be accessed transorally and ligated with minimal dissection. Ligation works by inducing gland atrophy from functional obstruction to reduce saliva production, and it blocks salivary flow immediately, resulting in reliable reduction in saliva volume. For management of the parotid glands, ligation is highly preferable because parotidectomy is a major operation involving considerable risk to the facial nerve trunk. Parotid duct ligation was initially performed in combination with submandibulectomy, but the ligation procedure has since been expanded to include the submandibular ducts as well (4-duct ligation). Common complications include mild temporary swelling and discomfort. Studies of 4-duct ligation have reported drooling improvement rates of more than 64%. Common complications include mild temporary swelling and discomfort. Duct clipping and laser photocoagulation have been investigated as potential procedural variations of ductal ligation, aiming to decrease surgical time and the extent of dissection even further. Submandibular ductal ligations result in higher rates of sialoliths (salivary stones) because of more mucous saliva, with the higher calcium content and viscosity of submandibular gland saliva, as well as the upward slanting course of Wharton's duct, causing retention of particulates. Less common complications include sialoceles (cystic collections of saliva typically in the cheek at the point of the parotid duct ligation) and ranulas in the floor of the mouth from inadvertent disruption of sublingual glands during ligation of the submandibular ducts.

In cases of chronic aspiration associated with pulmonary compromise, effective control of salivation is even more critical. When measures to decrease saliva production are not sufficient, tracheostomy, laryngotracheal separation, and laryngectomy may be required to prevent recurrent pneumonias. However, with advances in the treatment of drooling over the past several decades, these procedures are rarely necessary.

■ Conclusion

Drooling in the pediatric patient is a complex problem with many potential etiologies, and treatment requires an understanding of the underlying causes and a multidisciplinary approach to the treatment and possible complications of drooling. Treatment options range from behavioral changes to medications to botulinum toxin injections and to surgery, but many of the treatment options have side effects that must be considered along with the potential for an improvement in drooling. Patients derive the most benefit from an individualized approach to their drooling to remove correctable causes, avoid irreversible procedures and known adverse effects when possible, and address the potential risk of aspiration.

■ Selected References

Bachrach SJ, Walter RS, Trzcinski K. Use of glycopyrrolate and other anticholinergic medications for sialorrhea in children with cerebral palsy. *Clin Pediatr (Phila)*. 1998;37(8):485–490

Benson J, Daugherty KK. Botulinum toxin A in the treatment of sialorrhea. *Ann Pharmacother*. 2007;41(1):79–85

Blasco PA, Stansbury JC. Glycopyrrolate treatment of chronic drooling. *Arch Pediatr Adolesc Med*. 1996;150(9):932–935

Borg M, Hirst F. The role of radiation therapy in the management of sialorrhea. *Int J Radiat Oncol Biol Phys*. 1998;41(5):1113–1119

Bothwell JE, Clarke K, Dooley JM, et al. Botulinum toxin A as a treatment for excessive drooling in children. *Pediatr Neurol*. 2002;27(1):18–22

Camp-Bruno JA, Winsberg BG, Green-Parsons AR, Abrams JP. Efficacy of benztropine therapy for drooling. *Dev Med Child Neurol*. 1989;31(3):309–319

Chang CJ, May-Kuen Wong AA. Intraductal laser photocoagulation of the bilateral parotid ducts for reduction of drooling in patients with cerebral palsy. *Plast Reconstr Surg*. 2001;107(4):907–913

Chanu NP, Sahni JK, Aneja S, Naglot S. Four-duct ligation in children with drooling. *Am J Otolaryngol*. 2012;33(5):604–607

Crysdale WS. Management options for the drooling patient. *Ear Nose Throat J*. 1989; 68(11):820, 825–826, 829–830

El-Hakim H, Richards S, Thevasagayam MS. Major salivary duct clipping for control problems in developmentally challenged children. *Arch Otolaryngol Head Neck Surg*. 2008;134(5):470–474

Freudenreich O. Drug-induced sialorrhea. *Drugs Today (Barc)*. 2005;41(6):411–418

Garrett JR, Proctor GB. Control of salivation. In: Linden RWA, ed. *The Scientific Basis of Eating*. Basel, Switzerland: Karger; 1998:135–155

Grewal DS, Hiranandani NL, Rangwalla ZA, Sheode JH. Transtympanic neurectomies for control of drooling. *Auris Nasus Larynx*. 1984;11(2):109–114

Hockstein NG, Samadi DS, Gendron K, Handler SD. Sialorrhea: a management challenge. *Am Fam Physician*. 2004;69(11):2628–2634

Jongerius PH, Joosten F, Hoogen FJ, Gabreels FJ, Rotteveel JJ. The treatment of drooling by ultrasound-guided intraglandular injections of botulinum toxin type A into the salivary glands. *Laryngoscope.* 2003;113(1):107–111

Jongerius PH, van den Hoogen FJ, van Limbeek J, Gabreëls FJ, van Hulst K, Rotteveel JJ. Effect of botulinum toxin in the treatment of drooling: a controlled clinical trial. *Pediatrics.* 2004;114(3):620–627

Jongerius PH, van Tiel P, van Limbeek J, Gabreëls FJ, Rotteveel JJ. A systematic review for evidence of efficacy of anticholinergic drugs to treat drooling. *Arch Dis Child.* 2003;88(10):911–914

Khan WU, Islam A, Fu A, et al. Four-duct ligation for the treatment of sialorrhea in children. *JAMA Otolaryngol Head Neck Surg.* 2016;142(3):278–283

Klem C, Mair EA. Four-duct ligation: a simple and effective treatment for chronic aspiration from sialorrhea. *Arch Otolaryngol Head Neck Surg.* 1999;125(7):796–800

Lewis DW, Fontana C, Mehallick LK, Everett Y. Transdermal scopolamine for reduction of drooling in developmentally delayed children. *Dev Med Child Neurol.* 1994;36(6):484–486

Mahadevan M, Gruber M, Bilish D, Edwards K, Davies-Payne D, van der Meer G. Botulinum toxin injections for chronic sialorrhoea in children are effective regardless of the degree of neurological dysfunction: a single tertiary institution experience. *Int J Pediatr Otorhinolaryngol.* 2016;88:142–145

Mier RJ, Bachrach SJ, Lakin RC, Barker T, Childs J, Moran M. Treatment of sialorrhea with glycopyrrolate: a double-blind, dose-ranging study. *Arch Pediatr Adolesc Med.* 2000;154(12):1214–1218

Mullins WM, Gross CW, Moore JM. Long-term follow-up of tympanic neurectomy for sialorrhea. *Laryngoscope.* 1979;89(8):1219–1223

Pena AH, Cahill AM, Gonzalez L, Baskin KM, Kim H, Towbin RB. Botulinum toxin A injection of salivary glands in children with drooling and chronic aspiration. *J Vasc Interv Radiol.* 2009;20(3):368–373

Reddihough D, Johnson H, Staples M, Hudson I, Exarchos H. Use of benzhexol hydrochloride to control drooling of children with cerebral palsy. *Dev Med Child Neurol.* 1990;32(11):985–989

Reed J, Mans CK, Brietzke SE. Surgical management of drooling: a meta-analysis. *Arch Otolaryngol Head Neck Surg.* 2009;135(9):924–931

Scully C, Limeres J, Gleeson M, Tomás I, Diz P. Drooling. *J Oral Pathol Med.* 2009; 38(4):321–327

Talmi YP, Finkelstein Y, Zohar Y. Reduction of salivary flow with transdermal scopolamine: a four-year experience. *Otolaryngol Head Neck Surg.* 1990;103(4):615–618

Tscheng DZ. Sialorrhea: therapeutic drug options. *Ann Pharmacother.* 2002;36(11):1785–1790

Wilken B, Aslami B, Backes H. Successful treatment of drooling in children with neurological disorders with botulinum toxin A or B. *Neuropediatrics.* 2008;39(4):200–204

Wilkie TF. The problem of drooling in cerebral palsy: a surgical approach. *Can J Surg.* 1967;10(1):60–67

Wilkie TF, Brody GS. The surgical treatment of drooling: a ten-year review. *Plast Reconstr Surg.* 1977;59(6):791–797

CHAPTER 21

Chronic Cough in Children

David H. Darrow, MD, DDS, and Ian N. Jacobs, MD

▨ Introduction

Cough is one of the most common reasons patients seek medical attention. It accounts for 8.5% of all visits to a primary care clinician (PCC), causing financial burden for families because of time missed from work and medical expenditures. Most cases are caused by self-limited illnesses resulting from viral infections of the upper respiratory tract that resolve within 2 to 3 weeks. However, prolonged cough is a potential cause of discomfort for the child, anxiety for the parent, and sleep disturbance for both. Fear of a significant underlying pathology and the potential for injury are frequent parental concerns, and, indeed, chronic cough may portend a more serious disorder.

▓ Mechanism

Cough is the sudden and violent expulsion of air in late inspiration after the complete closure of the laryngeal sphincter. This results in the rapid expulsion of deep lung gaseous contents and facilitates clearance of abnormal secretions and infections, as well as expulsion of foreign bodies. Cough also prevents foreign material from entering the trachea in the first place.

Cough requires a neurologically competent larynx and pharynx as well as diaphragm and chest wall. Patients with vocal cord paralysis or loss of afferent sensation of the larynx may not have a competent cough and may be susceptible to aspiration and lower airway problems. Patients with diaphragmatic paralysis also may not be able to generate an effective cough.

Cough is mediated by the cough reflex arc (**Figure 21-1**). Cough receptors are found in varying concentrations in the mucosa of the entire respiratory tract, including the larynx, trachea, bronchi, pharynx, and nasal passages. Sensory fibers of the afferent limb, when stimulated by incidental contact or pressure with a foreign body or noxious agent, transmit impulses to the cough center in the medulla. Efferent

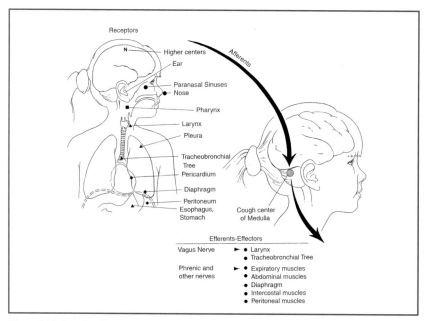

Figure 21-1. Cough reflex mechanism.

From Holinger LD, Sanders AD. Chronic cough in infants and children: an update. *Laryngoscope.* 1991;101(6 Pt 1):596–605, with permission from John Wiley & Sons.

impulses, in turn, travel from the medulla to the end organs, including the diaphragm, intercostal muscles, laryngeal adductors, and external chest wall muscles, via the vagus and phrenic nerves. This results in a violent Valsalva maneuver, which acts to expel debris or the noxious offending agent. The cough reflex is weak in premature neonates and develops by about age 5 years; this fact correlates with 5 years as the age at which accidental nut aspiration becomes less common.

> **Pearl:** Children younger than 5 years should not be fed nuts because their gag reflex is not yet mature enough to protect the airway against aspiration.

■ Clinical Assessment of the Child With Chronic Cough

The etiologies of cough are diverse and numerous (**Box 21-1**). As a result, it is critical that the PCC develop a conceptual framework for clinical and laboratory assessment of the child with cough.

HISTORY

Age

Patient age is one of the most important factors in determining the etiology of cough (**Box 21-2**). Among children from birth to 18 months of age, the most common causes of chronic cough are gastroesophageal reflux disease (GERD); congenital airway abnormalities such as tracheomalacia, laryngeal cleft, tracheoesophageal fistula (TEF) with direct aspiration, and long segment tracheal stenosis; and pertussis. In toddlers and young children, the most common cause of chronic cough is recurrent viral illness; in affected children, the illnesses are of typical duration, but the disease-free interval is very brief. Allergies, chronic sinusitis, cough-dominant asthma, cystic fibrosis, bronchitis, and pneumonia are also frequently encountered in this age group. In addition, this is the age group in which bronchial or other airway foreign bodies most commonly present. In school-aged children, cough-dominant asthma, infections (sinus and lung), psychogenic cough (habit cough), and allergies predominate as the causes of cough.

Box 21-1. Etiologies of Cough

Cough-Dominant Asthma	**Genetic**
Infections	Cystic fibrosis
Acute and chronic sinusitis	Immotile cilia syndrome
Adenoiditis	**Aspiration**
Adenovirus	Foreign body
Influenza	Gastroesophageal reflux disease
Pertussis	Saliva
Pneumonia	
Tuberculosis	
Congenital	**Psychogenic**
Congenital heart disease	**Neoplastic**
Laryngeal cleft	Airway hemangioma
Subglottic stenosis	Laryngotracheal papillomatosis
Tracheoesophageal fistula	Mediastinal tumor
Tracheomalacia	Neoplasms of the tracheobronchial tree
Vascular compression	
Vocal cord paralysis	
Environmental	
Cigarette smoke	
Pollution	

Box 21-2. Causes of Chronic Cough According to Age

Infants	**Older Children and Adolescents**
Airway anomalies	Allergy
GERD and feeding disorders	Bronchitis/bronchiolitis
Pertussis	Cough-dominant asthma
Toddlers and Young Children	Chronic sinusitis
Allergy	Cystic fibrosis
Airway foreign body	Psychogenic cough
Bronchitis/bronchiolitis	Pneumonia
Chronic sinusitis	Recurrent viral illness
Cough-dominant asthma	
Cystic fibrosis	
GERD	
Pertussis	
Pneumonia	
Recurrent viral illness	

Abbreviation: GERD, gastroesophageal reflux disease.

Character of Cough

Cough can be characterized on the basis of tonal qualities as well as the presence or absence of secretions. Barky cough is typical of subglottic disease (croup, subglottic stenosis, subglottic cyst, or hemangioma). Brassy cough is similar in tone but emanates more from the chest, suggesting tracheobronchial disorders (bronchitis, tracheomalacia, tracheal stenosis). In pertussis, a high-pitched "whoop" sound frequently follows the paroxysms of cough in the early stages of the disease. A wet or productive cough usually is present in pulmonary infections, bronchitis, chronic sinusitis, or any infection producing an abundance of mucus and secretions. A dry cough may be related to infections producing minimal secretions or to noninfectious processes, such as airway anomalies, cough-dominant asthma, airway foreign body, or habit cough. Unfortunately, studies suggest that parents have difficulty correctly characterizing wet and dry cough. Hemoptysis may suggest the presence of a neoplasm, a vascular anomaly, or severe inflammation.

Frequency, Duration, and Timing of Cough

In the absence of upper respiratory illness (URI) or other pathology, children will experience 10 or 11 cough episodes per day. Cough that is considered pathological should be substantially in excess of this number.

Although some infectious processes may last several weeks, it is critical that pathologies such as foreign bodies of the airway be discovered in a reasonable amount of time. As a result, cough persisting for more than 4 weeks should be considered chronic and merits more than clinical evaluation. Cough that recurs after appropriate therapy may warrant endoscopic evaluation for an underlying airway problem.

In newborns and infants, timing of the cough in relation to feeding may suggest a cause. Infants with laryngotracheal clefts or TEF typically cough *during* the swallow. Children with gastroesophageal reflux more commonly cough *after* feeding and when placed in a supine position.

As a rule, sleep generally suppresses cough. However, because nighttime is the quietest time of day, the presence of any cough at night is often unsettling to parents. Wet cough caused by postnasal drip may be exacerbated in the supine position. Conversely, habit cough will completely disappear during sleep.

Cough during URI may increase with exertion or exercise. However, cough present only during exercise is more typically associated with asthma or psychogenic etiology.

Pearl: Habit cough disappears completely during sleep.

Additional History

Additional information may be useful in identifying the etiology of a chronic cough. A history of endotracheal intubation, especially in a young child with a history of prematurity, suggests the presence of an acquired airway lesion. Parents of toddlers should be asked about circumstances that might suggest ingestion or aspiration of a foreign body. Symptoms of wheezing in association with chronic cough are common in very young children because of the small caliber of their airways; however, wheezing should also alert the PCC to the possibility of asthma. The PCC also should inquire about environmental irritants, such as tobacco smoke, that delay the resolution of cough and about any recurrent infections that might suggest an immune deficiency.

PHYSICAL EXAMINATION

The general appearance of the coughing child may provide some insight into the severity and cause of the problem. For example, the absence of cough during the office visit may prompt further inquiry into the actual frequency of cough and exacerbating factors. Children whose coughing ceases when asked to focus on other things during the examination are more likely to have habit cough. Tachypnea and stridor associated with cough are often immediately apparent on initial patient contact. Other patients may exhibit obvious signs of allergy or URI.

Anterior rhinoscopy may be performed using an otoscope with a large-diameter speculum. Findings of swollen, edematous mucosa and clear, watery rhinorrhea may suggest the presence of allergy, while mucoid or purulent secretions are associated with viral URI or sinusitis. Postnasal drip also may be evident on oropharyngeal examination. Nasal polyps are pathognomonic of cystic fibrosis.

Auscultation of the neck and chest yields important information about the condition of the lower airway and lungs. In cough caused by subglottic pathology, stridor can generally be appreciated over the neck. Decreased breath sounds over the chest may indicate an aspirated foreign body or consolidation due to infection. Wheezing is most suggestive of asthma, although foreign bodies and airway anomalies should be considered as well.

■ Additional Investigation

The history and clinical examination are useful in establishing the diagnoses shown in **Box 21-1** that are the most likely causes of chronic cough in a child. A clinical practice guideline from the American College of Chest Physicians proposes that these be further classified as *specific* or *nonspecific* causes of cough based on a set of indicators (**Box 21-3**). A specific cough is often wet and associated with underlying respiratory or systemic disease. The diagnosis often is made based on coexisting symptoms or laboratory findings suggestive of a particular disease. A nonspecific cough is defined as cough in the absence of these indicators; in such cases, the cough is the primary symptom and is usually dry. Individuals with nonspecific cough may also have a higher level of cough sensitivity, which can occur following routine viral URI.

The causes of chronic cough vary in prevalence among epidemiologic studies depending on the population studied. The most common etiologies are persistent bacterial bronchitis, asthma, gastroesophageal reflux, and upper airway cough syndrome, the latter referring to disorders including URI, allergy, and sinusitis in which the cough clears secretions of nasal origin from the larynx. Based on these data, it is reasonable for the PCC to begin empirical pharmacotherapy with antibiotics for possible bronchitis or sinusitis, or with a trial of inhaled corticosteroids to treat suspected asthma. Children who do not respond to treatment should undergo, at a minimum, chest radiography and spirometry.

Box 21-3. Indicators of Specific Cough in Children	
Daily, wet, or productive cough	Recurrent pneumonia
Auscultatory findings (wheeze or crackles)	Cardiac abnormalities (including murmurs)
Chronic dyspnea	Immune deficiency
Exertional dyspnea	Failure to thrive
Hemoptysis	Digital clubbing
Duration >6 months	Swallowing problems

Chang AB, Glomb WB. Guidelines for evaluating chronic cough in pediatrics: ACCP evidence-based clinical practice guidelines. *Chest.* 2006;129(1 Suppl):260S–283S.

Plain radiographs of the chest are useful for delineating infiltrates, radiopaque foreign bodies, and other types of infections. Inspiratory and expiratory views or lateral decubitus views also may show hyperinflation suggestive of a foreign aspiration with air trapping. Additional images of the neck may demonstrate subglottic pathology including stenosis, hemangiomas, or cysts.

Spirometry is indicated to identify disorders of reversible airway obstruction associated with cough. Testing is limited, in many cases, by the age of the patient, but it should be achievable in most children older than 3 years. When age or developmental status prohibits such testing, empirical treatment for asthma may be necessary.

> **Pearl:** Children with specific cough who do not respond to a trial of pharmacotherapy should undergo, at a minimum, chest radiography and spirometry.

EVALUATION OF SPECIFIC COUGH

Patients with signs and symptoms of respiratory disease, abnormalities on chest radiographs or spirometry, or cough characteristic of a particular disorder are considered to have specific cough and should undergo a directed evaluation. Diagnoses such as bronchiectasis, cystic fibrosis, and immune deficiency should be considered in children with chronic purulent cough. Computed tomography (CT) of the chest may be performed to demonstrate bronchiectasis, interstitial lung disease, or foreign bodies. It also may be useful in the diagnosis of chronic sinusitis but should be reserved for children with a consistent clinical picture in whom empirical medical therapy has failed. Patients with findings consistent with asthma should be treated empirically for 4 weeks and then reassessed. Diagnostic laboratory testing based on clinical indicators includes purified protein derivative (PPD), sweat chloride, and immunoglobulin titers.

Recommended testing for gastroesophageal reflux may vary among PCCs and might be delayed in favor of a trial of pharmacologic therapy, including histamine-2 receptor antagonists (H$_2$ blockers) or proton pump inhibitors. Such testing typically involves pH probes, impedance testing, or endoscopic evaluation. Upper gastrointestinal (GI) radiographic studies and nuclear scans are somewhat less useful, although swallow studies in infants who cough in association with feeding may demonstrate aspiration as a potential cause of the cough.

When the diagnosis behind chronic cough remains uncertain, referral to a pulmonologist or an otolaryngologist for endoscopy should be considered. In most cases, examination of the airway is performed under sedation using a flexible fiber-optic bronchoscope with side-port suction placed via a face mask or laryngeal mask airway. Mobility of the vocal folds is best assessed at this time and any airway anomalies are noted. Bronchoalveolar lavage is performed to obtain cultures and stains for bacteria (including mycobacteria), fungi, and viruses. Specimens are also obtained for quantitation of lipid-laden macrophages and to assay for pepsin, both of which are suggestive of aspiration due to reflux. Mucosal biopsy specimens may be obtained from the carina, bronchi, or nasal turbinates and sent for ultrastructural analysis of the cilia. Rigid airway endoscopy is less ideal for bronchial lavage but facilitates delivery of anesthesia and removal of any foreign bodies while providing a superior view of the airway. Upper GI endoscopy is often performed under the same anesthetic to obtain biopsy specimens of the esophagus that may suggest GERD or eosinophilic esophagitis, 2 common causes of cough. When recommended by the gastroenterologist, the procedure can be combined with impedance probes.

EVALUATION OF NONSPECIFIC COUGH

Children with no signs or symptoms of respiratory disease and normal findings on chest radiographs and spirometry have nonspecific cough. Because most cases of nonspecific cough are postinfectious, a 1- to 2-week period of additional observation is recommended prior to consideration of additional intervention. During this time, it is important to avoid environmental irritants that may prolong the inflammation of the airway or maintain a higher level of cough sensitivity. If cough persists, additional empirical treatment with inhaled corticosteroids or antibiotics is recommended. In children who remain unresponsive, a diagnosis of habit cough should be entertained; however, this is usually a diagnosis of exclusion, and referral to a pulmonologist is prudent.

> **Pearl:** Nonspecific cough is usually postinfectious and self-limited.

Treatment

Successful treatment of cough depends on an accurate diagnosis of the cause. Studies suggest that treatment algorithms (**Figure 21-2**) are useful in the assessment and management of chronic cough, and recent clinical practice guidelines advocate their use. Management of the myriad causes of cough is beyond the scope of this chapter; however, several disorders are worthy of brief discussion.

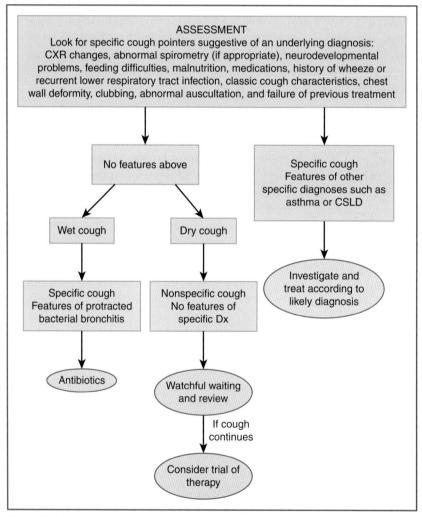

Figure 21-2. Algorithm for management of chronic cough.

Abbreviations: CSLD, chronic suppurative lung disease; CXR, chest radiograph; Dx, diagnosis.

From Chang AB, Robertson CF, van Asperen PP, et al. A cough algorithm for chronic cough in children: a multicenter, randomized controlled study. *Pediatrics*. 2013;131(5):e1576–e1583.

INFECTIONS OF THE LUNGS

Cough caused by lung infections may require prolonged courses of intravenous antibiotics as well as inhalational steroids and bronchodilators. *Streptococcus pneumoniae* and *Staphylococcus aureus* are common bacterial causes, although anaerobes may be present in cases of suspected aspiration. When sputum can be obtained, an accurate culture, Gram stain, and sensitivity may determine the optimal antimicrobial agent. Often, the disease must be treated empirically with broad-spectrum antibiotics and may take weeks to eradicate.

Other infectious etiologies include viral infections, *Mycoplasma pneumoniae, Bordetella pertussis,* and mycobacteria. Diagnosis of mycoplasma may be made based on specific IgM and IgG antibody production and cold agglutinins. *Bordetella* outbreaks are not unusual despite required vaccination programs. In the early phase of illness, rhinitis, conjunctivitis, low-grade fever, and mild cough are present. However, as the airway mucosa is infiltrated with lymphocytes and polymorphonuclear leukocytes, it begins to slough, leading to violent coughing paroxysms associated with a characteristic whoop. The disease may progress to complete respiratory failure in infants and young children. Treatment involves isolation to prevent further spread, especially from low-risk hosts to higher-risk hosts, and erythromycin (40 to 50 mg/kg/day), which is administered for at least 14 days. In infections caused by *Mycobacterium tuberculosis*, exposure results in few early symptoms, and respiratory symptoms usually progress slowly. Chest radiographic findings will remain negative even as the PPD converts to positive. Several months later, patients may develop progressive cough, malaise, and night sweats. Chest radiographs ultimately demonstrate lobar infiltrates, cavitary lesions, or military pattern. Treatment consists of a multidrug regimen.

COUGH-DOMINANT ASTHMA

The diagnosis of cough-dominant asthma is often difficult to make. The methacholine challenge test for bronchoprovocation is still occasionally performed in pulmonology practices, but more commonly the diagnosis is established based on the patient's response to bronchodilators and inhaled steroids. Treatment failures may be because of noncompliance with the medication regimen or failure to recognize and treat a secondary problem.

CHRONIC SINONASAL ILLNESS

Recurrent viral URI, recurrent acute sinusitis, chronic sinusitis, and allergic rhinitis may present with a moist, productive cough related to constant postnasal drip. In most children, chronic cough of sinonasal etiology results from frequent viral illness, with only brief periods of improvement or recovery. As a result, in children with chronic cough and rhinorrhea, it is imperative to try to ascertain whether the disorder improves at all within the typical 10- to 14-day duration of viral illness. Nasal saline irrigations may be useful in treating these self-limited cases. In recurrent acute or chronic sinusitis, a course of empirical antimicrobial therapy is usually indicated. Children whose condition fails to improve should be considered for referral to an otolaryngologist for endoscopic examination with or without cultures. In most refractory cases, adenoidectomy will be considered before CT scanning of the sinuses or sinus surgery is considered.

Symptoms of allergy should be distinguished from those of sinusitis based on systemic manifestations and quality of the rhinorrhea. Ultimately, affected children should undergo formal testing by an allergist or a trial of some combination of intranasal steroids, antihistamines, and leukotriene inhibitors.

GASTROESOPHAGEAL REFLUX AND FEEDING DISORDERS

Dietary modification, prokinetic agents, proton pump inhibitors, and H_2 blockers are used to treat GERD. Refractory cases may require surgery such as Nissen fundoplication or feeding assessment for postpyloric feeds.

Swallowing dysfunction may cause cough with chronic aspiration. Treatment strategies are based on the results of radiologic or endoscopic swallow evaluations or operative endoscopy. Certain feeding strategies such as thickening or avoidance of certain textures may minimize the cough. Surgery may be required if laryngeal cleft or TEF is present.

CONGENITAL AIRWAY DISORDERS

These disorders require endoscopic or open surgical repair and comprise the aberrant innominate artery with tracheal compression, laryngeal clefts, TEFs, subglottic stenosis, and tracheomalacia. Small laryngeal clefts (type 1) respond to endoscopic surgical closure; larger clefts and TEFs require open repair. The aberrant innominate artery requires aortopexy, which relieves the cough and lower airway symptoms. Subglottic stenosis requires intervention in severe cases.

HABIT COUGH AND PARADOXICAL VOCAL CORD DYSFUNCTION

Habit cough is usually related to stress and behavioral factors. The cough often begins with a viral syndrome but persists after improvement of the other symptoms. The cough is usually worse during the day and disappears at night. Biofeedback, breathing exercises, and psychological counseling may help. Benzonatate may help in refractory cases. In most cases, habit cough is self-limited.

Paradoxical vocal cord dysfunction is also typically stress related. It presents most commonly with stridor, but obstructive and cough-like symptoms may occur as well. Treatment is aimed at education through awareness, biofeedback, and stress relaxation. Specific breathing exercises with sniffing techniques can be performed with a speech/swallow specialist.

■ Selected References

Chang AB, Glomb WB. Guidelines for evaluating chronic cough in pediatrics: ACCP evidence-based clinical practice guidelines. *Chest*. 2006;129(1 Suppl):260S–283S

Chang AB, Oppenheimer JJ, Weinberger MM, et al; on behalf of the CHEST Expert Cough Panel. Use of management pathways or algorithms in children with chronic cough: CHEST guideline and expert panel report. *Chest*. 2017;151(4):875–883

Chang AB, Robertson CF, van Asperen PP, et al. A cough algorithm for chronic cough in children: a multicenter, randomized controlled study. *Pediatrics*. 2013;131(5): e1576–e1583

Denoyelle F, Leboulanger N, Enjolras O, Harris R, Roger G, Garabedian EN. Role of propranolol in the therapeutic strategy of infantile laryngotracheal hemangioma. *Int J Pediatr Otorhinolaryngol*. 2009;73(8):1168–1172

Donnelly D, Everard ML. 'Dry' and 'wet' cough: how reliable is parental reporting? *BMJ Open Respir Res*. 2019;6(1):e000375

Goldsobel AB, Chipps BE. Cough in the pediatric population. *J Pediatr*. 2010;156(3): 352–358

Holinger LD. In: Cotton RT, Myer CM III, eds. *Practical Pediatric Otolaryngology*. Philadelphia, PA: Lippincott-Raven Publishers; 1999:117–128

Holinger LD, Sanders AD. Chronic cough in infants and children: an update. *Laryngoscope*. 1991;101(6 Pt 1):596–605

Leigh MW, Zariwala MA, Knowles MR. Primary ciliary dyskinesia: improving the diagnostic approach. *Curr Opin Pediatr*. 2009;21(3):320–325

Mayerhoff RM, Pitman MJ. Atypical and disparate presentations of laryngeal sarcoidosis. *Ann Otol Rhinol Laryngol*. 2010;119(10):667–671

Meyer AA, Aitken PV Jr. Evaluation of persistent cough in children. *Prim Care.* 1996; 23(4):883–892

Milgrom H, Corsello P, Freedman M, Blager FB, Wood RP. Differential diagnosis and management of chronic cough. *Compr Ther.* 1990;16(10):46–53

Shaikh N, Wald ER, Pi M. Decongestants, antihistamines and nasal irrigation for acute sinusitis in children. *Cochrane Database Syst Rev.* 2010;(12):CD007909

CHAPTER 22

Aerodigestive Tract Foreign Bodies

Kristina W. Rosbe, MD, and Elizabeth A. Shuman, MD

Introduction
Epidemiology and Prevention
Signs and Symptoms
Imaging
Treatment
  Airway Foreign Body

Oropharyngeal Foreign
  Body
Esophageal Foreign
  Body
Recovery
Complications

▒ Introduction

Foreign body ingestion and aspiration are an important cause of morbidity and mortality in the pediatric population. Foreign bodies remain a diagnostic challenge because their presentation can vary from life-threatening airway compromise to subtle respiratory symptoms that often are misdiagnosed. A high level of clinical suspicion can prevent delays in diagnosis and complications related to these delays.

▒ Epidemiology and Prevention

Aerodigestive tract foreign bodies are the cause of approximately 150 pediatric deaths per year in the United States, and choking causes 40% of accidental deaths in children younger than 1 year. Most aerodigestive tract foreign bodies occur in children younger than 4 years. The high incidence of aerodigestive foreign bodies in children of this age is related to their increased mobility, introduction of adult food, high propensity for placing objects in their mouths, incomplete dentition, and immature swallowing coordination. Other populations at risk for esophageal foreign bodies include psychiatric patients, patients with underlying esophageal or neurologic disease, and edentulous adults. Coins are the most commonly swallowed foreign bodies in infants and toddlers (**Figure 22-1**); in older children and adults, fish or chicken bones may lodge in the oropharynx. Nuts and seeds are the most commonly aspirated foreign bodies (**Figure 22-2**). Fortunately, mortality

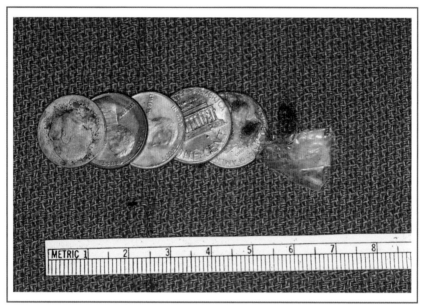

Figure 22-1. Coins are the most commonly swallowed foreign bodies in infants and children.

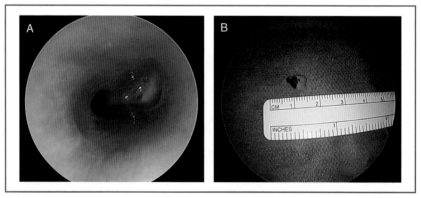

Figure 22-2. Right main bronchus obstruction. A, Almond fragment aspirated into right main bronchus. B, Extracted fragment.

is rare in foreign body accidents; however, the foreign bodies most commonly responsible in such cases are latex balloons.

The prevention of ingestion is the most important intervention for potential aerodigestive tract foreign body ingestions. The Consumer Products Safety Act was passed in 1979 and includes criteria for the minimum size of objects (>3.17 cm in diameter and >5.71 cm in length) allowable for children to play with; however, these regulations are not uniformly enforced. The small parts test fixture (SPTF) is a cylinder simulating the mouth (diameter) and pharynx (depth) with these dimensions (**Figure 22-3**). If an object can fit within the SPTF, it is considered a small part. Small balls are held to an even stricter standard given their high-risk shape; they must be 1.75 inches or larger for children younger than 3 years. The Consumer Product Safety Improvement Act of 2008 amended the Federal Hazardous Substances Act (FHSA) to include choking-hazard warnings in all media (eg, websites, catalogs) with direct means for purchase of objects for which a warning is required under the FHSA. Some suggest that even stricter dimensions should be adopted for the small part cylinder, which potentially could prevent at least 20% of the injuries and fatalities resulting from foreign body ingestions and aspirations in children. Young children should remain under constant adult supervision and be allowed to play only with age-appropriate toys. Small and hazardous objects should be safely stored so as not to be accessible to a newly mobile and curious child.

Some common foods, such as whole grapes, carrots, nuts, seeds, and hot dogs, are implicated in aspiration events, due, in part, to their shape and ability to obstruct without dissolving. Bright Futures offers guidance for prevention of choking on food, including ways to prepare high-risk foods to make them safer. Because many of the above policies have not been implemented to prevent choking on food, the American Academy of Pediatrics released a policy statement in 2010 aimed at government bodies, food manufacturers, parents, and physicians outlining regulations on choking hazards, with a particular emphasis on food products. These recommendations include the following:

- Label foods that pose a high choking risk
- Recall food products that pose a significant choking hazard
- Establish a national food-related choking-incident surveillance and reporting system
- Design new food and redesign existing food to minimize choking risk

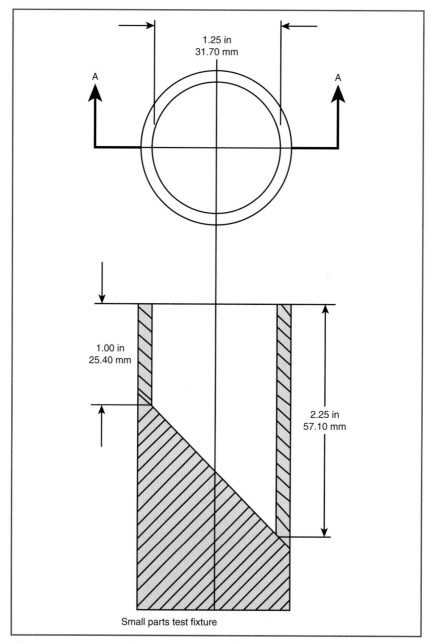

1.25 in
31.70 mm

A   A

1.00 in
25.40 mm

2.25 in
57.10 mm

Small parts test fixture

Figure 22-3. Small parts test fixture diagram. https://www.cpsc.gov/Business—Manufacturing/ Business-Education/Business-Guidance/Small-Parts-for-Toys-and-Childrens-Products.

- Provide choking-prevention counseling as part of anticipatory guidance by pediatricians, dentists, and other child health care professionals
- Teach cardiopulmonary resuscitation and choking first aid to parents, teachers, and child care providers

Food should be age appropriate and presented only in an observed setting. Furthermore, children with esophageal motility disorders or neurologic disorders should be encouraged to chew food slowly and completely to avoid esophageal impactions or aspiration.

■ Signs and Symptoms

A witnessed ingestion or aspiration episode should be brought to the attention of a physician. Information that is important to elicit from parents includes the approximate time of ingestion, any history of esophageal dysfunction, and severity and duration of swallowing and respiratory symptoms since the time of ingestion. When an unusual foreign body is aspirated or ingested, it may also be helpful to have parents bring in a similar object from home.

Typical signs and symptoms of esophageal foreign body ingestion include drooling, dysphagia, emesis, food refusal, and chest pain. Esophageal foreign bodies may also cause respiratory symptoms in a young child because of swelling in the wall shared by the trachea and esophagus. Airway foreign bodies may present with an episode of choking, gagging, and cyanosis followed by coughing, wheezing, or stridor. Physical examination may reveal asymmetric breath sounds or unilateral wheezing. However, the patient may be asymptomatic if air can pass through or around the foreign body, or when the reflexes fatigue after the foreign body has been present a long time. This can make diagnosis difficult, especially when the event was not witnessed.

> **Pearl:** A high index of suspicion should be maintained when evaluating children with a sudden onset of respiratory symptoms or with recurrent croup, asthma, chronic cough, or pneumonia without the expected response to treatment.

Imaging

Posteroanterior (PA) and lateral plain radiographs of the neck and chest are the imaging studies of choice. Radiopaque foreign bodies should be straightforward to diagnose, whereas organic and other radiolucent foreign bodies may be more difficult. Unilateral hyperinflation, localized atelectasis or infiltrates, mediastinal shift, and esophageal air trapping can be clues to the presence of a foreign body, even when no foreign body is visualized (**Figure 22-4**). Posteroanterior and lateral views should be obtained because they can help differentiate between esophageal and tracheal foreign bodies as well as provide clues regarding the type of foreign body. For example, the "halo" associated with button batteries on PA views is not always apparent. The clinician also should look for the characteristic "double contour" on lateral views in such cases (**Figure 22-5**).

Imaging studies should not be used to rule out the presence of a foreign body. High clinical suspicion or historical evidence (ie, witnessed ingestion or aspiration) warrants rigid endoscopy even if imaging study findings are normal. If plain radiographs are not diagnostic or the patient cannot cooperate for the imaging examination, airway fluoroscopy is sometimes used. This study has the advantage of demonstrating a dynamic view of the airway; however, it is dependent on the expertise of the radiologist performing the examination. In equivocal cases, the newer technology

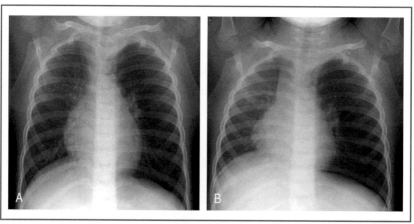

Figure 22-4. Inspiratory (A) and expiratory (B) radiographs of the chest demonstrating air trapping in the left lung.

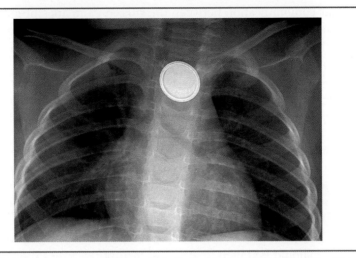

Figure 22-5. Button battery in esophagus. Note the "halo" near the rim, diagnostic of this foreign body. If not present, lateral radiograph may demonstrate a double contour.

in computed tomography provides rapid, high-definition imaging requiring only low-dose radiation, and allows for characterization of the shape and location of a foreign body. These studies can be performed without general anesthesia and may obviate the need for general anesthesia for diagnostic bronchoscopy to confirm the absence of a foreign body. Barium swallow is generally not indicated, and the presence of barium can make esophageal foreign body extraction more difficult.

■ Treatment

The treatment of choice for most aerodigestive tract foreign bodies is rigid endoscopic removal under general anesthesia. This procedure is carried out in the operating room with proper pediatric endoscopic equipment and pediatric anesthesiologists.

AIRWAY FOREIGN BODY

Most surgeons agree that an airway foreign body should be addressed at the time of presentation. That said, rigid bronchoscopy in a stable child with a subacute presentation may be deferred until the following morning when specialized personnel (ie, pediatric anesthesiologists) are present. Rapid-sequence induction techniques may be preferred if aspiration of stomach contents is a concern.

Clear communication between the surgeon and anesthesiologist is paramount regarding the appropriate depth of anesthesia for each step of the procedure. Spontaneous breathing during retrieval of an airway foreign body facilitates passage of a bronchoscope, prevents distal migration, and takes advantage of the natural increase in tracheal and bronchial cross-sectional area during inspiration. In addition, it lowers the risk of inability to ventilate should the foreign body strip off the extraction forceps during the procedure. After mask induction with an inhalational agent, topical lidocaine should be used to anesthetize the vocal folds. Direct laryngoscopy is performed and a rigid bronchoscope is introduced under direct vision. Once the bronchoscope has been introduced, the anesthesiologist may connect to the ventilation port. The foreign body is identified, secured against the tip of the bronchoscope, and removed with the scope as a unit. Care should be taken to avoid premature release of the foreign body because this can result in an obstructing laryngotracheal foreign body. Nuts and other foods may require multiple passes. Care should be taken to minimize mucosal trauma. Before completion, at least 1 more pass should be performed to evaluate for multiple foreign bodies and mucosal damage. Depending on the ease of extraction, the child may require a postoperative chest radiograph and close follow-up to rule out the development of pneumonia.

OROPHARYNGEAL FOREIGN BODY

Rarely, an oropharyngeal foreign body in an older, cooperative child, such as a fish bone impaling the tonsil, may be extracted when the patient is awake. Alternate methods of removal (eg, Fogarty or Foley catheters, bougienage, flexible endoscopes) have been used successfully at some facilities but are generally not recommended because of the difficulty in protecting the airway and controlling the foreign body with these methods.

ESOPHAGEAL FOREIGN BODY

The timing of esophageal foreign body removal can be debated based on the type and location of the foreign body, the elapsed time since ingestion, and the patient's age. An asymptomatic older child with a distal or midesophageal coin present for less than 24 hours and no history of esophageal disorders may be observed for 8 to 16 hours to see if the coin will pass. Meat tenderizers, muscle relaxants, and promotility agents have been used for esophageal foreign bodies in adults, but no evidence supports their use in pediatric patients. Spontaneous coin passage rates range widely from 9% to 77% in this patient population. In cases involving young children, foreign bodies present for longer than 24 hours, sharp metallic or caustic foreign bodies (eg, button batteries), and severe symptoms (eg, respiratory symptoms, discomfort, pooling, or intolerance of oral secretions) observation for spontaneous passage is not appropriate.

Disc or button battery ingestion demands immediate intervention by emergency department personnel and the otolaryngologist. When placed in contact with the electrolyte-rich mucosa, these batteries close a circuit and a caustic reaction ensues. Mucosal injury can happen immediately, with most severe injuries occurring approximately 2 hours after ingestion. To help slow the rate of injury from button batteries, the National Capital Poison Center Guidelines recommend the use of honey or sucralfate for ingestions detected within the last 12 hours: 10 mL every 10 minutes, up to 6 times before arrival to the hospital, and up to 3 times between hospital arrival and surgery. Avoid giving honey to children younger than 1 year of age. Suspected cases of button battery ingestion should trigger a hospital's trauma protocol, facilitating urgent removal in the operating room to avoid mucosal erosion or perforation. A poster (**Figure 22-6**) created by the National Button Battery Task Force, a joint effort of the American Academy of Pediatrics, the American Broncho-Esophagological Association, and the American Academy of Otolaryngology-Head and Neck Surgery, provides management guidance.

■ Recovery

If the foreign body is removed easily without mucosal trauma, the child can be extubated and discharged from the recovery room if he or she is able to take adequate oral intake. If the foreign body has been present for an unknown length of time and there are signs of mucosal damage, the patient may require a longer period of postoperative observation. Dexamethasone (ie, Decadron) at a dose of 0.5 to 1.0 mg/kg intravenous may be administered in the operating room and continued postoperatively if significant edema is present. Chest radiography should be performed if there is evidence of a traumatic extraction and any concern about significant mucosal damage to rule out perforation and mediastinal air.

Most children make a full recovery without permanent sequelae from aerodigestive tract foreign body ingestion. Delays in the

Pediatric Button Battery Injuries
Information For Urgent Care and Emergency Department Medical Professionals

More than 3,000 button battery ingestions occur each year in the United States, and too many children have suffered significant injuries or died from button battery injuries. Many of these events are unwitnessed, so diagnosis can get delayed. Tissue injury and necrosis can occur within <u>hours</u>, and can lead to perforation of the esophagus or death.

- If any child presents or is transferred to you with a radio-opaque esophageal foreign body, review the x-ray images yourself. If you can't review the images directly, discuss the radiographic features of a button battery with the referring physician to be sure the diagnosis is correct.

- Children who have an unwitnessed ingestion of a button battery (or other foreign bodies) can present with non-specific viral symptoms; after performing a thorough history and physical examination, consider x-ray imaging to rule out.

- The care of a child with a button battery that is lodged within the body (esophagus, nose, ear canal, etc.) is considered an <u>emergency</u>. Please help expedite consultations for removal, including direct communication with consultants even while patient is being transported to your center.

- To help slow rate of injury, the National Capital Poison Center Guidelines recommend the use of honey or sucralfate (Carafate), for ingestions <12 hours, 10 mL every 10 minutes, up to 6 times pre-hospital, and up to 3 times between hospital arrival to OR. Avoid honey < 1 year of age.

- Complications days to weeks after esophageal battery removal can occur, including esophageal perforation, tracheoesophageal fistula, esophageal stricture, spondylodiscitis, aortoesophageal fistula and should be considered when patients have this history.

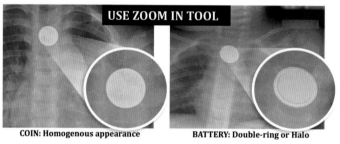

COIN: Homogenous appearance   BATTERY: Double-ring or Halo

The *National Button Battery Task Force*, affiliated with the American Academy of Pediatrics, the American Broncho-Esophagological Association, and the American Academy of Otolaryngology-Head and Neck Surgery, was formalized in 2012 with a focused mission statement: *A collaborative effort of representatives from relevant organizations in industry, medicine, public health and government to develop, coordinate and implement strategies to reduce the incidence of button battery injuries in children.*

Figure 22-6. National Button Battery Task Force poster.

diagnosis cause the most severe morbidity. Children who undergo a delayed or technically difficult extraction should be observed postoperatively in an inpatient setting until they no longer require airway support or can tolerate an age-appropriate diet.

■ Complications

Complications from aerodigestive tract foreign bodies result from the type of foreign body and duration of entrapment. Damage to the surrounding aerodigestive tract mucosa may result in granulation tissue formation, erosive lesions, and infection. Objects such

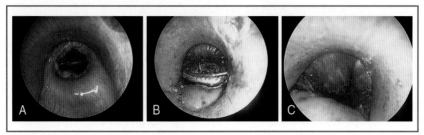

Figure 22-7. Endoscopic removal of button battery from the esophagus. A, View of battery prior to instrumentation. Note the eschar due to superficial necrosis; small bubbles at surface demonstrate ongoing electrolytic reaction. B, Battery after eschar removal and prior to extraction. C, Residual burns in esophageal wall where battery rim contacted mucosa.

as button batteries can cause mucosal erosion in as little as 6 hours from the time of ingestion (**Figure 22-7**). The risk of complications increases with the length of time the foreign body remains in place. The initial complications from a laryngeal or bronchial foreign body can be severe, including cyanosis, respiratory distress, and even respiratory arrest and death. A ball-valve effect can occur with a partially occluding bronchial foreign body, causing hyperexpansion of the affected lung. If complete bronchial occlusion is present, total or partial lung collapse can occur. Late complications of bronchial foreign bodies include granulation tissue formation, pneumonia, empyema, bronchial fistula, and pneumothorax. In the case of esophageal foreign bodies, late complications include granulation tissue formation, mucosal erosions, esophageal perforation, tracheoesophageal fistula, esophageal-aortic fistula, and mediastinitis.

■ Selected References

American Academy of Pediatrics Committee on Injury, Violence, and Poison Prevention. Prevention of choking among children. *Pediatrics*. 2010;125(3):601–607

Anfang RR, Jatana KR, Linn RL, Rhoades K, Fry J, Jacobs IN. pH-neutralizing esophageal irrigations as a novel mitigation strategy for button battery injury. *Laryngoscope*. 2019;129(1):49–57

Betalli P, Rossi A, Bini M, et al. Update on management of caustic and foreign body ingestion in children. *Diagn Ther Endosc*. 2009;2009:969868

Crysdale WS, Sendi KS, Yoo J. Esophageal foreign bodies in children: 15-year review of 484 cases. *Ann Otol Rhinol Laryngol*. 1991;100(4 Pt 1):320–324

Digoy GP. Diagnosis and management of upper aerodigestive tract foreign bodies. *Otolaryngol Clin North Am*. 2008;41(3):485–496, vii–viii

Donnelly LF, Frush DP, Bisset GS III. The multiple presentations of foreign bodies in children. *AJR Am J Roentgenol.* 1998;170(2):471–477

Hagan JF, Shaw JS, Duncan PM, eds. *Bright Futures: Guidelines for Health Supervision of Infants, Children, and Adolescents.* 4th ed. Elk Grove Village, IL: American Academy of Pediatrics; 2017

Lin VY, Daniel SJ, Papsin BC. Button batteries in the ear, nose and upper aerodigestive tract. *Int J Pediatr Otorhinolaryngol.* 2004;68(4):473–479

Pitiot V, Grall M, Ploin D, Truy E, Ayari Khalfallah S. The use of CT-scan in foreign body aspiration in children: a 6 years' experience. *Int J Pediatr Otorhinolaryngol.* 2017;102:169–173

Reilly JS. Prevention of aspiration in infants and young children: federal regulations. *Ann Otol Rhinol Laryngol.* 1990;99(4 Pt 1):273–276

Reilly JS, Walter MA, Beste D, et al. Size/shape analysis of aerodigestive foreign bodies in children: a multi-institutional study. *Am J Otolaryngol.* 1995;16(3):190–193

Waltzman ML, Baskin M, Wypij D, Mooney D, Jones D, Fleisher G. A randomized clinical trial of the management of esophageal coins in children. *Pediatrics.* 2005; 116(3):614–619

Zaytoun GM, Rouadi PW, Baki DH. Endoscopic management of foreign bodies in the tracheobronchial tree: predictive factors for complications. *Otolaryngol Head Neck Surg.* 2000;123(3):311–316

CHAPTER 23

Pediatric Tracheostomy

Nicole Murray, MD

▣ Introduction

The history of tracheostomy goes back much further than one might think. The Talmud describes the insertion of a reed through a newborn's trachea to help breathing in 400 AD. The first well-documented tracheostomy was performed in 1546, but the procedure did not gain medical acceptance for hundreds of years. In 1799, President George Washington died of asphyxiation, likely caused by supraglottitis, while 3 physicians debated the potential consequences of the procedure that could have saved his life. The recognition of tracheostomy as a vital intervention finally came during the diphtheria epidemic at the turn of the 20th century during which the lives of many people, especially children, were saved by the surgery.

Despite improved acceptance of tracheostomy, it was accompanied by a high complication rate, and the procedure was reserved for children with infections and obstructing masses of the upper airway. However, in the 1960s, as long-term endotracheal intubation became increasingly common in the resuscitation of preterm infants, so did the development of subglottic stenosis, and tracheostomy is now considered a critical intervention in the treatment of these patients.

Although attitudes toward tracheostomy have evolved considerably over the centuries, many clinicians still consider tracheostomy as a "last resort." In fact, while it is true that surgeons often perform a tracheostomy if there are no other good options, in many situations the procedure is performed electively and preemptively to avoid potential obstruction of the airway. It also is true that childhood with a tracheostomy today can be more mainstream than ever before (**Figure 23-1**). All physicians who decide to perform a tracheostomy appreciate that it has vast quality-of-life implications for a family, as well as for the global medical care of a child. In this chapter, we will discuss not only the procedure and its indications but also the maintenance and quality-of-life implications of tracheostomy with which the primary care clinician (PCC) should be familiar.

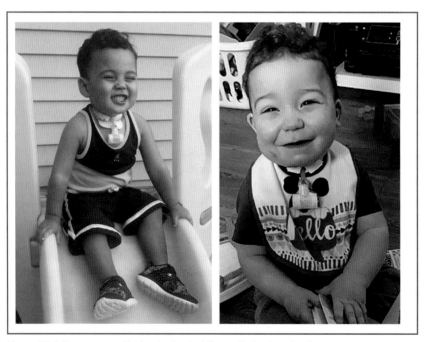

Figure 23-1. Happy, normally developing toddlers with tracheostomies.

▓ Incidence

Tracheostomy rates among infants and children remain low. Studies suggest that approximately 2% of infants and children in a prolonged intensive care unit (ICU) setting will receive a tracheostomy. Half of all children who receive a tracheostomy are younger than 6 months. However, most tracheostomies are placed for prolonged ventilation and are not short-lived. Without a doubt, compared with children of decades past, today's child with a tracheostomy is younger and more chronically ill and has the tracheostomy for a longer period.

▓ Indications for Tracheostomy

Pediatric tracheostomy is performed for 3 main reasons: facilitation of prolonged mechanical ventilation, relief of airway obstruction, and improved pulmonary toilet. Many children have some combination of these issues. In a recent report of 500 pediatric tracheostomies performed over 30 years at a tertiary children's hospital, cardiopulmonary disease was the most common medical indication. In such cases, the tracheostomy provides a conduit for oxygen and improves delivery of continuous positive airway pressure, bilevel positive airway pressure, and long-term mechanical ventilation. This indication, while accounting for 14% of tracheostomies in the first 25 years of the study, was the indication for the procedure in 39% over the past 5 years. These children generally had their tracheostomy placed at about 6 months of age.

The next most frequent indication for pediatric tracheostomy is to bypass airway obstruction. Affected patients may have either congenital laryngotracheal obstruction or acquired laryngotracheal obstruction such as tracheobronchomalacia or subglottic stenosis. This group of children also includes those with congenital obstruction higher in the airway, such as that seen with Pierre Robin sequence caused by micrognathia and glossoptosis. In the aforementioned study, this group consistently accounted for 32% of cases. These children usually received their tracheotomies at younger than 5 months, making them generally the youngest to have the procedure. Such children usually have airway obstruction that cannot immediately be corrected caused by age, anatomy, comorbidities, or family-related issues.

The third most common medical indication for tracheostomy in infants and children is neurologic impairment. The proportion of tracheostomies performed in this patient group has decreased over the past 30 years from 43% to 26%. These patients usually require the procedure for pulmonary toilet or mechanical ventilation. Patients in the pulmonary toilet group generally have an absent gag reflex, with or without other global neurologic deficits, that leads to chronic aspiration. These children are generally older, with a median age of 2.3 years at the time of tracheostomy.

Some children with traumatic injuries, such as drowning, caustic ingestion, smoke inhalation, fractures, and motor vehicle injuries, also require short- or long-term tracheostomy. The proportion of cases in this group has been stable at 4% over the past 30 years. As one would imagine, this group has the widest age range, but most patients are older than 3 years.

> **Pearl:** Pediatric tracheostomy is primarily performed for relief of airway obstruction, facilitation of mechanical ventilation, and improved pulmonary toilet.

■ The Tracheostomy Procedure

In most children requiring the procedure, tracheostomy is brief and uncomplicated. Exceptions include patients with medical instability and those with anomalous or poorly defined neck anatomy or restricted cervical range of motion. In children, the procedure is nearly always performed in the operating room unless a patient absolutely cannot be moved. This ensures the involvement of the most qualified personnel and the availability of equipment that would potentially be necessary to urgently secure an airway. The procedure is often performed in conjunction with preoperative endoscopic assessment of the airway.

Once examination of the airway is complete, the patient is positioned with the head extended and a roll beneath the shoulders. In most cases, the goal is to place the tube about 3 tracheal arches (previously called rings) below the cricoid cartilage. The airway is palpated for landmarks such as the cricoid cartilage, thyroid cartilage, and sternal notch, and the planned incision is diagrammed on the neck (**Figure 23-2**). The incision may be vertical or horizontal because the eventual scar after tracheostomy tube removal will have the same appearance. After the incision is made, dissection through the subcutaneous tissues identifies the strap muscles. These are separated in the midline and, if necessary, the thyroid isthmus is divided,

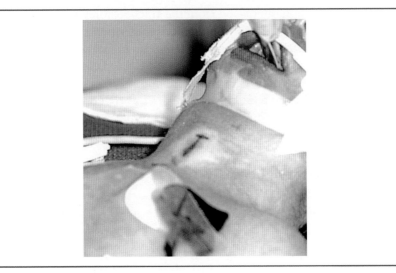

Figure 23-2. Skin markings prior to tracheostomy. Horizontal line marks cricoid cartilage, vertical line marks incision over upper trachea, and marking underneath pad on chest denotes sternal notch.

thus exposing the tracheal wall (**Figure 23-3A**). Of particular interest to the PCC are the "stay sutures" that are placed in the tracheal wall at the midpoint of the planned tracheal incision (**Figure 23-3B**). These sutures serve to reexpose the opening in the event of inadvertent decannulation during the perioperative period. Also of importance to the PCC is placement of protection to reduce perioperative skin breakdown, particularly in neonates. A variety of pads and tracheostomy ties are available for this purpose. After the tracheal incision,

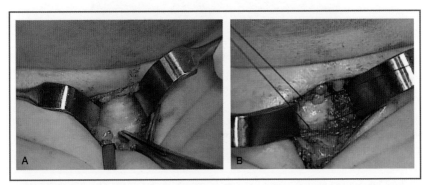

Figure 23-3. A, Tracheal wall exposed by separation of strap muscles and division of thyroid isthmus. B, "Stay sutures" placed on either side of planned vertical incision in midline of trachea.

sutures are occasionally placed from the tracheostomy to the skin to "mature" the stoma, simplify the tube replacement, and reduce the risk of creating a false tract in the event of accidental decannulation (**Figure 23-4**). The tube selected is based on the patient's age and airway size, the need for a cuff for ventilation or airway protection, and the need for an extended external shaft to reduce obstruction by the chin. Occasionally, the tube is sutured in place for several days for extra security until the first tube change.

■ Tracheostomy Tube Complications

Perioperative complications from tracheostomy include bleeding, pneumothorax, accidental decannulation, tube obstruction, improper tube selection with ventilation issues, and breakdown of skin under the connector or flanges. While the first two are avoided by meticulous surgery, the remainder are avoided by fastidious care by the pediatric ICU team and nursing and respiratory care practitioners with daily wound inspection and maintenance of head extension. Dressings and dressing changes may be recommended by the operating surgeon as well.

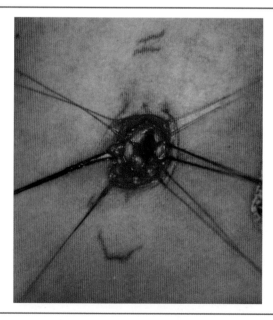

Figure 23-4. Sutures at stoma prior to tracheostomy tube placement. The 2 black sutures are nonabsorbable "stay sutures," while the 4 brown sutures are absorbable chromic sutures approximating the tracheal wall to the skin.

After discharge from the hospital, caregivers of infants and children with a tracheostomy are well trained to recognize and handle a complication. While most questions are directed toward the surgeon, PCCs should also be familiar with complications to effectively assist parents and caregivers.

AIRWAY OBSTRUCTION

The most dangerous complication of tracheostomy is *tube occlusion,* or loss of the airway. This may be the result of accidental tube decannulation, mucus plugging, or granuloma formation.

Accidental Decannulation

Accidental decannulation is defined as an inadvertent dislodgement of the tracheostomy tube, which is an airway emergency. If accidental decannulation occurs in the first 5 to 7 postoperative days, before stomal healing is complete, the tube may not be easily reinserted into the existing location, or it may be passed into the surrounding soft tissues, creating a "false tract." If the patient cannot breathe at all through the nose and mouth, the tracheostomy tube must be correctly repositioned for the child to breathe. For this reason, most surgeons keep children who have been recently tracheotomized in an ICU or a step-down unit until the stoma is well healed, so that skilled staff can arrive rapidly in the event of emergency. Effective bag mask ventilation is the first step until more help arrives. If even this cannot be achieved, an urgent or emergent evaluation in the operating room may be required.

If accidental decannulation occurs as a late complication (after healing of the stoma), the parent or caregiver can usually replace the tube. Caregivers of children with tracheostomy tubes are trained to avoid panic, to position the patient ideally, to use lubricant, and to quickly replace the tube. If the tube does not pass, they will try again with a predesignated emergency tube, which is at least 1 size smaller and should pass more easily. If still unsuccessful, they should immediately activate emergency medical services (EMS) (ie, call 911) for assistance with emergent ventilatory needs. Caregivers will proceed to perform cardiopulmonary resuscitation (CPR) and rescue breathing while awaiting EMS for bag mask ventilation or intubation. Frequent episodes of late accidental decannulation, or "pop-outs," can be an indicator of several problems. One cause is inadequate securement of the tracheostomy tube around the neck. Caregivers of a child with a tracheostomy are trained to secure the tube tightly, allowing passage of the pinky finger beneath the ties. Another cause of accidental decannulation is normal linear growth of the chest. For example, a neonatal tracheostomy tube that fits a 3-month-old may become too short by the time the infant is 7 months old, necessitating replacement of the tube with a longer one (**Figure 23-5**).

Mucus Plugging

Mucus plugging generally can be resolved by suctioning or by an emergency tracheostomy tube change. In the early postoperative phase, before the tract has healed and the tube can be safely changed, adequate humidification and routine suctioning are the best steps to prevent the formation of dried secretions in the lumen of the tube. In the later postoperative phase, after stomal healing, mucus plugging is prevented by adding routine tracheostomy tube changes to these measures.

Granuloma Formation

Tube occlusion can result from distal granulomas that form as a result of rubbing of the tube against the tracheal wall, or as a result of tracheal wall trauma from aggressive suctioning past the tube tip. Granulomas can be diagnosed urgently by otolaryngologists or other clinicians skilled in flexible airway endoscopy by looking with a fiberoptic scope through the tracheostomy tube. Occasionally, the size of a

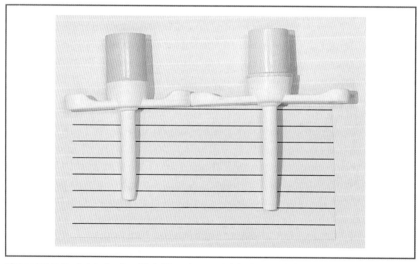

Figure 23-5. Pediatric (or "pedi"; left) and neonatal (or "neo"; right) tracheostomy tubes. Both are designated size 3.5 based on inner diameter, but pediatric tubes are longer. Choice of tube size is based on age, weight, torso length, and neck length, and tubes can be custom-made if necessary.

granuloma can be reduced by using a topical medication combining an antibiotic and a steroid, or the mass can be quickly bypassed with a change to a longer tube (**figures 23-6** and **23-7**). Weekly changes from a long tracheostomy tube to a shorter tube to avoid chronic pressure in 1 spot is an option that sometimes works as well. Some patients, such as those with mucopolysaccharidosis or scoliosis with a tortuous trachea, are prone to distal tracheostomy tube granulomas as a late complication, and maintenance of distal tracheostomy tube patency in these populations can be a challenge.

BLEEDING

Brisk red bleeding from the stoma or lumen of the tracheostomy tube should be evaluated immediately by endoscopy through the stoma to rule out the rare but usually lethal complication of erosion of the tracheostomy tube into a mediastinal vessel. This complication was more common with older tracheostomy cuffs that caused excessive pressure on the tracheal walls. Newer low-pressure cuffs have greatly reduced this problem. Most tracheal bleeding is mild and generally results from overly deep suctioning, stomal or distal granulation tissue, or pulmonary infection with friable tracheal or bronchial tissue. Suction trauma is generally evident on tracheoscopy as irritation and ulceration at the carina, resulting from repeated injury by a suction catheter. This problem resolves with cessation of deep suctioning. Stomal granulomas can be avoided or treated with improved local care to the stoma by using

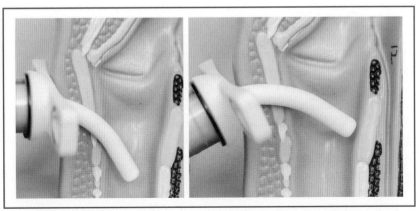

Figure 23-6. Side view of anatomical model demonstrating well-fitting tracheostomy tube (left) and poorly fitting tube (right). It should be noted that a tube that is too short can contact the back wall, resulting in both impaired ventilation and irritation to the tissue.

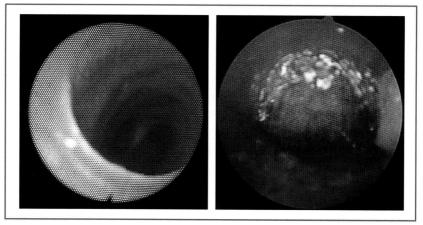

Figure 23-7. Flexible fiberoptic views through indwelling normal (left) and poorly positioned (right) tracheostomy tubes. On left, distal trachea and carina can be visualized. On right, only posterior tracheal wall can be seen, and there is potential for tube tip to cause a contact granuloma. This problem can be remedied by placement of a longer tube.

absorbent dressings and interventions to decrease movement, rubbing, and friction. Application of a topical steroid and antibiotic combination also works well. Occasionally, stomal granulomas must be cauterized or excised for definitive treatment. On occasion, bleeding is caused by infection or inflammation that may or may not be visible on tracheoscopy but may be inferred from the clinical picture and from a lack of other findings on tracheoscopy. In such cases, addressing the source of the infection or inflammation usually stops the bleeding.

STOMA PROBLEMS

Local stoma care is individualized. Different centers have different regimens, and within a center, patients and families may have widely varying preferences of and successes with one regimen over another. There is no single protocol to keep stomas healthy and free of inflammation, so families generally do what works for them. Most such regimens usually include wicking moisture or secretions from the skin around the stoma. Skin breakdown and ulceration are usually early complications in younger children resulting from excessive pressure of the tube connector or a flange against the skin (**Figure 23-8**). These can be avoided by attention to head positioning and wound care and use of beveled tubes and protective ties. A stomal infection may occur as an early postoperative complication or a late one and is indicated by erythema and discharge around the tracheostomy tube. An infection may require treatment with topical or systemic antibiotics. Stomal obstruction can

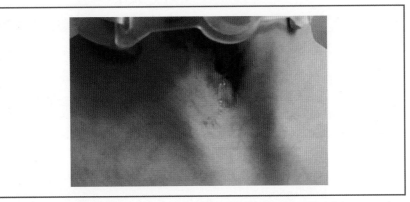

Figure 23-8. Ulceration of inferior aspect of stoma caused by pressure from tube connector. The risk of this complication can be reduced by using beveled tubes and avoiding flexion of the head or the neck.

occur from a stomal granuloma, keloid formation, or, rarely, stricture formation. If a keloid or granuloma is not causing problems, it may be left alone, but because an unobstructed stoma is critical for safe tracheostomy tube changes, many such masses must be treated. Granulomas that are bleeding or bulky can be treated with a topical steroid and antibiotic combination, better tracheostomy site care, cautery, or surgical removal (**Figure 23-9**). Obstructing keloids generally require surgical removal. Steroid injections may help prevent keloid recurrence.

OTHER COMPLICATIONS

Erosion of the tracheostomy tube through the posterior tracheal wall into the esophagus is a rare complication called a *tracheo-esophageal fistula* (**Figure 23-10**). It can be prevented by changing

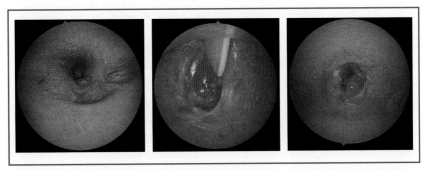

Figure 23-9. Stoma complications. Left photo shows normal unobstructed stoma with tube removed. Center photo demonstrates large stomal granuloma, seen to be significantly obstructive in photo on right of stoma with tube removed. This bulky granuloma was removed surgically.

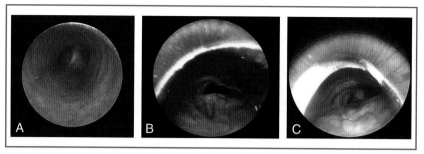

Figure 23-10. Tracheal complications. A, Normal tracheal mucosa caudal to stoma, with no ulceration or granulation. B, Posterior erosion of party wall with esophagus (center) caused by tracheostomy tube in patient with tracheomalacia. The flattened cartilaginous arches are a risk factor for this complication. C, Healing of erosion after changing shape and material of tube.

the tracheostomy tube to hit a different position on the back wall. This complication can be observed during bedside tracheoscopy by withdrawing the tracheostomy tube sufficiently to see the posterior tracheal wall that was covered by the tube. Alternatively, a tracheo-esophageal fistula can be seen during operative rigid or flexible bronchoscopy if performed through the mouth and larynx rather than through the tracheostomy tube.

▥ Life with a Tracheostomy

CHILDREN ARE NOT JUST LITTLE ADULTS

The PCC mantra, "Children are not just little adults," is certainly applicable to care of the child with a tracheostomy. Perhaps the most critical distinction is that young children cannot participate in their own tracheostomy care and, intentionally or unintentionally, they often hinder it. As examples, an infant's chin may occlude the tube, or a toddler may repeatedly try to self-decannulate or put every conceivable foreign body into the tracheostomy tube. Steps must be taken constantly to prevent devastating consequences. For this reason, caring for an infant or a child with a tracheostomy means constant "eyes on" from a caregiver trained in emergent tracheostomy replacement and CPR.

The smaller pediatric airway and neck also present several challenges that are not faced in teenagers or adults with a tracheostomy tube. First, in the adult airway, a tracheostomy tube generally provides an adequate airway while still leaving plenty of room around the tube for expired air to flow up through the vocal folds for phonation. In the pediatric airway, given the thickness of tube materials and the need to maximize tube size for adequate airflow, there is simply not much room left around the tube, particularly in infants. Thus, obstruction of the tube in an infant or a young child may result in a life-threatening emergency. Furthermore, with minimal airflow reaching the larynx, a young infant with a tracheostomy is often aphonic until some growth has created more space around the tube. Most infants and children can eventually produce a voice after tracheostomy, but some cannot. Not hearing an infant's cry may be surprising and disappointing to families. When tracheostomy is planned, families are counseled that voicing is a goal that will eventually be pursued by the medical team, including speech-language professionals, but that may take some time. Voicing will be discussed in more detail later in the chapter.

Second, adult tracheostomy tubes are manufactured with a changeable inner cannula to prevent obstruction by internal crusting of secretions. A child's tracheostomy tube has no room for an inner cannula. As a result, adequate humidification, suctioning, and frequent changes of the entire tube are critical.

Third, infant anatomy combines a short neck with chin rolls, which may lead to tracheostomy tube occlusion in certain positions. This can be mitigated by pediatric tracheostomy tube design with a longer external limb (**Figure 23-11**). The addition of a tracheostomy guard (also called a *basket*) or heat-moisture exchanger (HME) can also reduce this occurrence (**Figure 23-12**). As previously discussed, surveillance and upsizing of the tube with growth of the patient are necessary to avoid accidental decannulation.

> **Pearl:** An infant or a child with a tracheostomy must be under constant "eyes on" supervision by a caregiver who has tracheostomy supplies and is competent in emergency tracheostomy tube replacement and cardiopulmonary resuscitation.

THE ROLE OF THE CAREGIVER IN TRACHEOSTOMY CARE

Going home with an infant or a child with a tracheostomy tube may be daunting, but tracheostomy care is performed by thousands of families every day, and the skills can be learned by almost anyone. Prior to discharge of the child from the hospital, caregivers are trained to master routine tracheostomy maintenance, including

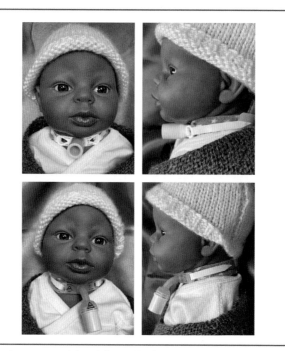

Figure 23-11. Tracheostomy training doll used for family and caregiver education. Top photos demonstrate a tracheostomy tube with a standard connector, and bottom photos show a tube with an extended external limb. In live infants and children, cervical soft tissues and short neck can cause obstruction of standard connector tube more than is apparent on doll.

cleaning of the tube, suctioning, peristomal skin care, and periodic tracheostomy tube changes, as well as emergency interventions such as emergency tracheostomy tube replacement and performance of age-appropriate CPR. The training is not intended to scare parents and caregivers but, rather, to inspire confidence in their own tracheostomy skills. After manikin training, the child serves as the training ground and the process takes place at a pace appropriate for the family. For this reason, many families are in the hospital for as long as a month postoperatively, and infants on a ventilator may stay considerably longer. The particular details of training and discharge requirements may vary, but most tracheostomy teams require the following for discharge:

- Two trained caregivers
- Home and portable monitors
- Emergency oxygen tank and Ambu bag

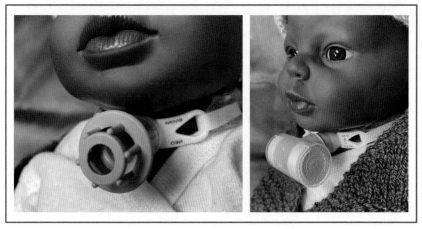

Figure 23-12. Training doll with a tracheostomy guard (left) and a heat-moisture exchanger (right). These devices can prevent the chin or clothing from obstructing the tube lumen.

- Home nursing
- Suction machine
- Home health company for equipment maintenance and supply
- Spare tracheostomy tubes, suctions, HMEs, tracheostomy ties
- A tracheostomy bag that is constantly available and contains a spare tube, an emergency downsize tracheostomy tube, and suction **(Figure 23-13)**

Unlike adults with a tracheostomy, an infant or a child with a tracheostomy must be under constant supervision by a caregiver who has, and is familiar with, tracheostomy supplies and is also competent in these procedures.

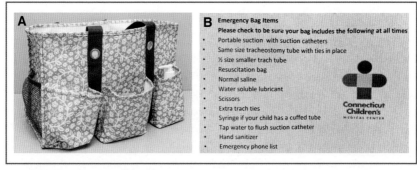

Figure 23-13. A, Tracheostomy bag supplied to patients upon discharge at Connecticut Children's Medical Center. B, Inset shows laminated inventory card on bag to aid families with restocking as supplies are used.

ACTIVITIES OF DAILY LIVING WITH A TRACHEOSTOMY TUBE

While life for a child with a tracheostomy has improved drastically over the past century, there are limitations, some obvious and some less apparent, that must be considered. For example, no water can get into the stoma or tracheostomy tube, so alterations in bathing are necessary, and certainly no swimming is allowed. Generally, sponge baths or very low water levels for bathing are recommended, and showers are prohibited. Small particles introduced into the tracheostomy tube are a potential problem, so beaches and sandy playgrounds are also generally avoided. Travel away from home, even for a short trip, involves bringing the tracheostomy bag, including all emergency supplies and suction, as well as the attendance of at least 2 competent caregivers. One caregiver cannot be expected to drive and, at the same time, maintain supervision of the child. Lastly, children breathing through a tracheostomy tube lose the natural immunologic defenses of the upper aerodigestive tract, while the tube facilitates access to the lungs for foreign materials and respiratory pathogens. As a result, the child with a tracheostomy is at increased risk of developing pulmonary infections, and caregivers must be vigilant of potential problematic exposures.

VOICING

Voice production requires air to be propelled from the lungs through the vocal folds, causing vibration and, thus, phonation. For newborns without a tracheostomy, this happens naturally, beginning with crying and followed by production of articulated sounds and, eventually, speech. For children with a tracheostomy, this process is longer and more difficult, but it can happen in most children in whom anatomy permits the air column to reach the larynx and who are otherwise developmentally capable. With a tracheostomy, airflow follows the path of least resistance; thus, in the infant airway, exhaled air will mainly flow through the tracheostomy tube, with very little air moving around the tube to reach the vocal folds. As a result, infants with tracheostomy tubes may have minimal or no phonation. However, with growth of the airway during childhood, the tube occupies less space, and children also learn to move their neck such that air may be directed through the vocal folds to generate sound. In selected patients, the process can be greatly assisted by using a speaking valve on the tracheostomy tube that allows air to pass in and out of the tracheostomy on gentle respiration but closes on forced expiration. Exhaled air is forced to flow around the tube and up through the vocal folds (**Figure 23-14**). Children with obstructive lesions above

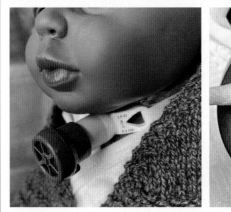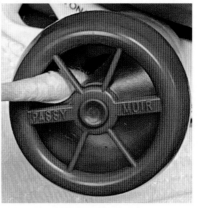

Figure 23-14. Training doll with speaking valve (left), as well as close-up of valve (right). Note the membrane (held open with cotton swab). The membrane is designed to allow air to enter and exit through the tube during quiet respiration. However, upon forceful expiration, such as that required for coughing or phonation, the membrane closes, forcing exhaled air around the tube and through the vocal folds to permit phonation and expulsion of secretions.

the tube such as high-grade subglottic stenosis or large suprastomal granulomas are able to exhale only through the tracheostomy tube and, therefore, cannot use the valve.

A child on a ventilator has an even greater challenge with voicing. The medical team (ie, otolaryngologist, pulmonologist, speech therapist, and respiratory therapist) can work together to determine if a child on positive pressure ventilation is a candidate for a speaking valve. Specialized in-line valves can be used if certain criteria are met.

- The child must tolerate having the tracheostomy cuff deflated, so that there is always a sufficient air leak for exhalation.
- The child must tolerate the increased work of breathing with the valve.
- The child's caregivers must understand and follow critical safety rules, including to never apply the valve with the tracheostomy cuff inflated. If this were to happen, the ventilator would deliver positive pressure breaths without the chance for exhalation, potentially causing pneumothorax, pneumomediastinum, and cardiorespiratory failure within minutes. Modern ventilators will sound an alarm at this increased pressure, but they will not stop delivering breaths, so caregiver intervention is required immediately to deflate the cuff or remove the valve.

Some children with a tracheostomy are unable to generate speech with or without a valve. In such cases, patients and their families use augmentative communication techniques such as sign language and/or assistive communicative devices such as a tablet. All children with a tracheostomy should be evaluated by a speech-language pathologist for assistance with communication.

FEEDING

Swallowing may be affected by a tracheostomy, but this is relatively uncommon in children. A proper swallow involves laryngeal elevation, which may be mildly impaired if the tracheostomy tube tethers the airway to the skin. Also, in infants and children, the esophagus may be somewhat compressed by the tube. Additionally, children who receive a tracheostomy for neurologic delays and aspiration, by definition, have swallowing dysfunction. Given the potential for feeding impediments, it may be surprising that most children who are developmentally able to swallow before a tracheostomy can still swallow well after a tracheostomy (**Figure 23-15**).

BREATHING

Generally, work of breathing is less with a tracheostomy because there is an appropriately wide airway and because the dead space of the glottis, pharynx, and nose are all bypassed and muscles of respiration have to move air a shorter distance. Poor work of breathing of some infants and children who are borderline candidates for mechanical ventilation is improved after a tracheostomy because of

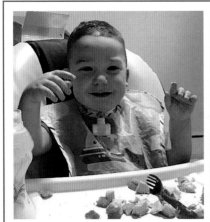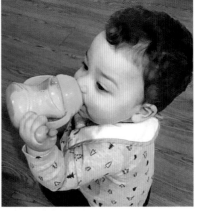

Figure 23-15. Toddler who depends on tracheostomy is able to feed happily and efficiently, without aspiration.

the elimination of dead space. However, patients with a tracheostomy are at a disadvantage in terms of cough and end-expiratory pressure maintenance. An effective cough is important for secretion clearance and is generated by a buildup of intrathoracic air pressure with subsequent explosive release. The presence of a tracheostomy means one cannot build up this pressure, and the cough is less effective. A speaking valve, if tolerated, can help as it restores the ability to build up subglottic pressure.

Maintenance of pressure is also necessary for proper alveolar pressure and small airway patency. A tracheostomy leads to an impaired ability to maintain positive end-expiratory pressure. In older children with strong healthy lungs, this may not be an issue. However, in an infant with some degree of tracheobronchomalacia, this loss may mean the child will need constant positive pressure ventilation after a tracheostomy, even if he or she did not need it beforehand. Setting realistic expectations for parents is always part of the preoperative discussion for tracheostomy in infants. Surgeons know that living with a tracheostomy is one thing and living with a ventilator is an entirely different thing, but the latter cannot always be avoided in small infants who need to develop more airway strength.

> **Pearl:** Most children with a tracheostomy can expect to achieve typical milestones such as communicating verbally and eating orally, although it may take longer for these children than their healthy counterparts. Working together, the family, the therapy team, and the medical team can achieve normality for these children.

■ Planned Decannulation

Otolaryngologists often start planning the steps necessary to decannulate at the time the tracheostomy is planned. Accomplishing decannulation is a long-term goal toward which the care team works in conjunction with the family. To start the process, the problem that required the tracheostomy must be sufficiently resolved. Subsequently, the tube is progressively downsized to a 2.5- or 3.0-mm diameter tube, followed by capping trials of increasing duration, solely performed while the patient is awake and under constant supervision. At some point in this process, operative bronchoscopy is performed to assess the airway for adequacy, including removal of any suprastomal granulomas (**Figure 23-16**) that might lead to failure. Once the tube can be capped all day without distress and the airway is deemed adequate for decannulation, the patient is admitted for observation in the ICU overnight. If there is minimal or no sleep apnea, the tube may be removed. At some centers, polysomnography is performed with the tracheostomy tube capped overnight to assess for respiratory distress. After successful decannulation, the stoma should close and leave a small circular scar. In some cases, it may remain open as a tracheocutaneous fistula that requires surgical closure (**Figure 23-17**). Until the stoma is closed, the patient continues to face airway risks from water or particulate matter and may continue to cough out mucoid secretions. A final inspection by the surgeon is required before the child is free to bathe normally, or perhaps to learn to swim.

▥ Conclusion

The history of tracheostomy, from reeds to George Washington to today, has allowed the development of the current standard of pediatric tracheostomy for acute or chronic problems. Primary care clinicians and the members of the tracheostomy care team can provide highly specialized and sophisticated care for infants and children who may need a tracheostomy for a short time or for a lifetime. After the child has been at home for several months to years, parents often

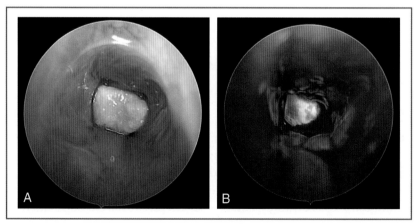

Figure 23-16. A, Suprastomal granuloma obstructs airway, precluding decannulation. B, Airway immediately after removal of the granuloma, with tracheostomy tube now visible. Patient is now a candidate for decannulation.

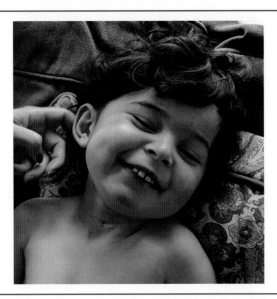

Figure 23-17. Child after resolution of severe tracheobronchomalacia and subsequent decannulation. Stoma remains open at this point but will often close with time or may be closed surgically.

become more knowledgeable about tracheostomies than many health care professionals, and they know what works for them. Therefore, family-centered care and shared decision-making are especially useful in this population. Today's pediatric tracheostomy population is younger and sicker than ever before, but the decision to perform a tracheostomy reflects the belief that even the smallest and most vulnerable child has a future worth fighting for.

■ Selected References

Das P, Zhu H, Shah RK, Roberson DW, Berry J, Skinner ML. Tracheotomy-related catastrophic events: results of a national survey. *Laryngoscope.* 2012;122(1):30–37

Gergin O, Adil EA, Kawai K, Watters K, Moritz E, Rahbar R. Indications of pediatric tracheostomy over the last 30 years: has anything changed? *Int J Pediatr Otorhinolaryngol.* 2016;87:144–147

Hartnick C, Diercks G, De Guzman V, Hartnick E, Van Cleave J, Callans K. A quality study of family-centered care coordination to improve care for children undergoing tracheostomy and the quality of life for their caregivers. *Int J Pediatr Otorhinolaryngol.* 2017;99:107–110

Lavin J, Shah R, Greenlick H, Gaudreau P, Bedwell J. The Global Tracheostomy Collaborative: one institution's experience with a new quality improvement initiative. *Int J Pediatr Otorhinolaryngol.* 2015;80:106–108

Mahida JB, Asti L, Boss EF, et al. Tracheostomy placement in children younger than 2 years: 30-day outcomes using the National Surgical Quality Improvement Program Pediatric. *JAMA Otolaryngol Head Neck Surg.* 2016;142(3):241–246

McGrath BA, Lynch J, Bonvento B, et al. Evaluating the quality improvement impact of the Global Tracheostomy Collaborative in four diverse NHS hospitals. *BMJ Qual Improv Rep.* 2017;6(1):1–8.

Mitchell RB, Hussey HM, Setzen G, et al. Clinical consensus statement: tracheostomy care. *Otolaryngol Head Neck Surg.* 2013;148(1):6–20

Watters KF. Tracheostomy in infants and children. *Respir Care.* 2017;62(6):799–825

Zhu H, Das P, Brereton J, Roberson D, Shah RK. Surveillance and management practices in tracheotomy patients. *Laryngoscope.* 2012;122(1):46–50

Zhu H, Das P, Roberson DW, et al. Hospitalizations in children with preexisting tracheostomy: a national perspective. *Laryngoscope.* 2015;125(2):462–468

SECTION 6

General

CHAPTER 24

Otolaryngological Disorders in Down Syndrome

Sally R. Shott, MD; Dorsey Ann Heithaus, MA;
and Anthony Sheyn, MD

Introduction
Chronic Otitis Media
    Epidemiology
    Presenting Signs and
      Symptoms
    Treatment Options
Hearing Loss: Audiologic
    Testing

Obstructive Sleep Apnea
    Syndrome
    Presenting Symptoms
    Management
Airway Abnormalities:
    Laryngeal and Tracheal
Chronic Rhinitis and Sinusitis
    Evaluation and Examination
    Treatment Options

▓ Introduction

Disorders of the ears, nose, and throat are common among children with Down syndrome (DS). The otologic problems observed include conductive hearing loss caused by the presence of chronic middle ear fluid, as well as sensorineural hearing loss. Management of these problems in children with DS may be further complicated by congenital ear canal stenosis. Obstructive sleep apnea (OSA) and sleep-disturbed breathing are also very common, occurring in as many as 60% of children as young as 3 to 4 years; this incidence increases as children grow older. The subglottic and tracheal airways of children with DS are smaller than those in other children of the same age. This is of particular importance if surgery requires endotracheal intubation of the airway for general anesthesia. Tracheomalacia, with stridor caused by partial collapse of the trachea with respiration, is not uncommon. Because of delay in development of the immune system and the midfacial hypoplasia with smaller nasal passages and smaller paranasal sinuses, young children are more prone to upper respiratory tract infections and rhinorrhea. This chapter will review the key management strategies for ears, nose, and throat–related disorders in children with DS.

■ Chronic Otitis Media

EPIDEMIOLOGY

Chronic middle-ear disease is common in DS, occurring in up to 95% of children. Etiologic factors include midface hypoplasia with a contracted nasopharynx, an abnormally configured eustachian tube, a higher incidence of upper respiratory infections caused by immaturity and delay in the immune system, and poor function of the tensor veli palatini muscle of the soft palate, the muscle responsible for opening and closing the eustachian tube.

The duration of eustachian tube dysfunction in DS is unknown, but it seems that middle ear disease continues much longer and to an older age than that in the general population. Studies demonstrate that aggressive medical and surgical management of chronic otitis media (OM) results in better hearing levels and a lower occurrence of tympanic membrane (TM) perforations and cholesteatoma.

PRESENTING SIGNS AND SYMPTOMS

Symptoms associated with acute OM in children with DS are no different from those in other children and include fever, pulling on ears, irritability, poor sleep, poor feeding, and otorrhea in the event of an acute perforation. Chronic middle ear fluid or negative middle ear pressure can present more insidiously, and affected children may have difficulty expressing associated symptoms such as aural fullness or hearing loss. Left untreated, these middle ear disorders may result in erosion of the ossicles and cholesteatoma, requiring extensive and aggressive surgical management. However, in children with DS, establishing a diagnosis of acute or chronic OM on physical examination can be more difficult than in other children. Up to 50% of newborns with DS have stenosis of the external auditory canals, often making visualization of the ear drum difficult or impossible. In addition, many affected children have developmental delay that complicates the office examination. As a result, there is a high incidence of underdiagnosis and undertreatment of middle ear disease in DS.

Because of the high incidence of OM with DS, it is recommended that these children undergo regular otoscopy by the primary care clinician (PCC). Patients with eustachian tube dysfunction resulting in severe retraction or retraction pockets, or chronic middle ear fluid causing potential hearing loss, should be referred to an otolaryngologist for evaluation and audiometric testing. When the ear canals are severely stenotic, the examiner's inability to adequately visualize the eardrum should not be trivialized if the child does not have classic symptoms of OM. Although the canals grow slowly during the first 3 years after birth, many children will need to have their cerumen removed and their ears examined by an otolaryngologist using more sophisticated techniques such as otomicroscopy and tympanometry to adequately rule out OM or TM retraction. In some cases, the ear canals may be so small that even tympanometry yields inaccurate results. Until the ear canals grow enough for the TMs to be easily visualized by otoscopy, children with ear canal stenosis should be examined by an otolaryngologist every 3 to 6 months. Surgery to correct the stenotic ear canals is rarely needed because the canals grow as the child grows.

TREATMENT OPTIONS

Children with DS fall outside the published guidelines for management of OM. However, similar to other children, initial treatment for acute OM is medical management with antibiotics. In addition, environmental risk factors such as exposure to cigarette smoke need to be discussed with the child's family and eliminated. It is important to stress that, because of delayed maturity of the immune system in children with DS, these risk factors place the child at an even higher risk of recurrent ear infections. When 3 to 4 ear infections are occurring within 6 months, or 5 to 6 within 12 months, insertion of pressure equalization (PE) tubes should be considered.

Because of more prolonged eustachian tube dysfunction, chronic OM and structural TM changes occur more frequently in children with DS. Poor ventilation resulting in hearing loss because of fluid that has not resolved within 3 months is also an indication for insertion of PE tubes. It has been shown through serial audiograms that children with DS with tubes in place have a 3.6 times higher chance of having normal hearing compared with children whose audiograms were done when tubes were not in place. In many cases, multiple sets of PE tubes may be needed for a child. Children with PE tubes in place should be seen by their otolaryngologist every 6 months for regular ear cleaning and evaluation of the status of the tubes. When PE tubes have extruded into the ear canal, they should be removed promptly to facilitate surveillance of the TM and middle ear.

Middle Ear Surveillance

The 2004 American Academy of Pediatrics (AAP) clinical practice guideline suggests that children should continue to have their ears monitored at least every 6 months as long as chronic retraction of the eardrums, ear effusions, or recurrent infections continue to be problematic. Subsequently, children with no evidence of OM in whom normal hearing has been established in both ears should undergo behavioral audiometric testing annually to rule out hearing loss that may develop from otherwise asymptomatic middle ear fluid. If the child has middle ear disease, testing should be performed again once the ears have cleared or tympanostomy tubes are placed to ensure that hearing is otherwise normal. A study by Lee et al showed that with aggressive medical surveillance and proactive surgical treatment of chronic ear disease, the need for more extensive otologic surgery can be minimized.

> **Pearl:** Children with DS who have ear canal stenosis should visit an otolaryngologist every 3 to 6 months for debridement, microscopic examination, and audiometric testing.

■ Hearing Loss: Audiologic Testing

Children with DS have a 3-times higher incidence of hearing loss secondary to chronic middle ear disease than other children with developmental delays. However, although most hearing loss in DS can be attributed to conductive pathology, data suggest that 4% to 20% of patients may have sensorineural or mixed hearing loss. Through evaluations of computed tomographic scans and magnetic resonance images (MRI), Blaser et al showed a high incidence of inner ear abnormalities in children with DS. Initial studies evaluating the incidence of hearing loss in children with DS reported rates as high as 78%.

As a result, children with DS should undergo an initial audiologic evaluation in the first month after birth in accordance with universal newborn screening and AAP recommendations. Initial audiologic evaluations during the newborn period are conducted by means of a screening auditory brain stem response (sABR) or an otoacoustic emissions (OAE) hearing test. Otoacoustic emissions are generated at the level of the cochlea and, thus, will miss more central dysfunction. They are also inaccurate in the presence of middle-ear fluid. The results are reported as "pass" or "refer" based on presentation of sound at a single amplitude, usually 25 decibel (dB), thus missing very mild sensorineural hearing loss. Screening auditory brain stem response testing evaluates hearing via neural pathways and can be performed without the child's cooperative participation. It is believed to be a superior test, as it can differentiate between sensorineural and moderate conductive hearing loss, and it can also be used for the detection of auditory neuropathy. However, standard sABR uses a broadband click stimulus containing mostly high-frequency sound that, like OAE, is set at a fixed intensity (eg, 20–25 dB) at a pass/fail level. Thus, a child with mild OM with effusion might pass an sABR, while low-frequency hearing loss can be missed.

When the initial OAE study results are abnormal, a second screen should be requested. If the results of the rescreen are also abnormal, reassessment by diagnostic ABR is indicated. When the initial screening is done by sABR with *abnormal* results, reassessment by ABR is also recommended. In both cases, definitive diagnostic ABR testing should be completed by age 3 months. Children with DS with *normal* results on a screening newborn OAE or sABR should be retested to confirm the results; while the AAP clinical practice guideline suggests retesting as young as 6 months of age, some state programs consider this result "pass with risk" and suggest repeated testing at between 12 and 24 months of age. Testing should be repeated every 6 to 12 months until normal hearing is established in both ears, with the former interval favored by the AAP.

> **Pearl:** Following abnormal results by means of OAE or sABR, reassessment by ABR is recommended. Definitive diagnostic ABR testing should be completed by age 3 months. Children with normal results on a screening newborn OAE or ABR are considered "pass with risk" and should undergo repeated testing before 24 months of age, preferably between the ages of 6 and 12 months.

Once normal hearing is confirmed bilaterally, behavioral testing is initiated. Behavioral testing may be performed in an open-room setting (sound field testing) or with headphones. Unfortunately, children younger than 3 years as well as many older children with DS are unable to be tested with headphones, and sound field testing does not provide audiometric information that is ear specific; consequently, a unilateral hearing loss could be missed. Therefore, the AAP suggests that behavioral testing continue every 6 months until the child is found to have normal hearing by ear-specific testing using insert/TDH earphones for at least 3 frequencies (500 Hz, 1,000 Hz, and 4,000 Hz) and normal speech awareness or speech reception threshold. Once these are achieved, annual audiologic testing can be initiated.

If a child fails the screening and diagnostic ABRs, he or she should be seen by an otolaryngologist who has experience working with children with DS. The otolaryngologist can then determine if medical or surgical interventions are indicated to treat or minimize hearing loss. After successful treatment, the child should undergo a repeated diagnostic ABR. Behavioral audiometry would be acceptable at this time if ear-specific information can be obtained.

Once the ear examination findings are normal, if a sensorineural hearing loss is identified, the child should be fitted with hearing aids as early as possible. These children are then followed up according to standards established for children with sensorineural hearing loss. The otolaryngologist should participate in long-term monitoring and management of the child's hearing loss and provide information and recommendations with regard to amplification, hearing-assistive devices, and surgical intervention. Amplification with hearing aids should be considered even if the hearing loss is mild, especially in view of data linking mild hearing loss with delays in educational, emotional, and language development. Similarly, statistically significant differences in IQ levels have been demonstrated between otherwise healthy children with mild hearing loss caused by OM and matched controls. These findings are of particular importance for children with DS, in whom expressive language skills are delayed compared with cognitive abilities, and in whom developmental problems associated with hearing loss may have a greater effect because of the associated mental and physical handicaps.

A policy statement regarding management of children with DS published in 2011 by the AAP Committee on Genetics recommends audiologic testing at birth and then every 6 months until ear-specific testing is achieved. A study by Maurizi et al showed that reliable, ear-specific results by behavioral audiometry could not be achieved in children with DS younger than 3½ years. Ear-specific testing was achieved only rarely in their study. This finding was confirmed by Shott et al, who found that only 12% of children with DS were able to undergo ear-specific testing at 3 years of age, and only 41% could be tested at age 4 years. Testing protocols should therefore be determined according to the child's developmental levels and not by chronologic age. The goal is to obtain ear-specific measurements of pure tones as well as speech awareness levels, and eventually speech reception levels and a determination of speech discrimination abilities. Therefore, hearing levels should be established by objective hearing tests such as ABR, and evaluations should continue every 6 months until ear-specific behavioral testing is achieved. If hearing is normal, annual follow-up hearing tests are adequate. More frequent audiologic evaluations are necessary in the presence of hearing loss.

■ Obstructive Sleep Apnea Syndrome

Studies report a 50% to 100% incidence of OSA in individuals with DS. A recent study by Heubi et al showed that in symptomatic children younger than 48 months with DS, 91% had OSA. Studies have shown that 60% to 70% of children with DS have abnormal sleep study findings by age 3½ to 4 years. Further evidence shows that these numbers increase as children grow older. In the study by Heubi et al, 91% of children with DS between 11 and 18 years of age also had OSA. In 50% of children, the OSA was moderate to severe. Fitzgerald et al reported a 97% incidence of OSA in children with DS aged 0.2 to 19 years who snored (mean age, 4.9 years). Predisposing factors include midface hypoplasia, mandibular hypoplasia, a relative macroglossia, medially displaced tonsils, adenoid sitting in a contracted nasopharynx and, thus, causing more obstruction, and hypotonia of the upper airway, with resultant collapse at multiple levels of the airway during sleep. Increased upper airway infections and nasal secretions, obesity, and hypotonia further contribute to oropharyngeal and hypopharyngeal collapse and obstruction with sleep. In addition, obesity and hypothyroidism, both common problems in DS, further predispose individuals to OSA.

Sleep-disordered breathing has been shown to affect cognitive abilities, behavior, and growth rate, as well as result in more serious consequences of pulmonary hypertension and cor pulmonale. Because of the high incidence of underlying congenital cardiac anomalies in individuals with DS, there is a higher risk of developing more severe complications. Abnormalities in the pulmonary vasculature also increase the risk of developing pulmonary hypertension.

Unfortunately, the ability of parents to predict sleep abnormalities in their children with DS has been shown to be poor. A sleep study, or polysomnography, continues to be the gold standard test from which to evaluate sleep-disordered breathing and sleep apnea. Because of the poor correlation between parental reporting and sleep study results, the AAP recommends a baseline sleep study or polysomnography for all children with DS by 4 years of age.

> **Pearl:** Children with Down syndrome should undergo baseline polysomnography by age 4 years.

PRESENTING SYMPTOMS

Starting at birth, PCCs should actively inquire about restless sleep, snoring, heavy breathing, uncommon sleep positions, frequent night-time waking, daytime sleepiness, apneic pauses, and behavioral problems associated with poor sleeping in their patients. Sleep positions should also be discussed, such as sleeping sitting up, sleeping with the neck hyperextended, or sleeping bent forward at the waist in a sitting position.

Although the focus of sleep-disturbed breathing tends to center around the tonsils and adenoid, other causes of obstruction, such as chronic rhinorrhea and congestion, nasal septal deviation, and nasal turbinate enlargement, need to be assessed and treated. If the oral examination shows edema of the posterior pharyngeal wall, thus decreasing the size of the posterior pharyngeal airway, gastroesophageal reflux (GER) or chronic postnasal drainage should be considered as the cause of these findings. Treatment with antireflux medications or decongestants, nasal steroid sprays, or antihistamines should be considered. Families should be counseled about the risk of sleep apnea because of obesity and the importance of weight control and need for continued exercise.

If there is any question of airway disturbances during sleep, the PCC should refer the child to an otolaryngologist to determine if a sleep study or surgical intervention is needed. In most cases, a sleep study or polysomnography is appropriate to evaluate the severity of the obstruction and to aid in preoperative planning, particularly if the tonsils and adenoid do not appear enlarged. Removal of enlarged tonsils and adenoids is the first-line surgical treatment for OSA in children with DS, as it is for all children. In children with DS, because of their midface hypoplasia and contracted nasopharynx, even mildly enlarged tonsils and adenoids may have a greater than expected effect with regard to airway obstruction. If the tonsils and adenoid do not appear enlarged, it has been suggested that a sleep study be performed to confirm that the child does *not* have sleep apnea.

If adenotonsillectomy is performed, the surgical team should endeavor to keep the child's neck in an anatomically neutral position throughout the entire procedure. Because of the high incidence of cervical spine abnormalities and atlanto-axial instability seen in DS, hyperflexion or hyperflexion of the neck could potentially lead to compression of the spinal cord. In most tonsil and adenoid surgeries, the neck is hyperextended while the tonsils are removed, but this is not done in those with DS. In the past, many recommended that flexion/extension radiographs of the neck be obtained prior to adenotonsillar surgery in all children with DS, but this is no longer commonly done because radiographs can miss the instability, and the cervical bones are not calcified until age 5 to 6 years. It is best to assume a cervical spine anomaly in *all* children with DS and take appropriate precautions for such children.

MANAGEMENT

Although adenotonsillectomy is the most common initial surgical intervention, studies have shown that residual airway obstruction after this surgery is possible, and further surgical and medical interventions may be needed. This has been shown to be more common than previously believed in typical children with OSA. In 2007, Mitchell reported a 10% to 20% incidence of persistent sleep apnea in a group of 79 children after adenotonsillectomy. Tauman et al, using a much more strict definition of surgical cure, reported complete normalization of all components evaluated in a sleep study in only 25% of the test population of "typical" children. This compares with the 5% total success rate reported in the study by Shott et al in which a similarly strict definition of *cure* was used in a group of children with DS. If cure is more akin to the definitions used in the study by Mitchell, almost 50% to 70% of the children with DS in this study continued to have OSA after adenotonsillectomy. All of these studies illustrate the need for postoperative evaluation of children with DS for residual sleep apnea after tonsil and adenoid surgery by means of a sleep study or polysomnography. Because of the higher rate of respiratory complications after removal of the tonsils and adenoid in children with DS, overnight observation in the hospital after this surgery is also recommended.

If residual obstruction is present despite tonsil and adenoid surgery, medical treatment with continuous positive airway pressure (CPAP) ventilation or supplemental oxygen remains an option. The authors have observed a compliance rate as high as 50% in children with DS who require CPAP. If the residual sleep apnea is in the mild range, studies suggest that effective treatment occurs with nasal steroids or with montelukast. Dental appliances to promote mandibular stabilization have also been shown to be helpful in cases of mild residual sleep apnea.

If persistent OSA is in the moderate-to-severe range, flexible naso-pharyngoscopy and laryngoscopy examination in the office is recommended to determine the site(s) of residual airway obstruction. This procedure aids in ruling out enlarged lingual tonsil tissue, residual or regrown adenoid tissue, and possible glossoptosis. Drug-induced sleep endoscopy (DISE) performed under a mild general anesthetic facilitates evaluation of the airway during sleep. Radiographic studies using cine-MRI studies also provide a dynamic evaluation of the site or sites of residual obstruction. Both DISE and cine MRI have shown that base-of-tongue obstruction from a combination of relative macroglossia and glossoptosis, enlarged lingual tonsils, and adenoid regrowth are some of the most common sites of residual obstruction in individuals with DS despite previous adenotonsillectomy.

Surgical options for persistent OSA in children with DS need to be tailored to each patient's pattern of obstruction. Surgical approaches currently used include lingual tonsillectomy, supraglottoplasty, uvulopalatopharyngoplasty, midline posterior glossectomy, genioglossus suspension and advancement, hyoid advancement, and craniofacial surgery, including mandibular and midface advancements. Because OSA can occur at multiple levels of the airway, multilevel and staged surgeries may be needed. Currently, successful treatment is in the range of 50% to 60%, and surgery is usually considered only after the child fails a trial of CPAP. In some cases, the surgery may not be fully successful, but it might improve the airway obstruction such that CPAP is better tolerated.

The hypoglossal nerve stimulator is one of the more recent surgeries being offered for treatment of OSA. Base-of-tongue obstruction is one of the most common sites of residual obstruction that persists after adenotonsillectomy. During sleep, this device stimulates the branches of the hypoglossal nerve that cause tongue protrusion.

In cases of severe sleep apnea with associated pulmonary hypertension, severe hypoxemia, or cardiac complications, tracheostomy may also need to be considered.

■ Airway Abnormalities: Laryngeal and Tracheal

In comparison to the general pediatric population, children with DS have smaller subglottic and tracheal airways. An association between DS, stridor, and subglottic stenosis is commonly discussed in the anesthesia literature. It has been shown that children with DS, when compared with other children matched for age and weight, require an endotracheal tube that is 2 sizes smaller when intubated appropriately, such that there is an air leak around the tube. The hypotonia seen in DS also affects the larynx and trachea, and laryngomalacia and tracheomalacia with associated stridor is not uncommon. Children with DS have more postoperative airway complications than typical children, usually caused by airway issues. The combination of the smaller airway, hypotonia, a high incidence of GER, and a high percentage of procedures in children with DS done under general anesthesia places them at higher risk for development of subglottic stenosis.

Although no ongoing monitoring is required, PCCs need to be aware of potential airway problems when their patient is scheduled for surgery, especially when intubation is expected to take place and if the child undergoes surgery in a center not accustomed to caring for children with DS. Recurrent croup should be treated aggressively, especially because the child's subglottic airway is likely smaller than usual. Treatment of GER should be considered, especially in cases of recurrent croup or if significant edema is seen in the posterior oropharynx. Mitchell found a high incidence of GER in a cohort of children with DS, and GER has been identified as a risk factor for recurrent croup. In addition, the incidence of GER is higher in children who have laryngomalacia. Although initial reports suggested a lower success rate in surgical treatment of subglottic stenosis in children with DS, more recent reports have shown success rates that are similar to those in other children.

Because of the higher potential for postoperative airway problems after general anesthesia, especially if intubation of the airway occurs, overnight hospitalization, following even a short procedure, should be considered in children with DS and is strongly advocated after adenotonsillectomy.

Owing to the higher incidence of airway anomalies such as laryngomalacia, tracheomalacia, and smaller subglottic airways, an otolaryngology consultation should be included when children with DS have recurrent croup, noisy breathing, or stridor.

■ Chronic Rhinitis and Sinusitis

The chronic rhinitis frequently seen in young children with DS has traditionally been dismissed as something that was "just part of DS" and was noted to improve as the child got older. However, chronic rhinitis in DS should not be accepted as an inevitable and untreatable condition, and specialty evaluation of refractory chronic rhinitis should be considered.

Radiographic studies have shown abnormal development of the frontal, maxillary, and sphenoid sinuses, including hypoplasia or lack of pneumatization of the paranasal sinuses. Similarly, midface hypoplasia in DS results in a smaller than usual nasal and nasopharyngeal airway and predisposes to stasis of secretions and poor ventilation. Delay in development of the immune system also contributes to the response to infectious rhinitis in children with DS. Saline nasal drops, sprays, and irrigations have long been used for treatment of chronic rhinitis and recently have been confirmed as effective treatment in adults. For children with midface hypoplasia and thus smaller than usual nasal passages, this treatment is invaluable. Further evaluation and treatment of chronic sinusitis should follow similar pathways as those that would be used in other children.

EVALUATION AND EXAMINATION

Patency of the nasal choanae should be confirmed in the newborn with DS or in the older child if this was not done previously by passing a size 8F suction catheter through each naris. If this is not possible, referral to an otolaryngologist may be needed to rule out an anatomical or congenital cause of the obstruction. Beyond the newborn age, examination of the nose will usually rule out nasal obstruction from foreign bodies, blockage from significant nasal crusting, or purulent rhinitis.

Other causes of nasal obstruction, such as adenoid hypertrophy and nasal turbinate enlargement, should also be considered. Symptoms consistent with environmental allergies should be discussed and allergy testing considered. This testing should include an assessment of the immune system, including immunoglobulin (Ig) G, (total and subclass levels), IgA, IgM, IgE, and titers to diphtheria, tetanus, and pneumococcus.

Primary care clinicians should educate parents about the need to eliminate any cigarette smoke exposure, as well as discuss with them the possibility of placing the child in smaller day care groups, especially in view of the delay in immune system development and higher incidence of upper respiratory infections in children with DS.

TREATMENT OPTIONS

Successful medical management of rhinitis and sinusitis in DS depends significantly on establishing the correct diagnosis. If nasal crusting and clear rhinitis is a problem, a trial of saline nose drops or spray used on a regular basis may result in improvement. In older children, empirical trials of decongestants or antihistamines may be considered; use of antihistamines that do not cross the blood-brain barrier and, therefore, are less sedating are suggested. If rhinitis is chronically purulent, treatment with antibiotics may be indicated.

If rhinitis continues despite medical management, referral to an allergist or otolaryngologist may be needed to refine medical management, including immunotherapy, topical therapies, intravenous immunoglobulin, and surgical intervention. Adenoidectomy with or without turbinate reduction may reduce nasal obstruction and rhinorrhea by improving nasal ventilation and reducing bacterial colonization of the nasopharynx. Studies have shown that adenoid regrowth after adenoidectomy is not uncommon in DS; as a result, persistence or recurrence of nasal obstruction after adenoidectomy should prompt a follow-up nasopharyngoscopy examination or lateral neck radiography to rule out adenoid recurrence.

▥ Selected References

American Academy of Family Physicians, American Academy of Otolaryngology-Head and Neck Surgery, American Academy of Pediatrics Subcommittee on Otitis Media With Effusion. Otitis media with effusion. *Pediatrics*. 2004;113(5):1412–1429

American Academy of Pediatrics, Joint Committee on Infant Hearing. Year 2007 position statement: principles and guidelines for early hearing detection and intervention programs. *Pediatrics*. 2007;120(4):898–921

Balkany TJ, Downs MP, Jafek BW, Krajicek MJ. Hearing loss in Down's syndrome. A treatable handicap more common than generally recognized. *Clin Pediatr (Phila)*. 1979;18(2):116–118

Balkany TJ, Mischke RE, Downs MP, Jafek BW. Ossicular abnormalities in Down's syndrome. *Otolaryngol Head Neck Surg (1979)*. 1979;87(3):372–384

Bess FH. The minimally hearing-impaired child. *Ear Hear*. 1985;6(1):43–47

Blaser S, Propst EJ, Martin D, et al. Inner ear dysplasia is common in children with Down syndrome (trisomy 21). *Laryngoscope*. 2006;116(12):2113–2119

Bonnet MH. The effect of sleep fragmentation on sleep and performance in younger and older subjects. *Neurobiol Aging*. 1989;10(1):21–25

Borland LM, Colligan J, Brandom BW. Frequency of anesthesia-related complications in children with Down syndrome under general anesthesia for noncardiac procedures. *Paediatr Anaesth*. 2004;14(9):733–738

Boseley ME, Link DT, Shott SR, Fitton CM, Myer CM, Cotton RT. Laryngotracheoplasty for subglottic stenosis in Down Syndrome children: the Cincinnati experience. *Int J Pediatr Otorhinolaryngol*. 2001;57(1):11–15

Bower CM, Richmond D. Tonsillectomy and adenoidectomy in patients with Down syndrome. *Int J Pediatr Otorhinolaryngol*. 1995;33(2):141–148

Brooks DN, Wooley H, Kanjilal GC. Hearing loss and middle ear disorders patients with Down's syndrome (mongolism). *J Ment Defic Res*. 1972;16(1):21–29

Bull MJ; American Academy of Pediatrics Committee on Genetics. Health supervision for children with Down syndrome. *Pediatrics*. 2011;128(2):393–406

Cone-Wesson B, Vohr BR, Sininger YS, et al. Identification of neonatal hearing impairment: infants with hearing loss. *Ear Hear*. 2000;21(5):488–507

Dahle AJ, McCollister FP. Hearing and otologic disorders in children with Down syndrome. *Am J Ment Defic*. 1986;90(6):636–642

Davies B. Auditory disorders in Down's syndrome. *Scand Audiol Suppl*. 1988;30:65–68

Diercks GR, Wentland C, Keamy D, et al. Hypoglossal nerve stimulation in adolescents with Down syndrome and obstructive sleep apnea. *JAMA Otolaryngol Head Neck Surg*. 2018;144(1):37–42

Dobie RA, Berlin CI. Influence of otitis media on hearing and development. *Ann Otol Rhinol Laryngol Suppl*. 1979;88(5 Pt 2 Suppl 60):48–53

Donaldson JD, Redmond WM. Surgical management of obstructive sleep apnea in children with Down syndrome. *J Otolaryngol*. 1988;17(7):398–403

Donnelly LF, Shott SR, LaRose CR, Chini BA, Amin RS. Causes of persistent obstructive sleep apnea despite previous tonsillectomy and adenoidectomy in children with Down syndrome as depicted on static and dynamic cine MRI. *AJR Am J Roentgenol*. 2004;183(1):175–181

Dyken ME, Lin-Dyken DC, Poulton S, Zimmerman MB, Sedars E. Prospective polysomnographic analysis of obstructive sleep apnea in Down syndrome. *Arch Pediatr Adolesc Med*. 2003;157(7):655–660

Fitzgerald DA, Paul A, Richmond C. Severity of obstructive apnoea in children with Down syndrome who snore. *Arch Dis Child*. 2007;92(5):423–425

Gershwin ME, Crinella FM, Castles JJ, Trent JK. Immunologic characteristics of Down's syndrome. *J Ment Defic Res*. 1977;21(4):237–249

Goldbart AD, Greenberg-Dotan S, Tal A. Montelukast for children with obstructive sleep apnea: a double-blind, placebo-controlled study. *Pediatrics.* 2012;130(3):e575–e580

Halstead LA. Role of gastroesophageal reflux in pediatric upper airway disorders. *Otolaryngol Head Neck Surg.* 1999;120(2):208–214

Harada T, Sando I. Temporal bone histopathologic findings in Down's syndrome. *Arch Otolaryngol.* 1981;107(2):96–103

Harley EH, Collins MD. Neurologic sequelae secondary to atlantoaxial instability in Down syndrome: implications in otolaryngologic surgery. *Arch Otolaryngol Head Neck Surg.* 1994;120(2):159–165

Heubi CH, Knollman PK, Meinzen-Derr J, Smith DF, Ishman SL, Wiley S, Shott SR. Obstructive Sleep Apnea in Infants and Toddlers with Down Syndrome. Oral presentation, American Society of Pediatric Otolaryngology, Austin, Texas. May 2019

Heubi CH, Meinzen-Derr J, Ishman SL, Smith DF, Wiley S, Shott SR. Utilization of Polysomnography in Children with Down Syndrome: Rate and Severity of Obstructive Sleep Apnea. Oral presentation, Society for Ear, Nose, and Throat Advances in Children (SENTAC) Annual Meeting. December 1, 2017

Holm VA, Kunze LH. Effect of chronic otitis media on language and speech development. *Pediatrics.* 1969;43(5):833–839

Jacobs IN, Gray RF, Todd NW. Upper airway obstruction in children with Down syndrome. *Arch Otolaryngol Head Neck Surg.* 1996;122(9):945–950

Jacobs IN, Teague WG, Bland JW Jr. Pulmonary vascular complications of chronic airway obstruction in children. *Arch Otolaryngol Head Neck Surg.* 1997;123(7): 700–704

Johnson JL, White KR, Widen JE, et al. A multicenter evaluation of how many infants with permanent hearing loss pass a two-stage otoacoustic emissions/automated auditory brainstem response newborn hearing screening protocol. *Pediatrics.* 2005;116(3): 663–672

Kheirandish-Gozal L, Bandla HP, Gozal D. Montelukast for children with obstructive sleep apnea: results of a double-blind, randomized, placebo-controlled trial. *Ann Am Thorac Soc.* 2016;13(10):1736–1741

Lal C, White DR, Joseph JE, van Bakergem K, LaRosa A. Sleep-disordered breathing in Down syndrome. *Chest.* 2015;147(2):570–579

Lee K, Richter G, Shott S. Hall, Choo D. Surgical management of otologic disease in Down syndrome patients. Abstract presented at American Society of Pediatric Otolaryngology, Orlando, FL, May 1, 2008

Levanon A, Tarasiuk A, Tal A. Sleep characteristics in children with Down syndrome. *J Pediatr.* 1999;134(6):755–760

Levine OR, Simpser M. Alveolar hypoventilation and cor pulmonale associated with chronic airway obstruction in infants with Down syndrome. *Clin Pediatr (Phila).* 1982;21(1):25–29

Marcus CL, Keens TG, Bautista DB, von Pechmann WS, Ward SL. Obstructive sleep apnea in children with Down syndrome. *Pediatrics.* 1991;88(1):132–139

Marcus CL, Lutz J, Carroll JL, Bamford O. Arousal and ventilatory responses during sleep in children with obstructive sleep apnea. *J Appl Physiol (1985).* 1998;84(6):1926–1936

Maurizi M, Ottaviani F, Paludetti G, Lungarotti S. Audiological findings in Down's children. *Int J Pediatr Otorhinolaryngol.* 1985;9(3):227–232

Merrell JA, Shott SR. OSAS in Down syndrome: T&A versus T&A plus lateral pharyngoplasty. *Int J Pediatr Otorhinolaryngol.* 2007;71(8):1197–1203

Miller JD, Capusten BM, Lampard R. Changes at the base of skull and cervical spine in Down syndrome. *Can Assoc Radiol J.* 1986;37(2):85–89

Mitchell RB. Adenotonsillectomy for obstructive sleep apnea in children: outcome evaluated by pre- and postoperative polysomnography. *Laryngoscope.* 2007;117(10):1844–1854

Mitchell RB, Call E, Kelly J. Ear, nose and throat disorders in children with Down syndrome. *Laryngoscope.* 2003;113(2):259–263

Mitchell V, Howard R, Facer E. Down's syndrome and anaesthesia. *Paediatr Anaesth.* 1995;5(6):379–384

Moos DD, Prasch M, Cantral DE, Huls B, Cuddeford JD. Are patients with obstructive sleep apnea syndrome appropriate candidates for the ambulatory surgical center? *AANA J.* 2005;73(3):197–205

Ng DK, Chan CH, Cheung JM. Children with Down syndrome and OSA do not necessarily snore. *Arch Dis Child.* 2007;92(11):1047–1048

Ng DK, Hui HN, Chan CH, et al. Obstructive sleep apnoea in children with Down syndrome. *Singapore Med J.* 2006;47(9):774–779

Pynnonen MA, Mukerji SS, Kim HM, Adams ME, Terrell JE. Nasal saline for chronic sinonasal symptoms: a randomized controlled trial. *Arch Otolaryngol Head Neck Surg.* 2007;133(11):1115–1120

Roizen NJ, Martich V, Ben-Ami T, Shalowitz MU, Yousefzadeh DK. Sclerosis of the mastoid air cells as an indicator of undiagnosed otitis media in children with Down's syndrome. *Clin Pediatr (Phila).* 1994;33(7):439–443

Rowland TW, Nordstrom LG, Bean MS, Burkhardt H. Chronic upper airway obstruction and pulmonary hypertension in Down's syndrome. *Am J Dis Child.* 1981;135(11):1050–1052

Sherry KM. Post-extubation stridor in Down's syndrome. *Br J Anaesth.* 1983;55(1):53–55

Shibahara Y, Sando I. Congenital anomalies of the eustachian tube in Down syndrome: histopathologic case report. *Ann Otol Rhinol Laryngol.* 1989;98(7 Pt 1):543–547

Shott SR. Down syndrome: analysis of airway size and a guide for appropriate intubation. *Laryngoscope.* 2000;110(4):585–592

Shott SR. Down syndrome: common ear, nose and throat problems. *Down Syndrome Quarterly.* 2000;5:1–6

Shott SR. Down syndrome: common otolaryngologic manifestations. *Am J Med Genet C Semin Med Genet.* 2006;142C(3):131–140

Shott SR, Amin R, Chini B, Heubi C, Hotze S, Akers R. Obstructive sleep apnea: should all children with Down syndrome be tested? *Arch Otolaryngol Head Neck Surg.* 2006;132(4):432–436

Shott SR, Donnelly LF. Cine magnetic resonance imaging: evaluation of persistent airway obstruction after tonsil and adenoidectomy in children with Down syndrome. *Laryngoscope.* 2004;114(10):1724–1729

Shott SR, Heubi C, Akers R. Hearing loss in Down syndrome—do PETs help? Abstract presented at Society for Ear, Nose and Throat Advances in Children, New Orleans, LA, October 2003

Shott SR, Joseph A, Heithaus D. Hearing loss in children with Down syndrome. *Int J Pediatr Otorhinolaryngol.* 2001;61(3):199–205

Southall DP, Stebbens VA, Mirza R, Lang MH, Croft CB, Shinebourne EA. Upper airway obstruction with hypoxaemia and sleep disruption in Down syndrome. *Dev Med Child Neurol.* 1987;29(6):734–742

Spina CA, Smith D, Korn E, Fahey JL, Grossman HJ. Altered cellular immune functions in patients with Down's syndrome. *Am J Dis Child.* 1981;135(3):251–255

Strome M. Down's syndrome: a modern otorhinolaryngological perspective. *Laryngoscope.* 1981;91(10):1581–1594

Tauman R, Gulliver TE, Krishna J, et al. Persistence of obstructive sleep apnea syndrome in children after adenotonsillectomy. *J Pediatr.* 2006;149(6):803–808

Venail F, Gardiner Q, Mondain M. ENT and speech disorders in children with Down's syndrome: an overview of pathophysiology, clinical features, treatments, and current management. *Clin Pediatr (Phila).* 2004;43(9):783–791

Yamaguchi N, Sando I, Hashida Y, Takahashi H, Matsune S. Histologic study of eustachian tube cartilage with and without congenital anomalies: a preliminary study. *Ann Otol Rhinol Laryngol.* 1990;99(12):984–987

CHAPTER 25

Vascular Anomalies

Tara L. Rosenberg, MD,
and David H. Darrow, MD, DDS

Introduction
Classification
Vascular Tumors
    Infantile Hemangioma
    Congenital Hemangiomas
    Kaposiform
    Hemangioendothelioma
    Tufted Angioma
    Pyogenic Granuloma

Vascular Malformations
    Lymphatic Malformations
    Venous Malformations
    Capillary Malformations
    Arteriovenous
        Malformations

▓ Introduction

The evaluation and management of vascular anomalies can be difficult because of confusing terminology, variations in clinical and radiographic presentation, and deficiencies in education about these lesions in many training programs. Inconsistent use of accurate terminology, lack of familiarity with clinical and radiographic characteristics, and inadequate exposure to patients with vascular anomalies can lead to errors in diagnosis and inappropriate treatment recommendations. However, an accurate and a thorough history and physical examination are key to diagnosing vascular anomalies and making an appropriate referral when necessary.

Vascular anomalies in children involve the head and neck approximately 60% of the time. They can affect important functions such as vision, hearing, and breathing. Some anomalies may be severely disfiguring, with significant psychosocial sequelae for patients and families.

■ Classification

In 1982, Mulliken and Glowacki suggested a classification system that categorized vascular anomalies as either *vascular tumors* or *vascular malformations* based on clinical history, histologic findings, and radiographic appearance. The most common vascular tumor is the infantile hemangioma (IH). Common vascular malformations include lymphatic, capillary, venous, and arteriovenous malformations (AVMs), which are named according to the type of vessels that make up the lesion. The International Society for the Study of Vascular Anomalies classification, initially drafted in 1996, was updated in 2018, and is the most widely used classification system for vascular anomalies. Using this classification system as a framework for evaluating vascular anomalies can improve diagnostic accuracy and lead to appropriate treatment recommendations.

■ Vascular Tumors

Vascular tumors are neoplasms that result from disordered angiogenesis. Infantile hemangiomas are by far the most common vascular tumor in infants and are the most common soft-tissue tumor of infancy. These will be discussed in detail in the sections to follow. Other vascular tumors discussed in this chapter include congenital hemangioma, kaposiform hemangioendothelioma (KHE), tufted angioma, and pyogenic granuloma.

INFANTILE HEMANGIOMA

Etiology

The pathogenesis of IHs is uncertain. In the recent past, it was suggested that they may be the result of transfer of placental cells to the fetus. The presence of glucose transporter 1 (GLUT1), which also is found in placenta but not in other vascular lesions and the increased risk of IHs after chorionic villus sampling support this hypothesis. However, the absence of villous architecture and trophoblastic elements makes ectopic placental tissue a less likely explanation. A more plausible theory is that IHs result from aberrant proliferation and differentiation of pluripotent progenitor cells that migrate to locations that enhance the growth of placenta-like tissue.

Epidemiology

The incidence of IHs is approximately 4% to 5%. Risk factors include prematurity, low birth weight, multigestational pregnancy, female gender, white race, advanced maternal age, and history of chorionic villus sampling during the first trimester. Infantile hemangiomas are typically single and sporadic. Only 3% of patients present with multifocal (more than 5) lesions. A few families exhibit an autosomal-dominant inheritance pattern.

Diagnosis and Natural History

Infantile hemangiomas can usually be diagnosed by history and physical examination alone. The age at which the lesion first appeared and changes in the size and appearance of the lesion over time usually lead the primary care clinician (PCC) to the correct diagnosis.

Infantile hemangiomas are not typically present at birth but usually appear during the first few months afterward. Their growth pattern is characterized by rapid proliferation, followed by involution of variable duration.

The proliferation phase begins immediately after the IH appears, usually in the first few weeks after birth. A period of rapid growth follows, with most growth completed by about 5 months of age. The involution phase usually begins at 6 to 12 months of age, with the results becoming more apparent as proliferation slows. Most of the regression occurs before 4 years of age, but it may continue for a few years more. During involution, the lesion becomes lighter, softer, and smaller. The vascular network is replaced with fibrofatty tissue and dense collagen. Infantile hemangiomas that leave a residuum that may appear as epidermal atrophy, telangiectasia, fibrofatty tissue, or excess skin. In such cases, the patient may benefit from laser treatment or surgery during the involution phase.

Physical Examination

The physical appearance of IHs can be described on the basis of depth and area. Lesions can be superficial, deep, or compound. Superficial lesions are usually red plaques or slightly raised lesions that do not involve deeper tissues (**Figure 25-1**). Deep lesions create a mass effect in soft tissues, and overlying skin typically has a bluish discoloration. Care must be taken in diagnosing deep lesions as IHs because some deeper blue-tinged lesions may actually be venous malformations or other vascular anomalies. Deep IHs typically have a fleshy quality and will not completely empty with compression. Compound IHs (**Figure 25-2**) have deep and superficial components. Infantile hemangiomas may be further characterized as focal or segmental. Segmental lesions (**Figure 25-3**) are often superficial and are more likely than focal lesions to have associated morbidity, most commonly ulceration.

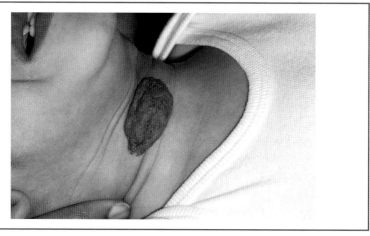

Figure 25-1. Superficial hemangioma. Such lesions may be raised and focal as seen, or flat and diffuse (segmental).

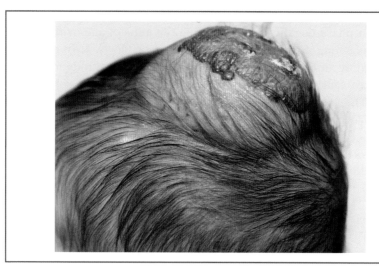

Figure 25-2. Compound hemangioma of the scalp, with both superficial involvement and deep involvement.

A small subset of children with IHs have congenital anomalies recognized as clinical associations. The most common is PHACE, which is a congenital vasculopathy with features of **P**osterior fossa defects, **H**emangiomas, cerebrovascular **A**rterial anomalies, **C**ardiovascular anomalies (most commonly **C**oarctation of the aorta), and **E**ye anomalies. Clefting of the sternum is also a common

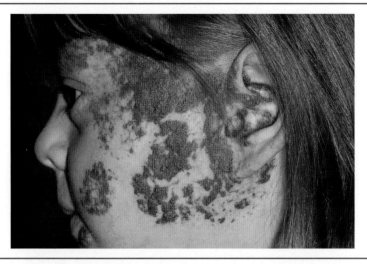

Figure 25-3. Superficial segmental hemangioma of the left side of the face.

finding. In PHACE, the IH is large and segmental, characteristically located on the face, scalp, or neck (**Figure 25-4**). Central nervous system sequelae include developmental delay, seizure, and/or stroke. Any infant with a large, facial segmental IH in a dermatome distribution should undergo a neurologic evaluation, an ophthalmologic examination, echocardiography, and magnetic resonance imaging (MRI) of the brain, neck, and chest with contrast as part of the evaluation for PHACE syndrome.

An IH of the airway should be suspected in infants with progressive stridor that is delayed in onset. Patients with these lesions are often erroneously diagnosed with recurrent croup because they respond well to steroids. Airway IHs are often associated with segmental IHs of the lower face, lip, oral mucosa, and/or anterior midline neck, especially in patients with PHACE. In such cases, early referral to an otolaryngologist for flexible fiberoptic laryngoscopy in the office and/or operative endoscopy is indicated.

> **Pearl:** Progressive development of stridor in a patient with a facial cutaneous hemangioma should prompt an airway evaluation.

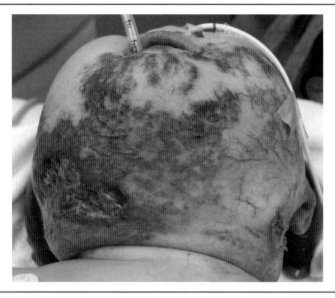

Figure 25-4. Large "beard distribution" segmental hemangioma with ulceration, typical of PHACE syndrome.

HISTOLOGIC EVALUATION

Lesions that require excision or biopsy may display immunohistochemical markers on the surface of the endothelium for diagnosis. Infantile hemangiomas stain positively for GLUT1 in the endothelium. This marker is not present in vascular malformations or congenital hemangiomas. Infantile hemangiomas also demonstrate multilaminated basement membranes not found in vascular malformations.

Imaging

Imaging usually is not required to diagnose IHs, but lesions with uncommon features or unusual histories may necessitate such evaluation. For cases in which the imaging is necessary to establish a diagnosis, Doppler ultrasound is cost-effective and easily performed in infants without the need for sedation and without the radiation risk associated with other imaging modalities. Ultrasound also may be indicated for patients with 5 or more cutaneous IHs because such patients are at higher risk for visceral IHs. This modality is 84% sensitive and 98% specific in diagnosing IHs when lesions demonstrate high vessel density ($>5/cm^2$) and high Doppler shift (>2 kHz).

For assessment of extent of the lesion, MRI is the study of choice. On MRI, IHs appear as hypervascular soft-tissue masses with flow voids and are typically lobulated and clearly separated from surrounding muscle. During involution, fibrofatty tissue is seen as increased areas of high-intensity foci. Unfortunately, MRI in infants typically requires general anesthesia.

> **Pearl:** While patients with multiple hemangiomas are at increased risk of developing visceral lesions, many visceral lesions can be followed with serial imaging and may not require intervention.

Complications

Many IHs resolve without sequelae. In some anatomical locations, complications will be more likely. Lesions near the eye may cause visual deficits, and those involving the airway may threaten breathing. Complications are most commonly seen in the early to mid-proliferating phase when growth is most rapid. Ulceration, obstruction, bleeding, infection, heart failure, and physical deformity can also be seen.

Ulceration occurs in up to 16% of IHs (**Figure 25-5**), typically in areas with significant moisture or friction, such as the lips, neck

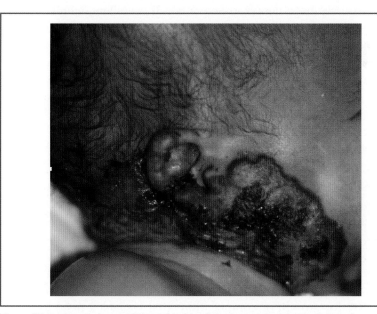

Figure 25-5. Ulcerated area of the right side of the face and neck. Ulceration always leaves a scar.

skin folds, and diaper area. Segmental lesions are 8 times more likely to ulcerate than focal lesions. Ulcers are usually painful and may be accompanied by reduced oral intake. Bleeding may occur with ulceration, but is usually easily controlled with pressure, and ulceration nearly always leaves behind scarred skin. Management is with barrier dressings, topical anesthetics, systemic β-blockers, and sometimes surgical excision.

Obstruction of the visual axis or auditory canal can lead to changes in vision or hearing. Periorbital lesions carry a high risk of serious complications, including ptosis, amblyopia, and astigmatism. Because of this, periocular lesions warrant close evaluation and early treatment, usually with systemic medical therapy. Lesions that are difficult to diagnose must be imaged to distinguish them from lymphatic malformations, neurofibroma, rhabdomyosarcoma, and neuroblastoma.

Bilateral lesions affecting the external auditory canal are rare but may produce conductive hearing loss severe enough to hinder speech and language development.

After age 3 years, as body image begins to develop, significant psychosocial sequelae may be observed. Children aged 3 to 5 years with head and neck IHs may feel that others do not value them as highly as children of the same age without such lesions. Negative psychosocial effects also have been demonstrated in family members of children with head and neck IHs. Family members are frequently subjected to questions or comments from friends and other family members and even from complete strangers. They may have to field questions about child abuse. Families notice that other people tend to stare at, ignore, or avoid children with IHs. Bullying or cruelty can lead to withdrawal, anger, or aggression in patients with vascular anomalies.

Management

Patients with high-risk IHs should be referred to a hemangioma specialist for evaluation and management. Features of head and neck lesions requiring immediate referral are listed in **Box 25-1.** However, one must keep in mind that proliferation of IH is an active process, and therefore any head and neck IH at least 1 cm in diameter, especially those in infants younger than 4 months of age with the potential to evolve, should also be considered for referral. Those IHs that do not meet these criteria should still be actively monitored by the PCC for growth or complications that suggest a need for intervention. The indications for intervention are listed in **Box 25-2,**

> ## Box 25-1. Referral Criteria for Infantile Hemangiomas of the Head and Neck
>
> Periorbital lesions
> Lesions of the central face and ears
> Segmental or ulcerating lesions
> Lesions associated with stridor
> Lesions over 4 cm in size
> Number of lesions (5 or more)

> ## Box 25-2. Indications for Intervention
>
> Emergency treatment of potentially life-threatening complications
> Urgent treatment for existing or imminent functional impairment, pain, or bleeding
> Evaluation to identify important structural anomalies potentially associated with infantile hemangiomas
> Elective treatment to reduce the likelihood of long-term or permanent disfigurement

and factors to consider when deciding the timing and type of treatment are shown in **Box 25-3.**

Medical Therapy

Although systemic corticosteroids were the primary medical therapy for IHs during the latter half of the 20th century, β-blockers have largely replaced them in this role. Widescale use of β-blocker therapy commenced after a 2008 case series reported that patients with cardiac manifestations of their lesions who had been treated with propranolol experienced regression of their IHs. The manner in which propranolol works in IH treatment is not completely understood, but

> ## Box 25-3. Factors to Consider for Timing and Type of Treatment
>
> Age of the patient
> Growth phase of the lesion
> Location and size of the lesion
> Degree of skin involvement
> Severity of complications and urgency of intervention
> Potential for adverse psychosocial consequences
> Parental preference
> Physician experience

proposed mechanisms of action include vasoconstriction, inhibition of angiogenesis, downregulation of matrix metalloproteinases and interleukin-6, regulation of the renin-angiotensin system, and inhibition of nitric oxide production.

Many authors have reported high success rates treating IHs with propranolol (**Figure 25-6**). The medication is administered orally at relatively low doses (maximum, 3–3.4 mg/kg/day depending on the formulation) until the lesion or lesions are clearly no longer proliferating. Contraindications to propranolol therapy include cardiogenic shock, sinus bradycardia, hypotension, heart block greater than first degree, heart failure, asthma/reactive airway disease, and known hypersensitivity to the drug. Special precautions have been suggested for children with PHACE syndrome who have high-risk intracranial vascular anomalies. Common adverse effects of propranolol include sleep disturbance, cold hands and feet, diarrhea, and bronchial hyperreactivity. Rare adverse effects include bradycardia and hypotension, which are generally asymptomatic, and severe hypoglycemia, which may be associated with decreased responsiveness or seizures. The medication typically is taken with meals and withheld during periods of illness to reduce the likelihood of hypoglycemia. Rebound growth after discontinuation of therapy is reported at 5% to 25%; as a result, some PCCs wean propranolol over a number of weeks to months.

Topical use of timolol, a β-blocker used to treat glaucoma, has demonstrated efficacy in the treatment of thin, superficial IHs. The medication is usually applied twice a day. Timolol 0.5% gel-forming solution has less systemic absorption than timolol in solution formulation.

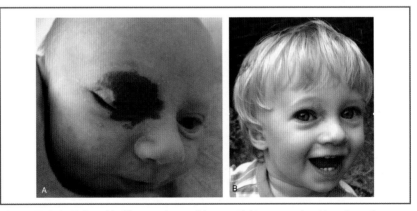

Figure 25-6. A, Right orbital hemangioma with potential to cause visual impairment. B, Same orbital lesion after 13 months of propranolol therapy.

With the advent of β-blockers in IH treatment, corticosteroids are now rarely used for systemic management. In the past, steroids were used based on their antiangiogenic properties, but they are associated with frequent and significant risks, and are now generally used only in cases of propranolol treatment failures. Rarely, intralesional steroids may be used as an adjunct to systemic therapy to reduce the size of bulky lesions.

Laser Therapy

Laser therapy may be useful in reducing the surface color of IHs. In the β-blocker era, laser is used primarily in the treatment of residual telangiectasia after the IH has mostly involuted. The pulsed dye laser has a wavelength of 595 nm, which is close to the absorption peak of oxyhemoglobin (577 nm) and is therefore the workhorse laser for this purpose. Laser is not effective in treating the deeper component of compound lesions, as its penetration is only 1 mm.

Surgical Treatment

Early surgical therapy (within the first year after birth) is reserved primarily for lesions with severe acute complications not responding to medical therapy. The most common complication requiring early surgical intervention is obstruction, affecting vision, hearing, or respiration (**Figure 25-7**). Delaying more elective surgery until after infancy allows the lesion time to involute, becoming smaller and less vascular, and reduces the risks of anesthetic morbidity, blood loss, and iatrogenic injury. Other reasonable indications for excision of an IH during infancy include a focal lesion in a favorable location or elective surgery leaving a scar that would be the same if the lesion were removed after involution. Late surgical intervention, when involution is complete,

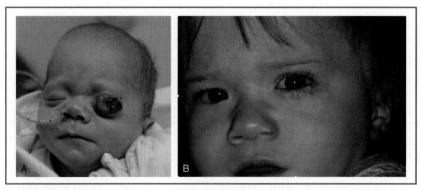

Figure 25-7. A, Ulcerating hemangioma of the left lower eyelid, causing severe pain and obstructed vision. B, Patient after excision of hemangioma.

is aimed at correcting abnormal contouring and distortion related to fibrofatty tissue and atrophy of affected skin. Because most hemangiomas do not improve significantly beyond age 4 years, surgery prior to this age should be considered to correct the deformity before self-esteem and long-term memory are well established.

CONGENITAL HEMANGIOMA

Congenital hemangiomas are present at birth. They can be divided into rapidly involuting congenital hemangioma and noninvoluting congenital hemangioma types. A third type of congenital hemangioma, known as partially involuting congenital hemangioma, has recently been described. Congenital hemangiomas do not undergo a rapid proliferation phase after birth because they are fully formed at birth. Rapidly involuting congenital hemangiomas are raised with a blue or violet color and are often surrounded by a hypopigmented halo. Regression begins early and is usually complete at between 6 and 14 months of age. Noninvoluting congenital hemangiomas are well-circumscribed solitary lesions with a reddish pink plaque, central telangiectasia, and hypopigmentation around the rim. They grow with the child and persist into adulthood. Both rapidly involuting and noninvoluting lesions are negative for GLUT1 on histologic staining.

KAPOSIFORM HEMANGIOENDOTHELIOMA

Kaposiform hemangioendotheliomas are rare in the head and neck. They occur anywhere on the body and are benign lesions with a significant lymphatic component. They generally are cutaneous nodules with a purple color that extend into deeper tissues. Most lesions appear before age 2 years and may be present at birth. They occur with equal frequency in boys and girls. Biopsy may be required to make a diagnosis. This lesion, and not IH, may be associated with Kasabach-Merritt phenomenon, a life-threatening condition related to platelet trapping within the lesion that results in significant thrombocytopenia. Magnetic resonance imaging demonstrates a hypervascular tumor involving multiple tissue layers with poorly defined margins. Occasionally, lesions may be multifocal.

TUFTED ANGIOMA

Tufted angiomas tend to be more localized than KHEs and appear as pink or red macules with papules. They occur with equal frequency in boys and girls. More than half appear before age 5 years, and

15% are congenital. As with KHE, biopsy is often required for diagnosis. These lesions can also produce the Kasabach-Merritt phenomenon.

PYOGENIC GRANULOMA

A pyogenic granuloma may be easily mistaken for an IH. While common during childhood, pyogenic granulomas are uncommon during the first year after birth. Pathogenesis of pyogenic granuloma is not well understood. They are often associated with minor trauma and may represent an exaggerated vascular proliferation in response to local irritation. They are usually raised and pedunculated, but occasionally may be sessile (**Figure 25-8**). They bleed easily even with mild trauma because of a large feeding vessel. Histologically, pyogenic granulomas are nearly identical to IHs with endothelial proliferation and vascular spaces, although they appear more lobular. Conservative local excision is usually curative, though other treatment options are available.

■ Vascular Malformations

Vascular malformations are present at birth and can contain arterial, venous, or lymphatic vessels. Some lesions are composed of a combination of blood vessel types. These lesions result from errors in vasculogenesis. Lesions are often associated with local soft-tissue or

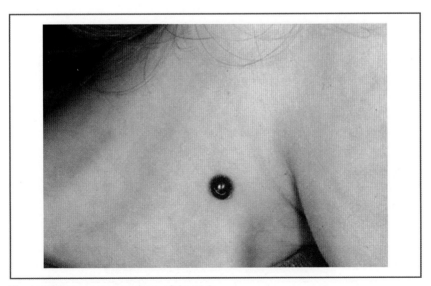

Figure 25-8. Pyogenic granuloma of the neck.

bony overgrowth. Malformations are one-tenth as common as infantile hemangiomas.

LYMPHATIC MALFORMATIONS

Etiology and Epidemiology

Lymphatic malformations (LMs) are conglomerates of abnormal lymphatic channels resulting in the accumulation of lymph in dilated cystic spaces. Estimates of incidence vary, but these lesions may be as common as 1 in 2,000 to 4,000 live births. Most LMs are found in the head and neck (**Figure 25-9**), and they are equally distributed among males and females. Approximately 50% of LMs are noted at birth, and symptoms present in 90% of patients by 2 years of age. With most pregnancies now closely monitored by ultrasound, many LMs are identified prenatally. Lesions occur sporadically, likely as a result of de novo somatic mutations.

Diagnosis and Natural History

Lymphatic malformations typically present as a skin-colored or blue-tinged mass involving the face or neck. If they are composed of many microcysts, LMs are usually noncompressible, but lesions consisting of 1 or 2 macrocysts are doughy to the touch. The lesions are nontender unless they have been recently inflamed. Such inflammation typically occurs as a result of trauma or

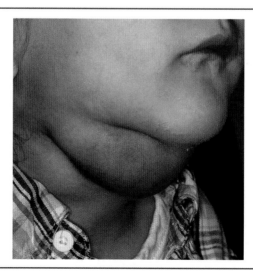

Figure 25-9. Inflamed lymphatic malformation of the neck.

infection. The overlying skin or mucosa may be involved; in such cases, there often are surface lymph vesicles that become hemorrhagic when inflamed. Lymphatic malformations tend to expand over time but seem to be less active in adulthood. A physical examination and imaging are usually adequate for diagnosis; biopsy is not ordinarily required.

Imaging and Staging

Although LMs are frequently imaged with both computed tomography (CT) and MRI, MRI provides superior detail of the extent of the lesion and its relationship to surrounding structures. T1-weighted MRI shows nonenhancing muscle signal intensity, and T2-weighted images show a high-signal-intensity lesion without feeding or draining vessels. Computed tomography reveals a fluid-density lesion that does not enhance. Both MRI and CT allow distinction between microcystic and macrocystic lesions, the latter of which have cystic spaces measuring 2 cm or more.

Staging is based on the relationship to the hyoid and on laterality. Stage 1 is unilateral and infrahyoid. Stage 2 is unilateral and suprahyoid. Stage 3 is unilateral suprahyoid and infrahyoid. Stage 4 is bilateral suprahyoid. Stage 5 is bilateral suprahyoid and infrahyoid.

Complications

Complications due to LMs most commonly are associated with suprahyoid lesions. Airway compromise can occur via extrinsic compression or intrinsic involvement of the tongue, larynx, or other structures in the airway, often necessitating tracheotomy. Those involving the tongue can cause obstruction, but they may also interfere with articulation and swallowing at a minimum, and with severe malocclusion and dentofacial deformity in severe cases. Large lesions may be associated with lymphocytopenia affecting T, B, and natural killer cells. Bony overgrowth usually is observed, but in some cases bone loss occurs, particularly in Gorham disease as lymphatic vessels replace bony structures.

Lymphatic malformations—especially suprahyoid microcystic lesions—are particularly prone to infection. Swelling associated with infection may compromise feeding and respiration. Infections are treated with broad-spectrum antibiotics. Systemic corticosteroids may help resolve compressive or obstructive sequelae associated with infection.

Treatment

The goal in treating LMs should be preservation or, when necessary, restoration of functional and esthetic integrity. Severe or life-threatening functional impairment requires prompt treatment. If there is no significant functional deficit, treatment may be delayed to allow the patient to grow.

Observation is appropriate for some lesions. Macrocystic lesions, especially those in the posterior neck, may be observed and, rarely, regress spontaneously. Small lesions without functional deficit also may be observed. However, trauma or infection can lead to rapid enlargement.

Sclerotherapy is most useful in treating macrocystic lesions. Sclerosing agents include doxycycline, bleomycin, OK-432 (picibanil), and ethanol, although the latter carries a significant risk of neuro-toxicity. Bleomycin has been associated with pulmonary fibrosis and interstitial pneumonia in treatment of malignancy, but these adverse effects are minimized by keeping the total lifetime dose below 400 units. Erythema, pain, fever, and skin blistering sometimes are seen. Macrocystic lesions generally respond well to sclerotherapy, while microcystic lesions demonstrate a complete response rate of only 14% and a partial response rate of 50%.

Surgery continues to be the most effective treatment modality. Macrocystic lesions, whether suprahyoid or infrahyoid, are often amenable to resection. However, infiltrative microcystic lesions are much less easily resected, especially if they are bilateral or supra-hyoid, or if they compromise the aerodigestive tract. These lesions are more likely to require tracheostomy and gastrostomy. Rates of surgical complications for some lesions, particularly large, mixed suprahyoid lesions, are high. Complications include cranial nerve injury, bleeding due to great vessel injury, infection, and airway compromise. Complete excision should be performed whenever possible, but extensive lesions may require subtotal excision to protect vital structures. Nerve injury may be minimized by using appropriate nerve monitoring.

Systemic medication has become an important adjunct in the management of LMs. Sirolimus, a mammalian target of rapamycin inhibitor used for immunosuppression in patients undergoing trans-plantation, blocks downstream protein synthesis and demonstrates antitumoral and antiangiogenic activity. Several large series suggest efficacy in treatment of LMs, but optimal dosing and duration of therapy have not yet been established. In addition, there are some reports of induction of lymphomas and skin cancers. Nevertheless, sirolimus seems to be solidifying its place in the management of large and/or unresectable LMs.

VENOUS MALFORMATIONS

Etiology and Epidemiology

Venous malformations (VMs) arise from defective development of veins in selected areas. These lesions consist of dilated and dysfunctional venous channels and are characterized by defects in the smooth muscle layer of the vessels. More than 90% of VMs occur sporadically, but some may be inherited and may be linked to a mutation in the tyrosine kinase protein receptor. Approximately 40% of these lesions appear in the head and neck region.

Diagnosis and Natural History

Venous malformations are present at birth, but they may not be visible at birth. When there is cutaneous or superficial soft-tissue involvement, the lesions are blue and compressible (**Figure 25-10**). Deeper lesions may not be evident on inspection but demonstrate characteristic enlargement due to venous filling when the head is below the level of the heart or during a Valsalva maneuver. While clinical presentation alone is often sufficient to make the diagnosis, patients with deeper lesions may require imaging or needle aspiration to confirm the diagnosis.

Venous malformations gradually become larger and may become painful, especially when the affected body part is lowered and fills with venous blood or when they develop intralesional thrombi. They also may become more symptomatic in response to trauma, intervention, infection, or hormonal influences.

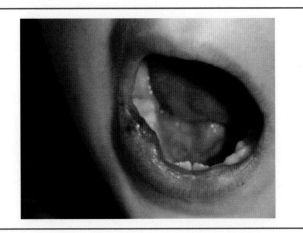

Figure 25-10. Venous malformation of the right lower lip. A purple color is typical of these lesions.

Like LMs, VMs are best imaged via MRI for purposes of establishing the extensiveness and relationship to surrounding structures. Magnetic resonance imaging reveals a bright signal on T2-weighted signals and hypointensity on T1. Phleboliths are a common finding on imaging and are noted as signal voids on MRI and as calcifications on CT and plain radiographs (**Figure 25-11**). Computed tomography often is not diagnostic, and MRI may be required to confirm the diagnosis.

Biopsy usually is not required to make the diagnosis. However, if biopsy is performed, histologic evaluation shows venous and lymphatic elements. On ultrasound, VMs demonstrate slow blood flow.

Complications

Complications are similar to those seen with LMs. Airway compromise can occur as a result of involvement of the tongue, larynx, or other structures in the airway. Oral lesions can be easily traumatized and will ooze briskly should this occur. Tongue VMs can cause obstruction and problems with speech and swallowing. As with LMs, malocclusion and dentofacial deformity in severe cases may result from chronic tongue protrusion. About 50% of patients

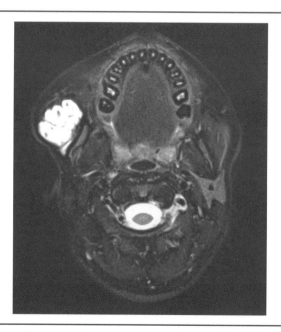

Figure 25-11. Magnetic resonance imaging demonstrating venous malformation of the right buccal fat space. Flow voids in the mass are due to phlebolith formation.

develop localized intravascular coagulation that, owing to trauma or surgery, can evolve into disseminated intravascular coagulation when D-dimers are severely elevated and fibrinogen levels are very low.

Treatment

Conservative management of head and neck VMs includes elevation of the head when in bed, and management of thrombosis-related pain using low-dose aspirin and nonsteroidal anti-inflammatory drugs. Superficial VMs may be treated with the long-pulse neodymium:yttrium-aluminum-garnet (Nd:YAG) laser. Deeper lesions are managed with sclerotherapy (usually sodium tetradecyl sulfate or bleomycin), surgical resection, or both. Preoperative embolization displaces blood from the lesion, facilitating the surgery. Surgery alone may be considered first-line treatment for some smaller VMs. Sirolimus has been used with some success in the management of complex or otherwise untreatable VMs.

CAPILLARY MALFORMATIONS

Etiology and Epidemiology

Capillary malformations are commonly referred to as *port-wine stains* (PWSs). The lesions consist of dilated postcapillary venules resulting from unopposed parasympathetic influence on the vessels. Histologic evaluation of a PWS shows a plexus of dilated blood vessels at a depth of 100 to 1,000 µm (in the upper dermis). The overlying epidermis is histologically normal. Port-wine stains are seen in 0.3% to 0.5% of children and occur equally in boys and girls. They are frequently found on the face or neck (**Figure 25-12**) and can have a significant psychosocial effect.

Diagnosis and Natural History

Port-wine stains are frequently seen on the midface and upper face. Lesions with V1 or V2 distribution are seen in Sturge-Weber syndrome. Lesions with significant eyelid involvement should raise suspicion for this syndrome, and MRI imaging to rule out leptomeningeal involvement is warranted. In such cases, evaluation by an ophthalmologist to rule out glaucoma is appropriate. Lesions are present at birth and become darker, thicker, and more nodular over time. The surface skin lesions have a poorly understood influence on the underlying soft and bony tissues, causing tissue hyperplasia. This results in significant orodental changes in V2 lesions and facial asymmetry for all facial lesions.

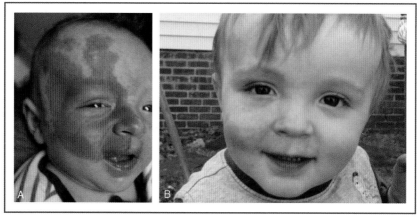

Figure 25-12. A, Capillary malformation (port-wine stain with right V1 and V2 distribution). B, Malformation after treatment with pulsed dye laser.

Complications

Complications from capillary malformations are rare and are primarily related to the tissue hyperplasia and oral cavity changes described earlier. In advanced cases, small blebs may develop on the surface of the lesions and bleed intermittently.

Treatment

Historically, skin grafting, radiation, dermabrasion, cryosurgery, tattooing, and electrotherapy have been used to treat PWS. However, because of poor cosmetic outcomes and associated risks, none of these modalities is currently considered appropriate therapy for PWS.

Although no curative therapy exists, current treatment consists of serial treatments with the pulsed dye laser. Using light at a wavelength of 585 to 595 nm allows selective photothermolysis of abnormal blood vessels seen in PWS by targeting oxyhemoglobin and deoxyhemoglobin. Because melanin is a barrier to pulsed dye laser, patients with darker skin may be more difficult to treat. Cobblestones and blebs may be excised as necessary.

ARTERIOVENOUS MALFORMATIONS

Etiology and Epidemiology

Of all vascular malformations, AVMs can be the most dangerous and difficult to manage because of their high flow, bleeding risk, and infiltrative nature. Arteriovenous malformations develop from somatic mutations causing perivascular instability and vascular infiltration. The lesions contain an abnormal precapillary connection between arteries and veins and histologically demonstrate arterio-venous shunts and dilated capillary beds. The lesions are rare but, among vascular lesions, they are associated with the greatest morbidity and mortality.

Arteriovenous malformations occur 1.5 times more often in females than in males. Lesions appearing at birth or during child-hood are equal among males and females, but lesions occurring after puberty are seen 4 times as often in females.

Diagnosis and Natural History

In 59% of cases, AVMs are present at birth. Ten percent appear in childhood, 10% in adolescence, and 20% in adulthood. They fre-quently involve the midface. Early AVMs may be mistaken for IHs, but do not demonstrate involution. The lesions tend to go through 4 stages. The first is dormancy; during this stage, the lesion may be mistaken for other vascular lesions. These malformations demonstrate cutaneous blush and warmth. Expansion, the second stage, often occurs during adolescence. During expansion, lesions demonstrate bruit or audible pulsation. Intraluminal hydrostatic pressure associ-ated with the arterial component seems to predispose these lesions to expansion at a much greater rate than that of other vascular malfor-mations. It has been suggested that arteriovenous communications dilate surrounding veins. Destruction and heart failure are the final 2 stages and are discussed later in the section on Complications.

Lesions demonstrate high flow, enlarge over time, and can occur anywhere in the head and neck. They often involve the cheek or auricle. Lesions frequently are pulsatile, and a bruit may be pres-ent. On arteriography, early venous filling is diagnostic of these lesions. Magnetic resonance imaging demonstrates the extent of the lesion and allows for treatment planning. Computed tomographic angiography provides excellent detail of vascular architecture and can guide treatment as well. These lesions may progress rapidly, so diagnostic workup should be completed in a timely fashion. The physical examination and imaging usually provide the diagnosis. A biopsy of an AVM can produce significant blood loss and should be avoided.

Complications

During the destruction stage (stage 3), lesions are painful and ulcerative. They may lead to life-threatening hemorrhage or infec-tion. Ischemia secondary to arterial steal can cause pain and skin breakdown. In stage 4, high-output cardiac failure may occur early, even in infancy. These lesions may undergo rapid change during puberty, trauma, surgery, or pregnancy. Once symptoms develop, they persist or worsen until the lesion is treated. Lesions can involve bone, especially the mandible and maxilla, and can create significant deformity.

Treatment

Treatment typically consists of embolization followed by surgery. Lesions are prone to recurrence, so the treatment plan must be carefully considered. Arteriovenous malformations undergoing subtotal excision or proximal ligation may suddenly expand. Extensive lesions may require free-tissue transfer for reconstruction after complete resection.

Deciding which lesions to treat and the timing of treatment remains controversial for some lesions. Discrete stage 1 lesions can be removed relatively easily. Treating these lesions early may eliminate the need for higher-risk or urgent treatment later. Treatment success has been shown to be higher in stage 1 lesions. Stage 2 and 3 lesions, which may be painful, rapidly enlarging, or ulcerating, warrant timely treatment because they may progress to cause more serious and potentially life-threatening complications. Deciding when or if to treat extensive stage 1 lesions is more difficult because surgery may be disfiguring and have a significant effect on normal function. Complete resection may not be possible, leading to high rates of recurrence, and currently it is not possible to predict which lesions will ultimately progress to stage 2 or 3.

■ Selected References

Adams DM, Trenor CC III, Hammill AM, et al. Efficacy and safety of sirolimus in the treatment of complicated vascular anomalies. *Pediatrics*. 2016;137(2):e20153257

Beck DO, Gosain AK. The presentation and management of hemangiomas. *Plast Reconstr Surg*. 2009;123(6):181e–191e

Boscolo E, Bischoff J. Vasculogenesis in infantile hemangioma. *Angiogenesis*. 2009;12(2):197–207

Ceisler EJ, Santos L, Blei F. Periocular hemangiomas: what every physician should know. *Pediatr Dermatol*. 2004;21(1):1–9

Darrow DH, Greene AK, Mancini AJ, Nopper AJ; American Academy of Pediatrics Section on Dermatology, Section on Otolaryngology-Head and Neck Surgery, Section on Plastic Surgery. Diagnosis and management of infantile hemangioma: executive summary. *Pediatrics*. 2015;136(4):786–791 de Serres LM, Sie KC, Richardson MA. Lymphatic malformations of the head and neck: a proposal for staging. *Arch Otolaryngol Head Neck Surg.* 1995;121(5):577–582

Dubois J, Patriquin HB, Garel L, et al. Soft-tissue hemangiomas in infants and children: diagnosis using Doppler sonography. *AJR Am J Roentgenol.* 1998;171(1): 247–252

Gampper TJ, Morgan RF. Vascular anomalies: hemangiomas. *Plast Reconstr Surg.* 2002;110(2):572–585

Itinteang T, Tan ST, Guthrie S, et al. A placental chorionic villous mesenchymal core cellular origin for infantile haemangioma. *J Clin Pathol.* 2011;64(10):870–874

Kelly KM, Choi B, McFarlane S, et al. Description and analysis of treatments for port-wine stain birthmarks. *Arch Facial Plast Surg.* 2005;7(5):287–294

Kelly ME, Juern AM, Grossman WJ, Schauer DW, Drolet BA. Immunosuppressive effects in infants treated with corticosteroids for infantile hemangiomas. *Arch Dermatol.* 2010;146(7):767–774

Kilcline C, Frieden IJ. Infantile hemangiomas: how common are they? A systematic review of the medical literature. *Pediatr Dermatol.* 2008;25(2):168–173

Kohout MP, Hansen M, Pribaz JJ, Mulliken JB. Arteriovenous malformations of the head and neck: natural history and management. *Plast Reconstr Surg.* 1998;102(3):643–654

Konez O, Burrows PE. An appropriate diagnostic workup for suspected vascular birthmarks. *Cleve Clin J Med.* 2004;71(6):505–510

Krowchuk DP, Frieden IJ, Mancini AJ, et al; American Academy of Pediatrics Subcommittee on the Management of Infantile Hemangiomas. Clinical practice guideline for the management of infantile hemangiomas. *Pediatrics.* 2019;143(1):e20183475

Léauté-Labrèze C, Dumas de la Roque E, Hubiche T, Boralevi F, Thambo JB, Taïeb A. Propranolol for severe hemangiomas of infancy. *N Engl J Med.* 2008;358(24): 2649–2651

Mulliken JB, Glowacki J. Hemangiomas and vascular malformations in infants and children: a classification based on endothelial characteristics. *Plast Reconstr Surg.* 1982;69(3):412–422

North PE, Waner M, Buckmiller L, James CA, Mihm MC Jr. Vascular tumors of infancy and childhood: beyond capillary hemangioma. *Cardiovasc Pathol.* 2006;15(6):303–317

Perkins JA, Chen EY. Vascular anomalies of the head and neck. In: Flint PW, Haughey BH, Lund VJ, et al, eds. *Otolaryngology Head & Neck Surgery.* 5th ed. Philadelphia, PA: Mosby; 2010

Perkins JA, Manning SC, Tempero RM, et al. Lymphatic malformations: review of current treatment. *Otolaryngol Head Neck Surg.* 2010;142(6):795–803.e1

Phung TL, Hochman M, Mihm MC. Current knowledge of the pathogenesis of infantile hemangiomas. *Arch Facial Plast Surg.* 2005;7(5):319–321

Railan D, Parlette EC, Uebelhoer NS, Rohrer TE. Laser treatment of vascular lesions. *Clin Dermatol.* 2006;24(1):8–15

Rosenberg TL, Suen JY, Richter GT. Arteriovenous malformations of the head and neck. *Otolaryngol Clin North Am.* 2018;51(1):185–195

Sandler G, Adams S, Taylor C. Paediatric vascular birthmarks: the psychological impact and the role of the GP. *Aust Fam Physician*. 2009;38(3):169–171

Sheth SN, Gomez C, Josephson GD. Pathological case of the month. Diagnosis and discussion: pyogenic granuloma of the tongue. *Arch Pediatr Adolesc Med*. 2001;155(9): 1065–1066

Smith SP Jr, Buckingham ED, Williams EF III. Management of cutaneous juvenile hemangiomas. *Facial Plast Surg*. 2008;24(1):50–64

Williams EF III, Stanislaw P, Dupree M, Mourtzikos K, Mihm M, Shannon L. Hemangiomas in infants and children: an algorithm for intervention. *Arch Facial Plast Surg*. 2000;2(2): 103–111

Index